Inflammatory Bowel Disease

Editor

SEAN J. LANGENFELD

SURGICAL CLINICS OF NORTH AMERICA

www.surgical.theclinics.com

Consulting Editor
RONALD F. MARTIN

December 2019 • Volume 99 • Number 6

ELSEVIER

1600 John F. Kennedy Boulevard • Suite 1800 • Philadelphia, Pennsylvania, 19103-2899

http://www.surgical.theclinics.com

SURGICAL CLINICS OF NORTH AMERICA Volume 99, Number 6
December 2019 ISSN 0039–6109, ISBN-13: 978-0-323-71047-3

Editor: John Vassallo, j.vassallo@elsevier.com
Developmental Editor: Casey Potter

Surgical Clinics of North America (ISSN 0039–6109) is published bimonthly by Elsevier Inc., 360 Park Avenue South, New York, NY 10010-1710. Months of publication are February, April, June, August, October, and December. Business and Editorial Offices: 1600 John F. Kennedy Blvd., Suite 1800, Philadelphia, PA 19103-2899. Periodicals postage paid at New York, NY and additional mailing offices. Subscription prices are $417.00 per year for US individuals, $845.00 per year for US institutions, $100.00 per year for US students and residents, $507.00 per year for Canadian individuals, $1071.00 per year for Canadian institutions, $536.00 for international individuals, $1071.00 per year for international institutions and $250.00 per year for Canadian and foreign students/residents. To receive student/resident rate, orders must be accompanied by name of affiliated institution, date of term, and the *signature* of program/residency coordinator on institution letterhead. Orders will be billed at individual rate until proof of status is received. Foreign air speed delivery is included in all *Clinics* subscription prices. All prices are subject to change without notice. POSTMASTER: Send address changes to *Surgical Clinics*, Elsevier Health Sciences Division, Subscription Customer Service, 3251 Riverport Lane, Maryland Heights, MO 63043. **Customer Service (orders, claims, online, change of address): Telephone: 1-800-654-2452 (U.S. and Canada); 314-447-8871 (outside U.S. and Canada). Fax: 314-447-8029. E-mail: journalscustomerservice-usa@elsevier.com (for print support); journalsonline support-usa@elsevier.com (for online support).**

Reprints. For copies of 100 or more, of articles in this publication, please contact the Commercial Reprints Department, Elsevier Inc., 360 Park Avenue South, New York, New York 10010-1710. Tel. 212-633-3874, Fax: 212-633-3820, E-mail: reprints@elsevier.com.

The Surgical Clinics of North America is also published in Spanish by McGraw-Hill Interamericana Editores S.A., P.O. Box 5-237 06500 Mexico D.F. Mexico; and in Portuguese by Interlivros Edicoes Ltda., Rua Comandante Coelho 1085, CEP 21250, Rio de Janeiro, Brazil; and in Greek by Paschalidis Medical Publications, Athens Greece.

The Surgical Clinics of North America is covered in *MEDLINE/PubMed (Index Medicus), EMBASE/Excerpta Medica, Current Contents/Clinical Medicine, Current Contents/Life Sciences, Science Citation Index,* and *ISI/BIOMED.*

Contributors

CONSULTING EDITOR

RONALD F. MARTIN, MD, FACS
Colonel (retired), United States Army Reserve, Department of Surgery, York Hospital, York, Maine

EDITOR

SEAN J. LANGENFELD, MD, FACS, FASCRS
Chief, Colon and Rectal Surgery, Associate Professor of Surgery, Associate Program Director, General Surgery Residency, Department of Surgery, University of Nebraska Medical Center, Omaha, Nebraska

AUTHORS

JAMES ANSELL, MD
Fellow, Division of Colon and Rectal Surgery, Mayo Clinic, Rochester, Minnesota

GRETA V. BERNIER, MD
Assistant Professor of Surgery, University of Washington School of Medicine, Seattle, Washington

KYLE G. COLOGNE, MD
Associate Professor, Surgery, Division of Colorectal Surgery, University of Southern California, Keck School of Medicine of USC, Los Angeles, California

DERRICK D. EICHELE, MD
Assistant Professor, Department of Internal Medicine, Division of Gastroenterology and Hepatology, University of Nebraska Medical Center, Omaha, Nebraska

SAMUEL EISENSTEIN, MD
Department of Surgery, UC San Diego Health System, La Jolla, California

ADINA E. FEINBERG, MDCM, FRCSC
Department of Colorectal Surgery, Digestive Disease and Surgery Institute, Cleveland Clinic, Cleveland, Ohio

PHILLIP FLESHNER, MD, FACS, FASCRS
Division of Colorectal Surgery, Cedars-Sinai Medical Center, Los Angeles, California

SEAN FLYNN, MD
Department of Surgery, UC San Diego Health System, La Jolla, California

MATTHEW A. FUGLESTAD, MD
Department of Surgery, University of Nebraska Medical Center, Omaha, Nebraska

MEGAN K. FULLER, MD
Department of Surgery, University of Nebraska Medical Center, Children's Hospital and Medical Center, Omaha, Nebraska; Boys Town National Research Hospital, Boys Town, Nebraska

DANICA N. GIUGLIANO, MD
Cleveland Clinic, Cleveland, Ohio

ROBERT N. GOLDSTONE, MD
Section of Colon and Rectal Surgery, Department of Surgery, Massachusetts General Hospital, Boston, Massachusetts

FABIAN GRASS, MD
Clinical Research Fellow, Division of Colon and Rectal Surgery, Mayo Clinic, Rochester, Minnesota

ERIC K. JOHNSON, MD, FACS, FASCRS
Professor of Surgery, Cleveland Clinic Lerner College of Medicine of Case Western Reserve University, Cleveland Clinic Colorectal Surgery, Mayfield Heights, Ohio

BRIAN R. KANN, MD, FACS, FASCRS
Senior Staff Surgeon and Associate Residency Program Director, Department of Colon and Rectal Surgery, Ochsner Medical Center, New Orleans, Louisiana

AARON L. KLINGER, MD
Resident, Department of Colon and Rectal Surgery, Ochsner Medical Center, New Orleans, Louisiana

ANGELA KUHNEN, MD
Lahey Hospital and Medical Center, Burlington, Massachusetts

JENNIFER A. LEINICKE, MD, MPHS
Assistant Professor, Department of Surgery, University of Nebraska Medical Center, Omaha, Nebraska

AMY L. LIGHTNER, MD
Digestive Diseases Institute, Associate Professor of Colon and Rectal Surgery, Cleveland Clinic, Cleveland, Ohio

LEA LOWENFELD, MD
Division of Colorectal Surgery, University of Southern California, Keck School of Medicine of USC, Los Angeles, California

NICHOLAS P. McKENNA, MD
Department of Surgery, General Surgery Resident, Mayo Clinic, Rochester, Minnesota

AMIT MERCHEA, MD
Assistant Professor of Surgery, Division of Colon and Rectal Surgery, Mayo Clinic, Jacksonville, Florida

RANDOLPH M. STEINHAGEN, MD
Chief, Division of Colon and Rectal Surgery, Professor, Department of Surgery, Icahn School of Medicine at Mount Sinai, New York, New York

JON S. THOMPSON, MD, FACS
Professor, Department of Surgery, Chief, Division of General Surgery, Shackleford Professor of Surgery, University of Nebraska Medical Center, Omaha, Nebraska

ADAM TRUONG, MD
Division of Colorectal Surgery, Cedars-Sinai Medical Center, Los Angeles, California

MICHAEL A. VALENTE, DO, FACS, FASCRS
Assistant Professor of Surgery, Department of Colorectal Surgery, Digestive Disease and Surgery Institute, Cleveland Clinic, Cleveland, Ohio

RENEE YOUNG, MD
Professor, Department of Internal Medicine, Division of Gastroenterology and Hepatology, University of Nebraska Medical Center, Omaha, Nebraska

KAREN ZAGHIYAN, MD, FACS, FASCRS
Division of Colorectal Surgery, Cedars-Sinai Medical Center, Los Angeles, California

Contents

Foreword: Irritable Bowel Disease   xiii

Ronald F. Martin

Preface: Inflammatory Bowel Disease   xvii

Sean J. Langenfeld

Inflammatory Bowel Disease Presentation and Diagnosis   1051

Sean Flynn and Samuel Eisenstein

A full understanding of the presentation and work-up of inflammatory bowel disease is necessary to ensure appropriate treatment of this complex disease. Crohn's disease and ulcerative colitis share many common clinical features but are treated very differently. This article covers the factors which contribute to IBD pathogenesis and presentation as well as the methods of diagnosis and work-up to ensure that the appropriate diagnosis is reached. This article also serves as a basis of understanding for the more complex aspects of the disease to be discussed in subsequent articles.

Endoscopy in Inflammatory Bowel Disease   1063

Aaron L. Klinger and Brian R. Kann

The roles of flexible endoscopy in the setting of inflammatory bowel disease include diagnosis, surveillance, and determining response to treatment and monitoring for the development of recurrence, dysplasia, or malignancy. Advanced techniques, such as chromoendoscopy and narrow band imaging, can be useful adjuncts when performing endoscopy in patients with inflammatory bowel disease. There are several roles for therapeutic endoscopy in the setting of inflammatory bowel disease, including endoscopic balloon dilation and endoscopic stricturotomy.

Preoperative Considerations in Inflammatory Bowel Disease   1083

Nicholas P. McKenna and Amy L. Lightner

Patients with ulcerative colitis and Crohn's disease often present to surgery malnourished and on combination immunosuppression. These factors affect operation selection and postoperative outcomes. Corticosteroids have a well-established detrimental effect on postoperative outcomes, whereas the impact of biologic agents is more controversial. In a patient exposed to these medications, and in the presence of other risk factors, temporary intestinal diversion is likely the best choice. Enteral nutrition may help optimize malnourished patients at high risk of adverse postoperative outcomes.

Postoperative Considerations in Inflammatory Bowel Disease 1095

Lea Lowenfeld and Kyle G. Cologne

Treatment of inflammatory bowel disease (IBD) is often multidimensional, requiring both medical and surgical therapies at different times throughout the course of the disease. Both medical and surgical treatments may be used in the acute setting, during a flare, or in a more elective maintenance role. These treatments should be planned as complementary and synergistic. Gastroenterologists and colorectal surgeons should collaborate to create a cohesive treatment plan, arranging the sequence and timing of various treatments. This article reviews the anticipated postoperative recovery after surgical treatment of IBD, possible postoperative complications, and considerations of timing surgery with medical therapy.

Surgical Management of Dysplasia and Cancer in Inflammatory Bowel Disease 1111

James Ansell, Fabian Grass, and Amit Merchea

Patients with inflammatory bowel disease are at an increased risk of cancer secondary to long-standing intestinal inflammation. Surgical options must take into account the significant risk of synchronous disease at other colonic sites. Ileal pouch anal anastomosis is a viable option for patients with ulcerative colitis, but this should be restricted to early cancers that are unlikely to require preoperative or postoperative radiation treatment.

Elective Abdominal Surgery for Inflammatory Bowel Disease 1123

Adina E. Feinberg and Michael A. Valente

Elective abdominal surgery for inflammatory bowel disease is common. Surgery for Crohn's disease is not curative, and treatment must be individualized to the disease process. Surgery for ulcerative colitis generally is curative but consideration of patient-specific factors is important for staging of the procedure and determining whether ileal pouch–anal anastomosis is appropriate.

Abdominal Emergencies in Inflammatory Bowel Disease 1141

Robert N. Goldstone and Randolph M. Steinhagen

Although improved medical therapies have been associated with decreased rates of emergent intestinal resection for inflammatory bowel disease, prompt diagnosis and management remain of utmost importance to ensure appropriate patient care with reduced morbidity and mortality. Emergent indications for surgery include toxic colitis, acute obstruction, perforation, acute abscess, or massive hemorrhage. Given this broad spectrum of emergent presentations, a multidisciplinary team including surgeons, gastroenterologists, radiologists, nutritional support services, and enterostomal therapists are required for optimal patient care and decision making. Management of each emergency should be individualized based on patient age, disease type and duration, and patient goals of care.

Anorectal Crohn's Disease 1151

Adam Truong, Karen Zaghiyan, and Phillip Fleshner

Medical treatment remains the mainstay of perianal disease management for CD; however, aggressive surgical management should be considered for severe or recurrent disease. In all cases of perianal CD, medical and surgical treatments should be used in tandem by a multidisciplinary team. Significant development has been made in the treatment of Crohn's-related fistulas, particularly minimally invasive options with recent clinical trials showing success with mesenchymal stem cell applications. Inevitably, some patients with severe refractory disease may require fecal diversion or proctectomy. When considering reversal of a diverting or end ileostomy, cessation of proctitis is the most important factor.

Other Surgeries in Patients with Inflammatory Bowel Disease   1163

Danica N. Giugliano, Greta V. Bernier, and Eric K. Johnson

Patients with inflammatory bowel disease (IBD) will often require abdominal surgical intervention for indications not directly related to their IBD. Because these patients often have a history of multiple previous abdominal operations and/or ostomies, they are at increased risk for incisional and parastomal hernias. They may also have develop symptomatic cholelithiasis, chronic pain, or desmoid disease. All of these potentially surgical issues may require special consideration in the IBD population.

Pediatric Inflammatory Bowel Disease: Special Considerations   1177

Megan K. Fuller

Pediatric inflammatory bowel disease may present differently than adult onset disease. It is important to consider a broader differential diagnosis in very early onset disease. Diagnostic and treatment decisions must consider the long term risks and benefits over a lifetime. Surgical triggers in children may include impaired growth and inability to wean from steroids in addition to standard adult indications. Effective transition of care to adult providers is a key to prevent flares and loss of follow-up.

Ileal Pouch Complications   1185

Jennifer A. Leinicke

Complications after ileal pouch surgery can result in poor pouch function and can have a significant negative impact on a patient's quality of life. Timely diagnosis and appropriate management of complications allows for the best chance of pouch salvage. Many complications require a multimodal approach. As with any reoperative surgery, the success of surgical revision or redo of an ileal pouch is highly dependent on the skill, judgment, and experience of the surgeon and requires an extremely motivated patient.

Genetic and Environmental Considerations for Inflammatory Bowel Disease   1197

Angela Kuhnen

Inflammatory bowel disease is a chronic inflammatory disorder of the gastrointestinal tract driven by an exaggerated immune response to luminal microbiota in susceptible individuals. It presents with a heterogenous pattern of clinical disease severity, location, and behavior. Understanding the interaction between the host genome, gut microbiome, and further environmental exposures in the development of IBD is in the early stages, and factors that trigger onset of disease in susceptible individuals remain unknown. This article addresses the genetic, microbial, and environmental influences on development of inflammatory bowel disease and the ability to manipulate these factors through surgery and medical therapy.

Inflammatory Bowel Disease and Short Bowel Syndrome   1209

Matthew A. Fuglestad and Jon S. Thompson

Short bowel syndrome/intestinal failure (SBS/IF) is a rare and debilitating disease process that mandates a multidisciplinary approach in its management. Inflammatory bowel disease (IBD), in particular Crohn's disease (CD), predisposes patients to development of SBS/IF. This review discusses SBS/IF from the perspective of IBD, with an emphasis on prevention and treatment in the setting of CD. The aims of this review are to emphasize the unique treatment goals of the newly diagnosed SBS/IF patient, and highlight the role of both medical and surgical therapies in the management of IBD-related SBS/IF, including intestinal transplantation.

Medical Management of Inflammatory Bowel Disease   1223

Derrick D. Eichele and Renee Young

Inflammatory bowel disease has become a growing concern worldwide. The chronic and progressive nature of inflammatory bowel disease poses significant challenges to the treatment and management of affected patients, straining health care resources. Therapeutic options and optimal management strategies have evolved dramatically. The treat-to-target strategy has shifted focus toward identifiable and attainable treatment targets and with the ability to optimize tight control. Advancements in our understanding of the pathophysiology led to therapeutic mechanisms that have a more narrowed focus toward gut-specific targets, improving safety profiles.

SURGICAL CLINICS
OF NORTH AMERICA

FORTHCOMING ISSUES

February 2020
Melanoma
Rohit Sharma, *Editor*

April 2020
Robotic Surgery
Julio A. Teixeira, *Editor*

June 2020
Surgical Oncology for the General Surgeon
Randy Zuckerman and Neal Wilkinson,
Editors

RECENT ISSUES

October 2019
Practicing Primary Palliative Care
Pringl Miller, *Editor*

August 2019
Surgical Management of Endocrine Disease
Rebecca S. Sippel and David F. Schneider,
Editors

June 2019
Management of the Foregut
Sushanth Reddy, *Editor*

SERIES OF RELATED INTEREST

Advances in Surgery
Available at: https://www.advancessurgery.com/
Surgical Oncology Clinics
Available at: https://www.surgonc.theclinics.com/
Thoracic Surgery Clinics
Available at: http://www.thoracic.theclinics.com/

THE CLINICS ARE AVAILABLE ONLINE!
Access your subscription at:
www.theclinics.com

Foreword

Irritable Bowel Disease

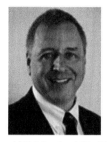

Ronald F. Martin, MD, FACS
Consulting Editor

It has been said that one can be judged by the company that one keeps. It has also been said that one cannot be judged guilty by association. So once again, aphorisms don't clarify matters too much for us. Still, both of those ideas can be true simultaneously under the correct circumstances. With whom we choose to associate does say much, though not all, about us. In the field of medicine, some of the same logic prevails. Once upon a time, there were surgeons and physicians, and their paths did not intersect much. Some of the distinction was based on the ability to perform some invasive procedure for the patient. Nowadays, what constitutes an invasive procedure is less obvious than it once was, and many disciplines, whether from the tradition of surgery or not, possess some capacity to perform invasive procedures. Also, what constitutes "invasive" when it comes to procedures has morphed into more of a continuum rather than a binary set of conditions.

As we progress in our knowledge and technology, certain trends are clear. One is that patient care is more likely to involve coordination of physician disciplines that derive from different historical pasts. This makes complete sense. A complex gastrointestinal surgeon is much more likely to have interaction with our gastroenterology colleagues and body image radiologists than perhaps with a neurosurgeon. Our cardiac surgery brethren are much more likely to spend time with our cardiology colleagues than with orthopedic surgeons. And so on. As a result, whom we "choose" to associate with is based on how our skillsets interact to deliver the (hopefully) best health care to our patients. Furthermore, that need for association and collaboration may change from patient to patient.

One other trend, or maybe better characterized as a persistent observation, is that we as a group get the behaviors that we incent. This is particularly true in medicine. There are many rewards to be offered in providing incentives for physicians. That said, the most powerful incentive that I have seen in effect is monetary compensation. Personally, I wish this were not true, and it certainly is not *always* true. Yet, it is true

Surg Clin N Am 99 (2019) xiii–xv
https://doi.org/10.1016/j.suc.2019.08.015
0039-6109/19/© 2019 Elsevier Inc. All rights reserved.

surgical.theclinics.com

often enough at this time. Anybody who has served in an administrative capacity could probably share tales of extreme concern over salary plans and individual compensation that she or he has seen or heard. Nowhere is the monetary impact more clearly seen in the behavior of physicians than when they are placed on a work Relative Value Unit (wRVU)-based compensation model. In my experience, this is especially true for procedure-based providers but still holds well for office-based providers. It is astounding to see how quickly one can arrange to have a patient seen when they need a procedure and how long it can take to be seen for an office visit.

I bring these topics up in tandem because the two ideas intersect at an interesting place, particularly as regards the care of patients with complex gastrointestinal maladies. Inflammatory bowel disease is one of the very great examples of how patients may find themselves in a position where they need to develop long-term relations with both their surgeon and their gastroenterologist. They may also need help from the many other disciplines and allied providers who are required to care for these complex patients. So, all of us involved in the care of these patients need to "associate" across the historical separations in medical care. Also, almost everybody in this framework is compensated in some different way.

I am not interested in discussing the benefits and failures of different compensation schemes at this time. There is no right answer anyway. However, what I would posit to you, dear reader, is that how we handle this question is important. If we are to develop strategic objectives to optimize health care and health care value for our patients and communities, then it should follow that all members of the team should be incented in such ways (not necessarily identically) to align each member's behaviors with the long-term success of the larger group. Much of what we can attach a wRVU to has merits in achieving our goals. That said, very large and important parts of what we collectively do have no wRVU associated with them. Care delivered during the "global period," time spent collaborating, time spent educating the physician force as well as other members of the team, time spent learning new technology, and countless other time-consuming tasks are invisible to many compensation schemes. This frequently provides a framework for people working at cross-purposes, which mainly diminishes overall efficiency and sometimes quality. One of the challenges for our current and future leaders will be to solve how to incent all to play roles that support the larger mission. If it were easy, it would have been done already. Despite that, it needs to be improved, as our current efficiency trajectory is probably not sustainable.

The historical divisions that evolved in the field of medicine are fading and shifting rapidly. Our organizations are merging and consolidating. While culture may start at the top, it has to be bought into all the way to the bottom or it will not sustain. It is said that people get the government they deserve. Likewise, all organizations get the behaviors they incent. What might be best for one organization might not work for another. Still, we must all try to find ways to align our organizational goals with the needs of our patients; after all, to serve them is why we exist. Examining whether we are doing that will be the first step to deciding what, if anything, needs to be changed.

One aspect of our field that I feel has not changed and it is hoped will not change is the degree to which we can and do rely on one another. I have reached out to Dr Langenfeld many times during my stewardship of this series. Each and every time, he has offered his expertise without hesitation, and every time he and his colleagues have delivered beyond expectation. We at the *Surgical Clinics of North America* remain deeply indebted to him and his colleagues for their excellent contributions to this series.

I hope this issue not only provides insight into the complexities of biology and treatment of inflammatory bowel disease but also sparks your interest into how you can integrate your local resources to improve your collective ability to deliver care.

Ronald F. Martin, MD, FACS
Colonel (retired), United States Army Reserve
Department of Surgery
York Hospital
16 Hospital Drive, Suite A
York, ME 03909, USA

E-mail address:
rfmcescna@gmail.com

Preface

Inflammatory Bowel Disease

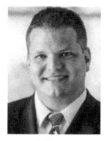

Sean J. Langenfeld, MD, FACS, FASCRS
Editor

This is my second round as a guest editor for the *Surgical Clinics of North America*. My first topic was colorectal cancer, which I described as "one of the deadliest and most common malignancies that patients encounter."[1] My second contribution focuses on diseases that are not nearly as common or deadly. However, they are, without a doubt, some of the most difficult and frustrating cases that a surgeon encounters.

Ulcerative colitis and Crohn disease are exceptionally challenging ailments for the patient and surgeon alike. There is significant heterogeneity in phenotype and disease severity, so symptoms and response to treatment are difficult to predict. Even in the best hands, the complication rates for inflammatory bowel disease (IBD) surgery are high, and the functional outcomes are guarded. Guidelines for management are infrequent, vague, and usually outdated. Despite the absence of reliable guidelines, emergencies are common; general surgeons are tasked with making swift management decisions, often in the middle of the night without the ability to "phone a friend."

There are 1000-page textbooks on IBD, so this issue is not meant to be comprehensive. Instead, my goal is to provide a practical and well-rounded overview of IBD that is useful for the practicing surgeon. To accomplish this, I was lucky enough to receive help from authors whose experience and expertise far exceed my own. They provide insight into IBD surgery that comes from years of seeing the "worst of the worst," and I am confident that you will find their work to be of the highest quality.

I want to thank the authors, who devoted their time and expertise to this issue. I would also like to thank the publishing team from Elsevier, who continue to show a unique level of organization and support. Last, I would like to thank Dr Ronald Martin for inviting me back for a second round as guest editor. He continues to impress

Surg Clin N Am 99 (2019) xvii–xviii
https://doi.org/10.1016/j.suc.2019.08.016
0039-6109/19/© 2019 Elsevier Inc. All rights reserved.

me with his dedication to surgical education, and the culture of editorial excellence that he demands.

Sean J. Langenfeld, MD, FACS, FASCRS
Department of Surgery
University of Nebraska Medical Center
983280 Nebraska Medical Center
Omaha, NE 68198-3280, USA

E-mail address:
sean.langenfeld@unmc.edu

REFERENCE

1. Langenfeld SJ. Preface. Surg Clin North Am 2017;97(3):xv–xvi.

Inflammatory Bowel Disease Presentation and Diagnosis

Sean Flynn, MD, Samuel Eisenstein, MD*

KEYWORDS

- Inflammatory bowel disease • Genetics • Environment • Endoscopy • Enterography

KEY POINTS

- The cause of inflammatory bowel disease (IBD) is multifactorial and includes genetic, host, and environmental factors working together.
- The presentations of Crohn's disease (CD) and ulcerative colitis (UC) are similar; however, UC is more likely to present with diarrhea and bleeding, whereas CD is more likely to present with watery diarrhea and vague symptoms.
- Endoscopic diagnosis is the gold standard and should involve a colonoscopy with intubation of the terminal ileum.
- Laboratory tests are only useful in aiding in the diagnosis of IBD when all other tests are equivocal because they have a low sensitivity and specificity to differentiate between CD and UC.
- Computed tomography enterography or magnetic resonance enterography (MRE) should be used in aiding in the diagnosis of IBD. MRE is likely a better choice because it does not involve ionizing radiation and is more sensitive in diagnosing perianal disease.

INTRODUCTION

Inflammatory bowel disease (IBD) is the continuum of diseases that comprise Crohn's disease (CD), ulcerative colitis (UC), and indeterminate colitis. The incidence of IBD has been increasing in virtually every industrialized country during the twenty-first century. To fully understand the disease, it is first critical to understand its origins, presentation, and diagnosis. This article covers these points and prepares for a nuanced discussion of management of this complex disease.

CAUSE

The cause of IBD is incompletely understood. There are genetic, environmental, and host-related factors that contribute to the development of gut inflammation. Genetic

Disclosure: The authors have no financial conflicts.
Department of Surgery, UC San Diego Health System, 3855 Health Sciences Drive #0987, La Jolla, CA 92093, USA
* Corresponding author.
E-mail address: seisenstein@ucsd.edu

components of IBD have long been recognized. Twins studies have shown an increased concordance for both CD and UC, with CD having up to a 58% concordance between monozygotic twins.[1] First-degree relatives of patients with IBD have also been shown to have a 5-fold increase in the risk of developing IBD.[2] More than 201 genetic mutations have been implicated in the development of IBD, and, based on genome-wide association studies, IBD is likely a polygenic process.[3] Within these genetic loci, there have been identified 41 CD-specific and 30 UC-specific genetic polymorphisms, but 137 loci are associated with both CD and UC (**Table 1**).[3] From 80% to 90% of identified loci associated with IBD are noncoding and likely represent epigenetic markers, microRNAs, and noncoding RNAs.[2]

The host adaptive immune response has also been implicated in the development of IBD. T cell–mediated responses are amplified in both CD and UC. In CD, inflammation is triggered by an amplified T-helper (Th) 1 and Th17 response; this leads to the secretion of proinflammatory cytokines interleukin (IL)-17, interferon gamma (IFN-γ), and tumor necrosis factor alpha (TNF-α), which then leads to a self-perpetuating cycle of inflammation. In UC, the response is Th2 mediated, leading to more efficient activation of B cells and natural killer T cells, and is mediated by IL-5 and IL-13.[2] Many of the genetic loci associated with IBD are also responsible for T-cell function.

The intestinal barrier is also intimately involved with host innate immunity. This environment consists of intestinal epithelial cells (enterocytes, goblet cells, neuroendocrine cells, Paneth cells, and M cells) and immune cells. Disturbance of this barrier has been shown to lead to IBD in animal models, such as in Muc2-deficient mice, which are unable to secrete mucin from goblet cells and spontaneously develop IBD.[4] Paneth cell defects, which have been shown to be mediated via gene abnormalities in NOD2, have been linked with the development of CD. NOD2 has been shown to be involved with autophagy and clearance of intracellular pathogens, and breakdown of this pathway is closely linked to the development of CD.[5] Antigen-presenting cells (APCs) in the mucosal barrier are also linked to the development of IBD. Patients with CD have been shown to have attenuated macrophage activity, which impairs

Table 1 Inflammatory bowel disease–associated genes	
UC-associated Genes	TNFRSF14, RFTN2, PLCL1, PRKCD, ITIH4, NFKB1, MANBA, SLC9A3, CARD11, GNA12, DLD, IRF5, JRKL, MAML2, FAM55A, FAM55D, ITGAL, ZFP90, CALM3, ADA, HNF4A
CD-associated Genes	PTPN22, ADAM30, UCN, FASLG, TNFSF18, SP140, ATG16L1, IL6ST, IL31RA, CPEB4, TAGAP, CEB5, JAZF1, RIPK2, LACC1, RASGRP1, SPRED1, NOD2, LGALS9, NOS2, GPX4, FUT2, HMHA1, IFNGR2, IFNAR1
IBD-associated Genes	TNFRSF18, TNFRSF4, TNFRSF9, IL23R, RORC, CD48, FCGR2A/B, FCGR3A, C1orf53, KIF21B, IL10, ADCY3, FOSL2, BRE, REL, SPRED2, IL18RAP, IL1R1, IFIH1, IL18RAP, IL1R1, GPR35, MST1, PFKB4, IL2, IL21, DAP, PTGER4, ERAP2, ERAP1, IBD5 locus, SPRY4, NDFIP1, IRGM, IL12B, DOK3, TRAF3IP2, TNFAIP3, PHACTR2, CCR6, RPS6KA2, ZPBP, IKZF1, SMURF1, EPO, TRIB1, JAK2, NFIL3, TNFSF15, CARD9, IL2RA, IL15RA, MAP3K8, CREM, CISD1, IPMK, TSPAN14, C10orf58, NKX2-3, TNNI2, LSP1, CNTF, LPXN, CD6, RELA, CCDC88B, CXCR5, MUC19, LOH12CR1, VDR, IFNG, SMAD3, GPR183, GPR18, ZFP36L1, FOS, MLH3, GPR65, GALC, CRTC3, SOCS1, LITAF, PRKCB, IL27, IRF8, CCL13,CCL2, ORMDL3, STAT3, TUBD1, RPS6KB1, SMAD7, CD226, TYK2, CEBPG, HCK, CD40, DNMT3B, CEBPB, ZNF831, CTSZ, ICOSLG, TNFRSF6B, LIF, OSM

neutrophil activity and permits more bacterial translocation across the gut.[2] Another type of APC, the dendritic cell, has been shown to accumulate in the lamina propria of the gut of patients with IBD. This impaired trafficking to lymphoid follicles prevents appropriate antigen sampling and immune activation.[6]

Although genetic susceptibility is a key feature in the development of IBD, it is clear that environmental factors are also key to the development of these diseases. This finding might explain why there are increases in IBD in places such as Asia and Africa, where, until recently, IBD was extremely rare. Dietary factors have been shown to contribute to the development of IBD across populations. Diets high in saturated fat and processed meats have been implicated in the development of IBD. High-fiber diets have been shown to decrease the risk of CD.[7] Medications that perturb the host microbiome (antibiotics, nonsteroidal antiinflammatories, contraceptives, and statins) have all been shown to increase the risk of development of IBD.[2]

A decrease in the diversity of the host microbiome has been linked with the development of IBD.[8] Most commonly there is a decrease in the population of Firmicutes and an increase in Proteobacteria and Bacteroidetes, which may lead to a decrease in the production of short-chain fatty acids and can impair T-regulatory cell and epithelial cell function. Other changes identified in the host microbiome include an increase in mucolytic bacteria leading to a breakdown in the epithelial barrier[9] as well as an increase of bacteria adherent to the intestinal epithelium, such as Proteobacteria, which in turn affects the permeability of the gut and alters the overall composition of the microbiome.[10]

EPIDEMIOLOGY

IBD is most common in Western countries, particularly those in northern Europe and North America. Approximately 1.6 million Americans are affected by IBD, with 785,000 patients with CD, and 910,000 with UC.[2] Both UC and CD have similar age and gender distributions, with most likely onset in the second or fourth decade of life and no particular gender predilection.[11] CD tends to affect patients slightly earlier in life, at an average age of 15 to 25 years old, whereas UC is more likely to set in between 25 and 35 years of age.[12] Historically these diseases most commonly afflicted white people, particularly those of Ashkenazi Jewish heritage. However, over the last decade the incidence has been increasing in both Asian and Hispanic populations. Studies have also shown that people who emigrate from low-prevalence regions to high-prevalence regions are at an increased risk of IBD, particularly in the children of these people who were then born in high-prevalence zones. As countries industrialize, their incidences of IBD increase. Similarly, those who live in urban centers are also more likely to be afflicted than those living in a rural setting.[11]

SYMPTOMS
Crohn's Disease

CD can involve any aspect of the gastrointestinal (GI) tract, from mouth to anus. Disease severity and location dictate the associated signs and symptoms, leading to a wide spectrum of clinical presentations. The classic hallmarks of CD include abdominal pain, watery diarrhea, and weight loss.[13,14] Abdominal pain is usually colicky and often persists for many years before diagnosis. It is frequently associated with, and relieved after, bowel movements. Because of the predilection for involvement of the terminal ileum, pain frequently localizes to the right lower quadrant. This pain can be acute and severe, often mimicking appendicitis. More often it is of insidious onset with flares and remissions. CD diarrhea is generally watery, but can be bloody. Bloody diarrhea is most often seen with colonic and rectal involvement.[15] Severe bleeding is rare, but can occur in 1% to 2% of patients.[16] Like the pain, diarrhea is often episodic and can also persist intermittently for many years before diagnosis. Patients with CD often have had significant weight loss by the time of their diagnosis. Weight loss is multifactorial as a result of chronic diarrhea, malabsorption, and anorexia derived from a fear of eating.

Inflammation of CD can evolve into a penetrating fistulous pattern or a fibrostenotic obstructing pattern. Intestinal fistulas occur in about 20% to 40% of patients with Crohn's.[17,18] Fistula formation can occur to any adjacent structure, including to the bowel, bladder, skin, or vagina. Enteroenteric fistulas are the most common form of luminal fistulizing disease. These fistulas may be clinically asymptomatic, but can contribute to malabsorption and diarrhea. Enterovaginal fistulas are the next most common and present with the passage of stool or gas through the vagina. Enterocutaneous fistulas, separate from perianal fistulas, result in drainage of enteric contents through the skin. Enterovesicular fistulas account for 3% of all fistulas.[17] Sinus tracts from transmural inflammation do not always lead to fistulas, but may also result in the development of intra-abdominal abscesses or phlegmon.

The fibrostenotic pattern of inflammation results in the development of strictures. Strictures can present with obstructive features, including abdominal pain, nausea, and vomiting. Presentation can be acute or chronic. Strictures can occur throughout the GI tract. Small bowel involvement and obstruction is most common, but gastric outlet obstruction, colonic obstruction, and anal strictures are also seen.

Up to one-third of patients with CD have perianal involvement.[19] The most common manifestations of perianal CD include fistulas, fissures, abscesses, and skin tags. Development of perianal fistulas is thought to represent a distinct disease phenotype. This phenotype is typically a more aggressive form of disease, and may necessitate different medical and surgical interventions.[20] The incidence of perianal fistulas increases with more distal GI involvement, being most closely associated with Crohn's colitis with rectal involvement.[21] Approximately 15% of patients have perianal fistula at the time of their diagnosis. The overall incidence of perianal fistulas ranges from 17% to 43%.[22,23]

Systemic symptoms are also often seen in CD. Fatigue is common as a result of the ongoing inflammation and malabsorption. Fevers are also often seen and are typically low grade. Higher fevers indicate a more severe inflammatory process, such as abscess formation or perforation. Up to half of patients also present with extraintestinal manifestations (**Table 2**).[24]

Ulcerative Colitis

Inflammation of UC is confined to the colonic mucosa, making symptoms less heterogeneous than in CD. However, UC still encompasses a wide spectrum of disease presentations and clinical courses because symptom severity is correlated to the extent of inflammation.[25] The Montreal classification system describes the extent of colonic involvement and is most often used to objectively classify disease extent and severity and can help guide clinical management.[26] Timing from onset of symptoms to diagnosis is usually shorter in UC than CD, often occurring over weeks to months as opposed to years.

The major feature of UC is diarrhea from rapid transit of intestinal contents through the inflamed colon. It is often postprandial and can be nocturnal as well. The severity of diarrhea is related to the extent of inflammation. Rectal inflammation leads to frequent, small-volume bowel movements, and is associated with the frequent passage of mucus. More proximal disease, up to pancolitis, results in more

Table 2
Extraintestinal manifestations of inflammatory bowel disease

Site	Manifestations	Incidence (%)
Dermatologic		2–34
	Erythema nodosum	10
	Pyoderma gangrenosum	1–12
Rheumatologic	Peripheral arthritis	5–20
	Spondylitis	1–26
	Symmetric sacroiliitis	<10
Ocular	Conjunctivitis	0.3–5
	Uveitis	
	Iritis episcleritis	
Hepatobiliary	Primary sclerosing cholangitis	2–5
	Autoimmune hepatitis	
	Hepatic steatosis	
	Cholelithiasis	
Renal	Nephrolithiasis	6–23
	Obstructive uropathy	
Cardiovascular	Hypercoagulable state (deep vein thrombosis, pulmonary embolism, stroke)	—
	Endocarditis	
	Myocarditis	
	Pleuropericarditis	
Bone	Osteoporosis	—
	Osteomalacia	

severe, larger-volume diarrhea with liquid stool. Blood is classically associated with UC, but is not always present, especially in cases of mild disease limited to distal involvement. Bloody diarrhea is present in most patients and the severity of bleeding is correlated to the extent of colonic involvement. Patients with more distal disease may only pass bloodstained mucus or small amounts of fresh blood. As the disease extends proximally, blood becomes mixed in with stool and can lead to grossly bloody diarrhea. Severe bleeding is seen in up to 10% of patients, with approximately 1% to 3% of the UC population experiencing at least 1 episode of massive hemorrhage that may necessitate surgical intervention.[27] Fulminant colitis or toxic megacolon are seen in approximately 15% of patients with UC. They can result in severe bleeding or colonic perforation, and also frequently surgical emergencies.

Other common features of UC include tenesmus and abdominal pain. Abdominal pain ranges from mild colicky pain to severe cramping with more extensive disease. Systemic symptoms of fatigue, fever, and weight loss may also be present. With longer disease courses, patients may develop colonic strictures, occurring in about 5% to 10% of patients, which can lead to obstruction and pain.[28] Clinicians must have high suspicion for underlying malignancy whenever strictures are encountered. Constipation is also possible with UC, and is most frequently seen in localized distal disease, which results in delayed transit and motility of the proximal bowel. Even with constipation, patients typically have frequent discharge of blood and mucus. Extraintestinal manifestations are also seen with UC, but are less common than with CD.

WORK-UP

Work-up and diagnosis of IBD begins with a detailed history and physical examination. It is important to rule out infectious causes with a history of recent travel and exposures. Drug history should be obtained, including nonsteroidal antiinflammatories and antibiotic use. Patients should also be assessed for risk factors, such as a family history of IBD or smoking.

CD is classically associated with right lower quadrant pain secondary to terminal ileitis, but abdominal pain may be located throughout the abdomen. Examination may also reveal a palpable mass related to intra-abdominal phlegmon or abscess. Rectal examination should be performed to assess for any perianal changes, such as fistulas, fissures, abscesses, or skin tags. Eccentrically located fissures are concerning for IBD.

Laboratory work may be normal, although anemia and thrombocytosis are common. Hypoalbuminemia and vitamin deficiencies can suggest malnutrition associated with IBD. Serologic markers should be sent and are discussed later. Stool studies, including ova and parasite, and *Clostridium difficile*, help rule out infectious causes.

ENDOSCOPIC DIAGNOSIS

Endoscopy remains the primary diagnostic modality in IBD. Any patient who is being worked up for IBD should undergo colonoscopy with intubation of the terminal ileum when possible. Segments of obvious disease should be biopsied and at least 2 biopsies should be taken from 5 sites, including the ileum and rectum. Biopsies should also be taken from normal-appearing tissue to help determine the full histologic extent of the patient's disease.[29] Often the pattern of disease helps experienced endoscopists differentiate between CD and UC as well as between a variety of other inflammatory enteropathies. It is important to remember that true granulomas are only seen in approximately of one-third of biopsies of patients with CD, so the absence of granulomas does not rule out CD. Classic findings on colonoscopy in IBD can be found in **Table 3** and the most common endoscopic disease severity scoring systems can be seen in **Table 4**.

Upper endoscopy is not recommended in the routine management of asymptomatic patients even though upper GI disease can be found in up to 16% of patients with CD.[30] Esophagogastroduodenoscopy is often performed because there is significant overlap between IBD symptoms and a variety of foregut disorders. When performed for IBD, it is recommended that 2 biopsies be taken of the stomach, esophagus, and duodenum.[31] Similarly enteroscopy, be it capsule or balloon assisted, should only be undertaken after imaging has confirmed the presence of small bowel disease that is inaccessible to traditional endoscopic techniques. When considering capsule endoscopy, it is important to assess for bowel patency first because there is a risk for capsule retention in up to 13% of patients undergoing this procedure.[32] This assessment can be done by magnetic resonance enterography (MRE) or by using a patency capsule whose passage can be monitored via plain radiograph, and that dissolves after 40 to 80 hours if not passed through a stricture. Capsule endoscopy identifies lesions that were missed on MRE in up to 71% of patients with CD[33]; however, these lesions rarely require intervention and often there are other sites of more accessible disease that can be monitored for treatment response.

LABORATORY EVALUATION

Numerous biomarkers have been identified to monitor the inflammatory process. These biomarkers are generally nonspecific and are better suited to tracking disease response once the diagnosis has been established than to establishing a new diagnosis.

Table 3
Endoscopic findings in inflammatory bowel disease

	UC	CD
Location	Colon: distal to proximal Isolated periappendiceal: 5% Relative rectal sparing: 10%–15% Backwash ileitis Patchy appearance: 33%–44%	±Colon ±Ileum Can be discontinuous: skip lesions
Mucosa	Loss of vascularity Erythema Mucosal granularity Friability Erosions Ulcers Pseudopolyps	Loss of vascularity Erythema Mucosal granularity Friability Erosions Ulcers Pseudopolyps Aphthous ulcers Cobblestoning
Biopsy	Crypt abscess Crypt branching Crypt shortening Thickened muscularis Mucin depletion Paneth cell metaplasia Increased lamina propria cellularity Basal plasmacytosis Basal lymphoid aggregates Lamina propria eosinophils	Granulomas: 33% Fibrosis Neural hyperplasia Normal mucin Inflammation extending into submucosa

C-reactive protein (CRP) is the most sensitive blood marker for inflammation. Inflammation causes tissue injury, which causes macrophages to secrete a cytokine cascade that ends in hepatic synthesis of CRP.[34] CRP levels can increase rapidly, with a 500-fold to 1000-fold increase compared with baseline within hours of the initial insult.[35] CRP is an appealing biomarker for inflammation because it has a short half-life of 19 hours, but it is nonspecific and levels can increase as a result of a variety of different tissue insults[34] as well as in the presence of smoking, obesity, and drug therapies. CRP has a high negative predictive value and a CRP level of 5 mg/dL has been shown to convey less than a 1% chance of active IBD.[36] However, CRP testing has also been shown to be negative in up to 30% of patients with endoscopically active CD[37] and is incapable of distinguishing between UC and CD.

Table 4
Endoscopic scoring systems in inflammatory bowel disease

Ulcerative Colitis	Crohn's Disease
Mayo endoscopic subscore	Simple endoscopic score in CD
0: Normal. No signs of inflammation 1: Mild. Erythema 2: Moderate. Friability or erosions 3: Severe. Spontaneous bleeding or ulceration	Ulcer: none (0), 0.1–0.5 cm (1), 0.5–2 cm (2), >2 cm (3) Ulcerated surface: none (0), <10% (1), 10%–30% (2), >30% (3) Affected surface: none (0), <50% (1), 50%–75% (2), >75% (3) Narrowing: none (0), single passable (1), multiple passable (2), impassable (3)
Scored 0–3	Sum of the 5 (0–56)

Fecal calprotectin (FC) is a direct marker of intestinal mucosal inflammation. This protein is derived from the cytosol of neutrophils and is the result of neutrophil degranulation.[38] Because of this, its levels can also be increased in the setting of diverticulitis, infectious colitis, intestinal neoplasms, cirrhosis, and with use of nonsteroidal antiinflammatories and proton pump inhibitors.[39] FC is stable for up to 7 days in stool samples. FC's utility as a diagnostic tool is based both on the value considered positive as well as the pretest probability for IBD. Bressler and colleagues[39] suggested clinicians consider that FC level less than 50 to 100 µg/g likely represents quiescent disease, FC level greater than 250 µg/g suggests inflammation, and FC level 100 to 250 µg/g is indeterminate.

Both CRP and FC have been used as markers of treatment response. However, they may directly respond to the therapy administered even if inflammation has not subsided. For example, IL-6 level decreases in a direct response to ustekinumab therapy and directly decreases CRP secretion, even if the medication is not controlling the patient's disease. A useful strategy for monitoring these biomarkers may involve looking at the two in conjunction with therapeutic drug levels, which has been shown to be more predictive of disease recurrence.[40]

Several biomarkers have also been identified in aiding in the diagnosis of IBD. Perinuclear antineutrophil cytoplasmic antibody (p-ANCA) positivity is found in 6% to 39% of patients with CD, 41% to 73% of patients with UC, and 0% to 8% of healthy controls.[41] This finding gives this biomarker a low specificity for diagnosing CD (19%), and its utility is in distinguishing UC from CD with a 52% sensitivity and 91% specificity.[42] Anti–*Saccharomyces cerevisiae* antibody (ASCA) is present in approximately 60% of patients with CD, but only 13% of patients with UC, and 3% of healthy controls, showing its sensitivity (72%) and specificity (82%) in diagnosing CD.[43] Up to 20% of healthy family members of patients with CD have also been shown to express ANCA, and various ethnic groups, in particular Asian populations with CD, have been shown to not test positive for ANCA.[41] Other antibodies that have been shown to be useful in differentiating between IBD subtypes are shown in **Table 5**.

Based on what has been learned about the biomarkers in **Table 5** and the genetics of IBD, several diagnostic panels have been developed. At present, the most widely used are the Prometheus panels (Prometheus Laboratories, Inc., San Diego, CA). The Crohn's Prognostic panel (also known as the IBD7) has been available since 2006 and tests for a combination of anti-flagellin, anti-outer membrane protein C, p-ANCA, and NOD 2 genetic variants. This test has not been well validated and positive results still require an endoscopy, so its main utility is helping push the diagnosis toward CD in the setting of endoscopic equivalency.

IMAGING MODALITIES

Although colonic and ileal disease can be identified endoscopically, the absence or presence of these disease patterns does not preclude disease in the remainder of the bowel. To assess the small bowel, either MRE or computed tomography enterography (CTE) should be performed. Both of these studies require the patient to drink a large volume of neutral contrast, which is used to distend the bowel to help highlight intraluminal disorders such as inflammation, strictures, ulcers, and cobblestoning. Cross-sectional imaging can also identify extraluminal findings such as fistulae and mesenteric thickening. Up to 50% of CD cases with a normal colonoscopy have abnormalities on cross-sectional imaging,[44] highlighting its utility in the diagnosis of CD.

CTE and MRE are both acceptable modalities for diagnosing small bowel inflammation in CD. A recent meta-analysis showed that the sensitivity and specificity

Table 5
Antibodies used in the diagnosis of inflammatory bowel disease

Antibody	Antigen	Utility
p-ANCA	Mycobacteria with H1	41%–73% of UC, 6%–39% CD, 0%–8% Controls
Anti-GP2	Glycoprotein 2	21%–45% of CD, 2%–19% UC
Anti–GM-CSF	GM-CSF	CD>>UC; represents more complex ileal disease
ASCA	Oligomannoside on S cerevisiae	60% CD, 13% UC, 13% controls
ACCA[a]	Chitobioside	CD: Sen 77.4%, Spec 90.6%
ALCA[a]	Laminariboside	CD: Sen 77.4%, Spec 90.6%
AMCA[a]	Mannobioside	CD: Sen 77.4%, Spec 90.6%
Anti-L	Anti-Laminarin	CD: Sen 18.0%, Spec 96.7%
Anti-C	Anti-Chitin	CD: Sen 10.3%, Spec 97.7%; marker for penetrating disease
Anti-OmpC	Membrane protein of E. Coli	24%–55% CD, 2%–24% UC, 5%–20% controls
Anti-CBir1	Flagellin CBir1	50%–56% CD, <6% UC, 8% controls
Anti-I2	Sequence I2	38%–60% CD, 2%–10% UC

Abbreviation: ACCA, anti-chitobioside carbohydrate antibody; ALCA, anti-laminaribioside carbohydrate antibody; AMCA, anti-mannobioside carbohydrate antibody; GM-CSF; granulocyte macrophage colony-stimulating factor; GP, glycoprotein; Sen, sensitivity; Spec, specificity.
[a] If 2 of 3 are positive, sensitivity for CD is 99.1%.

were 87% (95% confidence interval [CI], 78%–92%) and 91% (95% CI, 84%–95%), respectively, for CTE and 86% (95% CI, 79%–91%) and 93% (95% CI, 84%–97%), respectively, for MRE.[45] When determining which imaging modality is best for an individual patient, it is important to take the strengths and weaknesses of each modality into consideration. CTE involves administration of ionizing radiation to patients, which is important because disease monitoring usually occurs on a lifelong basis for patients with IBD and the cumulative dose of radiation can be significant across decades. In contrast, MRE often requires the patient to stay in a small, enclosed location for more than an hour, which can cause great anxiety in a subset of patients. MRI is also the best current technique to evaluate perianal disease, and, thus, patients being evaluated for perianal disease often have the MRE performed simultaneously. Because of the numerous imaging studies these patients require across their lifetimes, and because of the frequency of perianal evaluation, it is our practice to primarily use MRE. When considering a lifetime of imaging for these patients, it is also important to remember that it is difficult to compare MRI and computed tomography, and thus consistency across imaging studies is important for patient care.

Ultrasonography also avoids the use of ionizing radiation in the evaluation of the bowel. A combination of intravenous microbubble contrast and low-mechanical-index imaging mode or power Doppler makes evaluation of the entire bowel feasible. Ultrasonography is primarily used to diagnose bowel wall thickening and can help differentiate between inflammatory and fibrotic strictures. There is a great amount of intraoperator variability with this study and it is generally reserved for specialty centers. Ultrasonography has shown a sensitivity of 89% and a specificity of 94.3% in the assessment of patients with known CD but is less accurate in detecting proximal lesions.[46] Head to head with MRE, ultrasonography showed good concordance at identifying Crohn's lesions except when for fistulae, for which the concordance was poor.[47]

As previously mentioned, MRI is currently considered the most accurate imaging modality for perianal disease and has been shown to be 97% sensitive and 96% specific in the diagnosis of anal fistulae in CD.[48] Ultrasonography can also be a useful modality in diagnosing perianal disease, but the process is more invasive and operator dependent, so generally those patients who can undergo MRI of the pelvis are recommended to do so.

SUMMARY

There are many diagnostic considerations to be taken into consideration for patients suspected of having IBD. Diagnosis is primarily made with endoscopy and cross-sectional imaging showing intestinal inflammation. Ideally biopsy is obtained, and histology in conjunction with disease pattern confirms either CD or UC; however, if these findings are equivocal, there are specialized panels of biomarkers that are potentially useful in determining the correct diagnosis. Careful diagnosis is critical to ensuring appropriate treatment recommendations are made to ensure that patients have the best possible outcomes.

REFERENCES

1. Xavier RJ, Podolsky DK. Unravelling the pathogenesis of inflammatory bowel disease. Nature 2007;448(7152):427–34.
2. Ramos GP, Papadakis KA. Mechanisms of disease: inflammatory bowel diseases. Mayo Clinic Proc 2019;94(1):155–65.
3. Jostins L, Ripke S, Weersma RK, et al. Host-microbe interactions have shaped the genetic architecture of inflammatory bowel disease. Nature 2012; 491(7422):119–24.
4. Van der Sluis M, De Koning BA, De Bruijn AC, et al. Muc2-deficient mice spontaneously develop colitis, indicating that Muc2 is critical for colonic protection. Gastroenterology 2006;131(1):117–29.
5. Fritz T, Niederreiter L, Adolph T. Crohn's disease: NOD2, autophagy and ER stress converge. Gut 2011;60(11):1580–8.
6. Hart AL, Al-Hassi HO, Rigby RJ, et al. Characteristics of intestinal dendritic cells in inflammatory bowel diseases. Gastroenterology 2005;129(1):50–65.
7. Hou JK, Abraham B, El-Serag H. Dietary intake and risk of developing inflammatory bowel disease: a systematic review of the literature. Am J Gastroenterol 2011;106(4):563–73.
8. Frank DN, St Amand AL, Feldman RA, et al. Molecular-phylogenetic characterization of microbial community imbalances in human inflammatory bowel diseases. Proc Natl Acad Sci U S A 2007;104(34):13780–5.
9. Schultsz C, Van Den Berg FM, Ten Kate FW, et al. The intestinal mucus layer from patients with inflammatory bowel disease harbors high numbers of bacteria compared with controls. Gastroenterology 1999;117(5):1089–97.
10. Ahmed I, Roy BC, Khan SA, et al. Microbiome, metabolome and inflammatory bowel disease. Microorganisms 2016;4(2):20.
11. Molodecky NA, Soon IS, Rabi DM, et al. Increasing incidence and prevalence of the inflammatory bowel diseases with time, based on systematic review. Gastroenterology 2012;142(1):46–54.
12. Vatn MH, Sandvik AK. Inflammatory bowel disease. Scand J Gastroenterol 2015; 50(6):748–62.
13. Mekhjian HS, Switz DM, Melnyk CS, et al. Clinical features and natural history of Crohn's disease. Gastroenterology 1979;77:898.

14. Sawczenk A, Sandhu BK. Presenting features of inflammatory bowel disease in Great Britain and Ireland. Arch Dis Child 2003;88:995–1000.

15. Farmer RG, Hawk WA, Turnbull RB Jr. Clinical patterns in Crohn's disease: a statistical study of 615 cases. Gastroenterology 1975;68:627.

16. Greenstein AJ, Sachar DB, Gibas A, et al. Outcome of toxic dilatation in ulcerative and Crohn's colitis. J Clin Gastroenterol 1985;7:1.

17. Schwartz DA, Loftus EV Jr, Tremaine WJ, et al. The natural history of fistulizing Crohn's disease in Olmsted County, Minnesota. Gastroenterology 2002;122:875.

18. Louis E, Collard A, Oger AF, et al. Behaviour of Crohn's disease according to the Vienna classification: changing pattern over the course of the disease. Gut 2001; 49:777–82.

19. Tozer PJ, Whelan K, Phillips RKS, et al. Etiology of Perianal Crohn's disease: role of genetic, microbiological, and immunological factors. Inflamm Bowel Dis 2009; 15:1591–8.

20. Beaugerie L, Seksi P, Nuin-Larmurier I, et al. Predictors of Crohn's disease. Gastroenterol 2006;130:650–6.

21. Safar B, Sands D. Perianal Crohn's disease. Clin Colon Rectal Surg 2007;20:282.

22. Kelley KA, Kaur T, Tsikitis V. Perianal Crohn's disease: challenges and solutions. Clin Exp Gastroenterol 2017;10:39–46.

23. Hellers G, Bergstrand O, Ewerth S, et al. Occurrence and outcome after primary treatment of anal fistulae in Crohn's disease. Gut 1980;21:525–7.

24. Levine JS, Burakoff R. Extraintestinal manifestations of inflammatory bowel disease. Gastroenterol Hepatol 2011;7(4):235–41.

25. Sairenji T, Collins KL, Evans DV. An update on inflammatory bowel disease. Prim Care 2017;14:673–92.

26. Satsangi J, Silverberg MS, Vermeire S, et al. The Montreal classification of inflammatory bowel disease: controversies, consensus, and implications. Gut 2006;55: 749–53.

27. Becker JM. Surgical management of ulcerative colitis. In: MacDermott RP, Stenson WF, editors. Inflammatory bowel disease. New York: Elsevier; 1992. p. 599.

28. De Dombal FT, Watts JM, Watkinson G, et al. Local complications of ulcerative colitis: stricture, pseudopolyposis, and carcinoma of colon and rectum. Br Med J 1966;1:1442.

29. Mowat C, Cole A, Windsor A, et al. Guidelines for the management of inflammatory bowel disease in adults. Gut 2011;60:571–607.

30. Levine A, Koletzko S, Turner D, et al. ESPGHAN revised porto criteria for the diagnosis of inflammatory bowel disease in children and adolescents. J Pediatr Gastroenterol Nutr 2014;58:795–806.

31. Spiceland CM, Lodhia N. Endoscopy in inflammatory bowel disease: role in diagnosis, management, and treatment. World J Gastroenterol 2018;24(35):4014–20.

32. Kornbluth A, Colombel JF, Leighton JA, et al. ICCE. ICCE consensus for inflammatory bowel disease. Endoscopy 2005;37:1051–4.

33. Doherty GA, Moss AC, Cheifetz AS. Capsule endoscopy for small-bowel evaluation in Crohn's disease. Gastrointest Endosc 2011;74:167–75.

34. Pepys MB, Hirschfield GM. C-reactive protein: a critical update. J Clin Invest 2003;111(12):1805–12.

35. Volanakis JE. Human C-reactive protein: expression, structure, and function. Mol Immunol 2001;38(2–3):189–97.

36. Menees SB, Powell C, Kurlander J, et al. A meta-analysis of the utility of C-reactive protein, erythrocyte sedimentation rate, fecal calprotectin, and fecal

lactoferrin to exclude inflammatory bowel disease in adults with IBS. Am J Gastroenterol 2015;110(3):444–54.

37. Peyrin-Biroulet L, Reinisch W, Colombel JF, et al. Clinical disease activity, C-reactive protein normalisation and mucosal healing in Crohn's disease in the SONIC trial. Gut 2014;63(1):88–95.

38. Ministro P, Martins D. Fecal biomarkers in inflammatory bowel disease: how, when and why? Expert Rev Gastroenterol Hepatol 2017;11(4):317–28.

39. Bressler B, Panaccione R, Fedorak RN, et al. Clinicians' guide to the use of fecal calprotectin to identify and monitor disease activity in inflammatory bowel disease. Can J Gastroenterol Hepatol 2015;29(7):369–72.

40. Roblin X, Duru G, Williet N, et al. Development and internal validation of a model using fecal calprotectin in combination with infliximab trough levels to predict clinical relapse in Crohn's disease. Inflamm Bowel Dis 2017;23(1):126–32.

41. Zhou G, Song Y, Yang W, et al. ASCA, ANCA, ALCA and many more: are they useful in the diagnosis of inflammatory bowel disease? Dig Dis 2016; 34(1–2):90–7.

42. Prideaux L, De Cruz P, Ng SC, et al. Serological antibodies in inflammatory bowel disease: a systematic review. Inflamm Bowel Dis 2012;18:1340–55.

43. Annese V, Andreoli A, Andriulli A, et al. Familial expression of anti-Saccharomyces cerevisiae Mannan antibodies in Crohn's disease and ulcerative colitis: a GISC study. Am J Gastroenterol 2001;96:2407–12.

44. Samuel S, Bruining DH, Loftus EV, et al. Endoscopic skipping of the distal terminal ileum in Crohn's disease can lead to negative results from ileocolonoscopy. Clin Gastroenterol Hepatol 2012;10(11):1253–9.

45. Liu W, Liu J, Xiao W, et al. A diagnostic accuracy meta-analysis of CT and MRI for the evaluation of small bowel Crohn disease. Acad Radiol 2017;24(10):1216–25.

46. Calabrese E, Maaser C, Zorzi F, et al. Bowel ultrasonography in the management of Crohn's disease. a review with recommendations of an international panel of experts. Inflamm Bowel Dis 2016;22:1168–83.

47. Castiglione F, Mainenti PP, De Palma GD, et al. Noninvasive diagnosis of small bowel Crohn's disease: direct comparison of bowel sonography and magnetic resonance enterography. Inflamm Bowel Dis 2013;19:991–8.

48. Sahni V, Ahmad R. Which method is best for imaging of perianal fistula? Abdom Imaging 2008;33:26–30.

Endoscopy in Inflammatory Bowel Disease

Aaron L. Klinger, MD, Brian R. Kann, MD*

KEYWORDS

- Endoscopy • Crohn disease • Ulcerative colitis • Dysplasia surveillance
- Chromoendoscopy • Narrow band imaging

KEY POINTS

- The roles of flexible endoscopy in the setting of inflammatory bowel disease include diagnosis, surveillance, and determination of response to treatment and monitoring for the development of recurrence, dysplasia, or malignancy.
- Advanced techniques, such as chromoendoscopy and narrow band imaging, can be useful adjuncts when performing endoscopy in patients with inflammatory bowel disease.
- There are several roles for therapeutic endoscopy in the setting of inflammatory bowel disease, including endoscopic balloon dilation and endoscopic stricturotomy.

INTRODUCTION

Flexible endoscopy remains the gold standard in the evaluation of the patient with suspected inflammatory bowel disease (IBD), helping to confirm a correct diagnosis in 85% to 90% of cases.[1,2] Meticulous mucosal evaluation of the rectum, colon, and ileum during endoscopy with biopsies is an essential step in confirming a diagnosis of IBD. Endoscopy also plays a critical role in preoperative and postoperative surveillance, determining response to treatment, and monitoring for the development of recurrence, dysplasia, or malignancy. Advanced techniques, such as chromoendoscopy (CE) and narrow band imaging, can be useful adjuncts in certain circumstances. Additionally, there are several roles for therapeutic endoscopy in the setting of IBD.

SCREENING/BIOPSIES

The 2 main variants of IBD are ulcerative colitis (UC) and Crohn disease (CD). Prior to endoscopic evaluation, careful perianal examination should be performed in symptomatic patients, noting the presence or absence of anorectal findings that may

The authors have nothing to disclose.
Department of Colon and Rectal Surgery, Ochsner Medical Center, 1514 Jefferson Highway, New Orleans, LA 70121, USA
* Corresponding author.
E-mail address: brian.kann@ochsner.org

suggest CD, such as anal skin tags, atypical anal fissures, anal canal ulceration, perianal abscesses or fistulae, or anorectal strictures.[3] Although there may be subtle differences in the mucosal appearance of CD and UC, these often are difficult to differentiate grossly, even by an experienced endoscopist; thus, histopathology is essential to confirm a diagnosis. The first sign of tissue injury in UC is an increase in mucosal surface blood flow, resulting in erythema, edema, and vascular congestion, and is often described as having the appearance of wet sandpaper endoscopically. Crohn colitis classically appears as patchy segmental inflammation, occasionally with rectal sparing, whereas the distribution of UC is diffuse, beginning distally at the dentate line and progressing proximally in a contiguous fashion. As both diseases become more severe, advanced mucosal changes are seen, including cobblestoning, worsening friability and ulceration, edema, and pseudopolyp formation (**Figs. 1–3**). In rare instances, rectal sparing can be seen in the setting of UC, especially in pediatric patients or those with concomitant primary sclerosing cholangitis (PSC). Despite these differences, a distinct disease type cannot be classified endoscopically in approximately 10% of patients. These patients are determined to have unclassified IBD.[4]

The use of ileocolonoscopy with biopsies for the diagnosis of CD has a sensitivity of 81% and specificity of 77%.[5] Ileal intubation with biopsies should always be performed to assess for ileitis. Care must be taken to not confuse Crohn ileitis with backwash ileitis, which can be seen in up to 17% of patients with UC. Backwash ileitis typically involves a short segment of TI with mildly inflamed mucosa extending from the cecum and typically does not demonstrate ulceration, stenosis, or other signs of CD. Small bowel (SB) involvement is present in approximately 80% of patients with CD, and approximately one-third of patients with CD demonstrate isolated SB involvement.[6] Upper endoscopy, although recommended for all children with suspected IBD, is not performed routinely in adults, although it should be considered in symptomatic patients to identify the smaller subset (approximately 15%) of CD patients with esophagogastroduodenal disease.[7,8]

Strictures can be found in both CD and UC and must be carefully examined and biopsied when encountered (**Fig. 4**). Strictures may be identified in up to 11% of CD patients on initial endoscopic evaluation and can carry up to a 24% risk of malignancy in UC and a 6% risk in CD. Enterocolic, enterenteric, colovesical, and enterovesical fistulae also may be seen endoscopically as well in the setting of CD (**Fig. 5**).

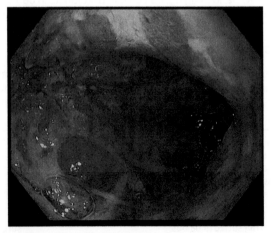

Fig. 1. Severe Crohn colitis with cobblestoning.

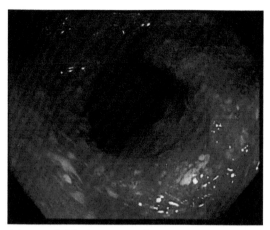

Fig. 2. Severe UC with superficial ulceration, edema, and mucosal friability.

ASSESSMENT OF DISEASE ACTIVITY

Beyond its role in the initial diagnosis of IBD, endoscopy also plays a crucial role in both determining severity of disease and monitoring response to treatment. The presence of mucosal healing has been associated with improved outcomes, including higher remission rates, decreased use of corticosteroids, decreased hospitalization, and lower risk of developing colorectal cancer (CRC).[9,10] Although mucosal healing is generally recognized as mucosa without ulceration or erosion, definitions of mucosal healing vary slightly for CD and UC; in patients with UC, mucosal healing is defined as a normal mucosal vascular pattern without friability and erosions, whereas mucosal healing in CD is defined as lack of visible ulceration.[11,12]

Several endoscopic scoring systems exist for both UC and CD; these vary in complexity and rely on endoscopic and physician assessment of disease severity. Of the endoscopic scoring systems used for the assessment of disease activity in

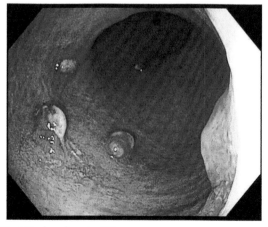

Fig. 3. Inflammatory pseudopolyps in UC.

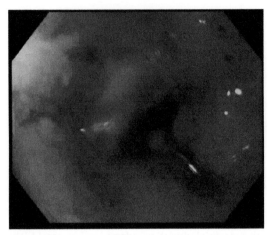

Fig. 4. Colonic stricture in CD.

the setting of UC, the Mayo Endoscopic Score (MES) and Ulcerative Colitis Endo-scopic Index of Severity (UCEIS) are the most commonly used. The MES is scored from 0 to 12 and is calculated based on stool frequency, presence and severity of rectal bleeding, mucosal appearance on endoscopy, and the physician's overall assessment of the patient's disease.[13] Since its introduction in 1987, the MES has been extensively studied; however, its objective nature allows for significant interob-server variation and limits its generalizability.[13]

The UCEIS contains a more detailed endoscopic assessment than the MES and assigns points based on the mucosal vascular pattern, presence of bleeding, and presence and severity of erosions and ulcers[14] (**Table 1**). Although this scale has been independently validated and has been shown to demonstrate satisfactory agreement between observers when viewing a procedural video, a recent Cochrane review[15] failed to fully validate it or any other UC scoring system. In addition, the distinction between mild, moderate, and severe disease is not clearly defined by the UCEIS.

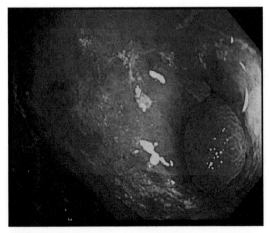

Fig. 5. Enterocolic fistula in CD.

Table 1	
The Ulcerative Colitis Endoscopic Index of Severity	
Vascular pattern	0 = Normal
	1 = Patchy obliteration
	2 = Complete obliteration
Bleeding	0 = None
	1 = Mucosal/coagulated
	2 = Luminal mild (free blood in the lumen)
	3 = Luminal moderate/severe (frank oozing)
Erosions/ulcers	0 = None
	1 = Erosions (<5 mm)
	2 = Superficial ulcer (>5-mm defects, fibrin covered but superficial)
	3 = Deep ulcer (deeper ulcers with slightly raised edges)

Adapted from Travis SP, Schnell D, Krzeski P, et al. Developing an instrument to assess the endoscopic severity of ulcerative colitis: the Ulcerative Colitis Endoscopic Index of Severity (UCEIS). *Gut.* 2012;61(4):535-542.

Several endoscopic scoring systems for CD have been created as well. The 2 most well studied are the Crohn's Disease Endoscopic Index of Severity (CDEIS) and the Simple Endoscopic Score for Crohn's Disease (SES-CD). The CDEIS evaluates mucosal patterns in the rectum, left colon, transverse colon, right colon, and ileum, and a score ranging from 0 to 44 is calculated. Its clinical use is somewhat limited, however, given that it is time consuming, requires specialized training, and significant interobserver variation in scores can occur.[16]

The SES-CD determines scores from 0 to 3 in the same 5 anatomic segments as the CDEIS, and at least 1 study has demonstrated acceptable intra/inter-rater reliability.[17] The Study of Biologic and Immunomodulator Naive Patients in Crohn's Disease trial found that a score decrease of at least 50% in either the CDEIS or SES-CD by week 26 of biologic treatment correlated with steroid-free remission at week 50.[18]

DYSPLASIA SURVEILLANCE

Long-standing IBD is a well-established risk factor for the development of CRC, which is responsible for up to 15% of all deaths in patients with IBD. Additionally, IBD (in particular UC) is the third highest risk factor for CRC, ranking only behind familial polyposis coli and hereditary nonpolyposis CRC. Unlike these familial/genetic syndromes, the cancer risk in IBD is related primarily to chronic mucosal inflammation. IBD-associated CRC does not typically follow the adenoma-carcinoma sequence but instead develops through an inflammation-dysplasia-carcinoma pattern.[19] This often results in an advanced stage at the time of diagnosis and poorer survival compared with sporadic CRC.[20] Specific cancer risks in IBD include colonic dysplasia, active inflammation, younger onset of disease, longer duration of disease, PSC, and the presence of inflammatory polyps. The risk of CRC with IBD-colitis has been estimated to be 2% at 10 years, 8% at 20 years, and 18% and 30 years. Other studies have shown, however, that 18% of IBD-associated CRC cases occur in patients with a less than 8-year history of IBD.[21] Given this increased risk, it is important for patients with IBD, in particular long-standing disease, to have regular endoscopic screening to detect dysplasia or discover cancer at an earlier, potentially more curable stage.

Older guidelines referred to endoscopically identified lesions in patients with IBD-colitis remote from an area of active colitis as *sporadic adenomas*, wheras those found in areas of inflammation were termed, *dysplasia-associated lesion or mass*. This terminology no longer is used and has been replaced with other descriptive terms, such as *visible*, for clearly identified lesions and, *invisible*, for lesions discovered in random biopsies. Likewise, the terms, *flat lesions* and *raised lesions*, have been abandoned, because these terms can be confused with the Paris classification of superficial colorectal mucosal lesions.[22]

In an effort to reduce CRC mortality in the setting of long-standing IBD-associated colitis, prophylactic total proctocolectomy was often recommended routinely in the past. With the increased availability of colonoscopy, a paradigm shift has occurred, favoring regular colonoscopic surveillance, reserving surgery for those with heightened cancer risk.[23] Endoscopic surveillance is cost effective and has been clearly shown to reduce the risk of CRC-associated death in IBD patients.[24-27] It is typically recommended to start colonoscopic screening in UC 8 years to 10 years after the onset of UC symptoms. The extent of disease should be clearly described at this time, because this determines the optimal follow-up period and estimates the risk of developing CRC risk. Disease is classified as extensive if it has progressed proximal to the splenic flexure, left-sided if it extends up to but does not include the splenic flexure, and proctosigmoiditis if it is limited to the rectum or sigmoid colon.[28]

The 2005 Crohn's and Colitis Foundation of America (CCFA) guidelines suggest follow-up examination intervals based on patients' individual risk factors. Those with extensive or left-sided colitis should be screened every 1 year to 2 years after a negative initial screen. After 2 negative examinations, the interval can be extended up to 3 years until disease has been present for 20 years, at which time surveillance should again be considered every 1 yera to 2 years.[23]

Traditional surveillance consists of mucosal evaluation with white light endoscopy (WLE), with targeted biopsies of visible lesions as well as random biopsies, because dysplasia may not always have a grossly abnormal appearance. Traditional surveillance for IBD patients with extensive colonic disease (beyond the splenic flexure in UC or involving at least one-third of the colon in CD) involves obtaining 4-quadrant biopsies every 10 cm throughout the colon. These specimens should be placed in separate jars by location, and any other visible or suspicious lesions should be biopsied and sent separately. For those with less extensive disease, biopsies should be taken at the proximal extent of disease and every 10 cm distally. In patients with UC, biopsies every 5 cm in the distal sigmoid and rectum may be considered in long-standing disease, because these areas have a higher frequency of CRC.[23]

Histologic interpretation should follow the definitions recommended by the 1983 IBD Dysplasia Morphology Working Group, which remains the standard for evaluation of surveillance specimens. Any biopsy with mucosal changes on histology that are indefinite for dysplasia or show low-grade dysplasia (LGD), high-grade dysplasia (HGD) (**Fig. 6**), or adenocarcinoma should be considered abnormal. CCFA guidelines call for histopathologic review and confirmation by an experienced gastrointestinal pathologist. Recommendations for follow-up endoscopic surveillance of dysplasia depend on whether a lesion is visible or invisible and also on the extent (low grade vs high grade) of dysplasia.[29]

In patients with UC, treatment of LGD identified in a random biopsy of grossly noninflamed mucosa remains controversial. Some studies suggest a 5-year risk of progression from LGD to HGD of 50% to 55%, although other studies dispute this.[23] There is also evidence that up to 20% of patients with LGD who undergo surgery may have an unrecognized synchronous cancer identified in the resected colon.[23] Given this CRC risk, offering proctocolectomy to patients with LGD in the setting of UC is a reasonable recommendation. Those who have more than 1 flat lesion with

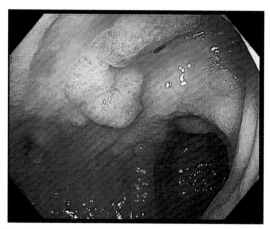

Fig. 6. Visible HGD in UC.

LGD on biopsy or who have flat LGD on 2 or more subsequent examinations should be strongly encouraged to have a proctocolectomy. For those patients who elect to continue surveillance rather than surgery, repeat endoscopic evaluation should be performed within 3 months to 6 months. Patients with lesions containing HGD, histologically confirmed by a pathologist with extensive experience in IBD, should be encouraged to undergo proctocolectomy given the high risk of synchronous and metachronous CRC.[23]

Visible lesions in UC may resemble sporadic adenomas and can be removed via traditional endoscopic polypectomy techniques. If removed from an area with grossly visible colitis, 4 biopsies should also be taken from the surrounding mucosa and sent separately. If these biopsies identify no additional dysplasia, repeat endoscopy should be performed at 6 months and at shortened intervals thereafter until no further active colitis is seen. If dysplasia is identified in biopsies of the mucosa surrounding the grossly visible lesion, proctocolectomy should be considered. Adenomatous polyps seen in areas without endoscopically visible evidence of colitis can be treated according to standard guidelines.[23]

Those patients with Crohn proctosigmoiditis are thought to have a CRC risk that approximates that of the general population and typically can be be screened according to standard colonoscopy guidelines, as long as disease is well controlled. If at any point colitis is identified on a biopsy proximal to 35 cm, even in grossly normal-appearing mucosa, or if disease becomes active, the patient should be entered into a UC-type screening protocol. Patients with more significant risk factors, such as PSC or significant family history, may require shorter intervals between endoscopic evaluation.[23] Patients with Crohn colitis and at least one-third colonic involvement and 8 years to 10 years of disease should be screened endoscopically for dysplasia or cancer, with targeted biopsies of grossly abnormal mucosa and 4-quadrant biopsies every 10 cm along the length of the colon and rectum. A negative examination with no evidence of dysplasia should be followed by repeat colonoscopy every 1 year to 2 years until 2 consecutive negative examinations have occurred, at which point examinations can be performed every 1 years to 3 years, as long as there is no evidence of dysplasia on biopsies. At 20 years of disease, the surveillance interval should be shortened to every 1 year to 2 years. The treatment of abnormal findings in Crohn colitis is identical to the treatment in UC.[23]

The utility of random biopsies has more recently been brought into question. van den Broek and colleagues[30] found UC-associated neoplasia to be macroscopically visible in 94% of colonoscopies and found only 1 patient over a 10-year period to have randomly detected neoplasia with clinical consequences. Watanabe and colleagues[31] randomly assigned UC patients to undergo targeted biopsies in addition to random biopsies versus targeted biopsies alone and found similar proportions of neoplasia in both groups, noting that the performance of targeted biopsies was more cost effective.

More advanced techniques have been developed to help detect lesions that otherwise might be missed on traditional WLE. CE utilizes various dyes (such as indigo carmine or methylene blue), which are misted via the colonoscope onto the colonic mucosa. Using a high-resolution or high-magnification endoscope, an endoscopist is then able to perform a detailed evaluation of the mucosal surface and potentially identify lesions that may not have been detected on WLE. The CCFA guidelines recognize CE and endorse its use but do not comment further. More recent guidelines from both the British Society of Gastroenterology and the American Society for Gastrointestinal Endoscopy (ASGE)/American Gastroenterological Association (AGA) advocate for the use of CE without random biopsies in the setting of IBD surveillance.[22,32] This technique has been gaining popularity since the early 2000s and, when performed by a trained, experience endoscopist, has been shown to allow for improved early diagnosis of adenomas and early cancers (**Fig. 7**).[33] The pit pattern classification developed by Kudo and colleagues[34] can be used to evaluate mucosal staining patterns and to help differentiate between neoplastic and nonneoplastic changes. A recent large Spanish study evaluated IBD patients first with traditional WLE followed by CE utilizing indigo carmine and found a dysplasia miss-rate of 43% using traditional WLE. Detection rates were similar between standard and high-definition optics, and they were similar between expert and nonexpert endoscopists. Furthermore, no significant learning curve in the use of CE was appreciated, further advocating for more widespread use.[35]

Many newer-generation endoscopic devices offer filters and algorithms that filter specific wavelengths of light in an attempt to mimic CE and better enhance the visualization of abnormal tissues. Several modalities of so-called virtual CE exist. Narrow band imaging filters out red and green light while enhancing blue light, allowing for better visualization of mucosal vasculature and helping to assess the degree of inflammation (**Fig. 8**). i-scan imaging (Pentax Medical, Montvale, NJ) consists of 3 algorithms designed to enhance mucosal features. A newer technique, confocal laser

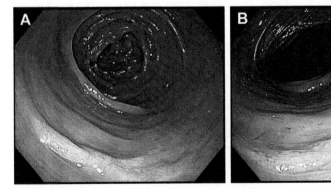

Fig. 7. Dysplastic lesion in CD viewed with white light high definition (HD) endoscopy (*A*) and with CE using methylene blue (*B*).

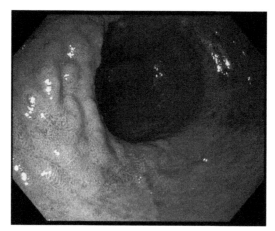

Fig. 8. Dysplasia in UC seen with narrow band imaging.

endomicroscopy, allows for real-time, 1000-times magnification of colonic mucosa and has been shown to be able to help differentiate between neoplasia, solitary adenoma, and benign regenerative changes (that may present in a similar fashion as dysplasia) with 97.8% accuracy. This technique uses intravenously administered fluorescent contrast and a specialized probe that can be passed through the working channel of an endoscope.[36–38] Although these newer techniques show promise, study outcomes are mixed, and dye-based CE currently remains the standard recommended technique for IBD surveillance.[27]

POSTOPERATIVE SURVEILLANCE IN THE INFLAMMATORY BOWEL DISEASE PATIENT
Ileoscopy/Proctoscopy After Subtotal Colectomy for Ulcerative Colitis

Since the introduction of tumor necrosis factor inhibitors and other biologic agents, operative rates for IBD have shown a significant decline.[39] Up to 30% of UC patients, however, still eventually require surgery for neoplasia or medically refractory disease.[40] Definitive surgery for UC involves a total proctocolectomy with either ileal pouch–anal anastomosis (IPAA) or end ileostomy (EI). In patients with severe/fulminant colitis, or those on high-dose corticosteroids, this procedure should be staged, first performing a subtotal colectomy with EI and Hartmann closure of the rectosigmoid stump. Lack of nutrients from luminal bacteria to the rectal mucosa can result in diversion proctitis in these patients who already have severely diseased mucosa in the remnant rectosigmoid. Patients may present with pelvic pain or discomfort, urgency, and bloody or mucoid discharge; endoscopic findings include extremely friable mucosa, exudates, edema, erythema, and ulceration.

Prior to construction of an ileal pouch after subtotal colectomy, ileoscopy may be considered to exclude SB CD. It is rare to see macroscopic disease in the absence of overt symptoms, so mucosal biopsy should be performed. Rarely, postcolectomy enteritis syndrome can occur after EI creation; endoscopically, this is characterized by diffuse mucosal inflammation, which should not be confused with the segmental inflammation seen in CD.

Pouchoscopy

After staged IPAA (with a diverting ileostomy), patients typically have a diverted pouch for anywhere from 6 weeks to 6 months. Lack of nutrients absorbed from luminal content can result in diversion pouchitis similar to that seen with a diverted Hartmann stump, which is characterized endoscopically by mucosal erythema, edema, friability, erosions, and ulceration. Diversion pouchitis typically resolves once the diverting ileostomy has been closed and intestinal continuity has been restored. Topical treatments, such as mesalamine suppositories, can temporize symptoms in patients who are not thought to be at an appropriate point for stoma closure.

Pouchoscopy also serves several diagnostic and therapeutic roles for functional ileal pouches after diverting ileostomy closure. These include diagnosis of mechanical or inflammatory complications, surveillance for neoplasia, and endoscopic management of complications. Mechanical complications include obstruction due to strictures (which can occur anywhere from the afferent limb inlet to the anal anastomosis), pouch angulation, pouch twisting, or pouch prolapse. Pouch leaks can be acute or chronic in nature and most commonly occur at the tip of the J or at the anastomosis. Anastomotic leaks can be associated with pouch vaginal fistulas or presacral sinuses.[40] Although pouch leaks typically are diagnosed via contrast enema, pouchoscopy often is utilized to identify the site and size of the leak to help determine optimal treatment.

Pouchoscopy is the main diagnostic tool for the evaluation of inflammatory IPAA complications, including pouchitis, cuffitis, and CD of the pouch. Up to half of all IPAA patients have at least 1 episode of pouchitis, and a majority of them have at least 1 additional episode within 2 years of the initial episode. Symptoms of pouchitis vary and can include mild to severe pelvic or perianal discomfort, increased stool urgency and frequency, tenesmus, abdominal cramping, and rarely bleeding.[41] Because these symptoms are nonspecific and do not always correlate with endoscopic or histologic findings, diagnosis of pouchitis should be made via a combination of clinical symptoms, endoscopic findings, and histologic evaluation of mucosal biopsies.[42] Endoscopic evaluation for pouchitis should include careful inspection of the pouch, the afferent ileum, and the rectal cuff. Biopsies can be helpful and should be performed even if the mucosa appears normal to exclude microscopic disease. Endoscopic features of pouchitis include friability, exudates, erythema, ulceration, and/or bleeding.

Two scores exist to diagnose and assess severity of pouchitis. The pouchitis disease activity index (PDAI) is the most commonly used scoring system and consists of three 6-point scales: clinical symptoms, endoscopic findings, and histologic changes of acute inflammation (**Table 2**).[43] Active pouchitis is defined as a score greater than or equal to 7. A modified PDAI was proposed by Shen and colleagues,[44] eliminating the need for histologic evaluation of the mucosa, and was found to have similar sensitivity and specificity to the PDAI, avoiding the added cost and time required to wait for pathology results. The pouchitis activity score is similar to the PDAI but also includes evaluation of histologic features of chronic inflammation. This score classifies disease as mild adaptive pouchitis, moderate pouchitis, or severe pouchitis.[45]

Patients who demonstrate symptoms concerning for pouch obstruction should undergo pouchoscopy, taking care to evaluate the anastomosis, the pouch body, the inlet, and the afferent limb. Anastomotic stricture may be identified on digital examination and often can be dilated digitally or endoscopically. On inspection of the pouch body, the endoscopist should note the course of the pouch staple line and the presence or absence of the characteristic owl's eyes configuration formed by the confluence of the afferent pouch inlet and blind efferent limb of the J-pouch. Disruption of this configuration is associated with a high risk of pouch failure and also can be seen with pouch torsion, pouch ischemia, or CD of the pouch. Difficulty intubating the pouch inlet due to sharp angulation or prolapse can suggest afferent limb syndrome.[46,47]

Table 2
Pouchitis disease activity index

Criteria	Score
Clinical	
Stool frequency	
Usual postoperative frequency	0
1–2 stools/d > postoperative usual	1
3 + stools/d > postoperative usual	2
Rectal bleeding	
None or rare	0
Present daily	1
Fecal urgency or abdominal cramps	
None	0
Occasional	1
Usually	2
Fever (temperature >37.8°C)	
Absent	0
Present	1
Endoscopic inflammation	
Edema	1
Granularity	1
Friability	1
Loss of vascular pattern	1
Mucous exudates	1
Ulceration	1
Acute histologic inflammation	
Polymorphonuclear cell infiltration	
Mild	1
Moderate + crypt Abscesses	2
Severe + crypt Abscesses	3
Ulceration per low-power field (mean)	
<25%	1
25%–50%	2
>50%	3

From Sandborn WJ, Tremaine WJ, Batts KP, Pemberton JH, Phillips SF. Pouchitis after ileal pouch-anal anastomosis: a Pouchitis Disease Activity Index. Mayo Clin Proc. 1994;69(5):409-415.

Several endoscopic therapies may be used to manage IPAA complications. Strictures can be treated with balloon dilation or needle-knife stricturotomy.[48] Likewise, presacral sinuses can be opened and drained using a needle knife. J-pouch tip or anastomotic leaks can be treated using an over-the-scope clip, such as the OTSC system (Ovesco, Cary, North Carolina), as long is there is percutaneous counterdrainage of the presacral cavity.[49] More recently, endoscopic-assisted endoluminal vacuum-assisted therapy has been reported to be an effective means of managing anastomotic leak after IPAA.[50]

Cuffitis refers to microscopic or macroscopic inflammation of the rectal cuff, which is the residual distal rectum located between the pouch anastomosis and the dentate line. Microscopically, the rectal cuff is lined by rectal columnar mucosa, distinct from the villous mucosa of the pouch or the squamous epithelium of the anatomic anal canal. Cuffitis typically refers to inflammation of the residual rectal mucosa specifically in patients who have undergone a stapled ileal pouch anastomosis without mucosectomy, although it can occasionally occur in occult remnant mucosa after mucosectomy. Cuffitis classically presents with anal bleeding, anal discharge, tenesmus, increased urgency and frequency, and anorectal pain with bowel movements. Pouchitis or CD of the pouch can often present in a similar fashion as cuffitis, although bleeding typically is seen more frequently in cuffitis. On pouchoscopy, cuffitis appears as rectal cuff inflammation distal to the anastomosis without pouch mucosal inflammation (**Fig. 9**); biopsies of the pouch should show no signs of inflammation, whereas cuff biopsies show ulceration with neutrophil infiltration.[51]

CD remains a relative contraindication for IPAA, because patients have significant risk for postoperative complications that may ultimately lead to pouch failure. For this reason, CD in patients with an IPAA typically is diagnosed postoperatively after restorative proctocolectomy for presumed UC or indeterminate colitis; a delayed diagnosis of CD can occur in up to 13% of patients in this setting. Associated signs and symptoms include anal fistulae, abscesses, strictures, other perianal disease, pain, tenesmus, and increased urgency/frequency. Symptoms of pouch CD may be confused with other inflammatory disorders, such as pouchitis or cuffitis. Diagnosis is confirmed both endoscopically and histologically. Pouchoscopy may reveal loss of the normal mucosal vascular pattern, mucosal ulcers, friable/hemorrhagic mucosa, and/or pseudopolyps (**Fig. 10**). The location of disease may aid in establishing a diagnosis of CD in an ileal pouch, especially if mucosal inflammation or ulceration is present in the afferent limb proximal to the pouch inlet, which can be suggestive of CD. Endoscopic biopsies should be obtained, because the presence of submucosal granulomas histologically may be suggestive of CD. Care should be taken to avoid biopsies immediately adjacent to the pouch staple line, because foreign body granulomas unrelated to CD may be identified as part of the normal response to surgical staples.[51,52]

Dysplasia is rare but can occur after IPAA, having been reported both in the residual rectal cuff and in the pouch itself. Risk factors for cuff dysplasia are similar to risk factors overall for dysplasia in the setting of UC, namely longer duration and increased

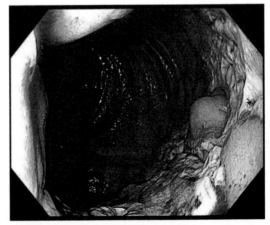

Fig. 9. Cuffitis. Note the normal appearance of the pouch mucosa.

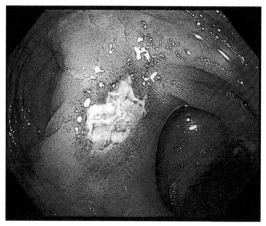

Fig. 10. Ulceration concerning for CD in a J-pouch.

severity of disease, family history of CRC, and PSC. Patients with dysplasia or malignancy in surgically resected bowel also are at increased risk for cuff malignancy. Intrapouch neoplasia is rare; risks include prior CRC related to UC, history of backwash ileitis, chronic pouchitis, and PSC. Most cases of IPAA-associated dysplasia seem to arise from the anal transition zone, and mucosectomy does not seem protective. In a review of more than 3200 patients who underwent restorative proctocolectomy with IPAA at the Cleveland Clinic, the incidence of pouch neoplasia was 0.9% at 5 years and 5.1% at 25 years.[53] A recent large Danish study reported an incidence of 0.12% at a median follow-up period of 12.9 years.[54] In this same study, the risk of cancer after IPAA was found to be identical to that of a case-matched comparison cohort.

Despite the low risk of developing cancer after IPAA, multiple organizations continue to recommend regular pouch surveillance. The European Crohn's and Colitis Organisation and British Society of Gastroenterology both suggest pouchoscopy every 5 years for average-risk patients and annual pouchoscopy with biopsies for patients with risk factors, such as prior dysplasia, type C histologic changes (persistent atrophy and severe inflammation), PSC, or prior CRC.[5] Although both the AGA and ASGE lack specific guidelines for pouch surveillance, a survey of American gastroenterologists and colorectal surgeons found that a majority of respondents felt that pouch surveillance with biopsies of the pouch body and cuff/transition zone is necessary.[55,56] A protocol published by McLaughlin and colleagues[57] recommends annual surveillance pouchoscopy with biopsies in those with dysplasia or cancer in the original resection specimen. In other patients, pouchoscopy with biopsies is recommended 1 year postoperatively after IPAA; after this, surveillance pouchoscopy with biopsies is suggested every 3 years in those with type C mucosal changes, chronic pouchitis, PSC, and a diagnosis of UC made more than 10 years prior. The authors' practice is to perform an initial pouchoscopy at 1 year after IPAA. In low-risk patients with a normal initial pouchoscopy, continued surveillance pouchoscopy is performed every 2 years to 3 years thereafter; in high-risk patients or those with the presence of LGD, the surveillance interval is shortened to yearly.

Endoscopic Surveillance After Surgery for Crohn Disease

Although there are no widely accepted guidelines for postoperative endoscopic surveillance in CD, initial postoperative colonoscopy typically is performed 6 months to

12 months after surgery. This allows for evaluation for early postoperative recurrence and early optimization of postoperative medical therapy.[58]

The Rutgeerts score, developed in 1990, is a useful tool for evaluation of the severity of recurrent endoscopic disease in postoperative CD patients (**Table 3**).[59] This scale specifically evaluates the appearance of the neoterminal ileum after ileocolic resection, because this is where inflammatory changes and recurrence typically occurs. The score, which ranges from 0 to 4, looks at the number of aphthous lesions present, mucosal inflammation, and other features, such as ulceration, luminal narrowing, and nodularity. Scores of 0 to 1 indicate endoscopic remission and have a low risk of clinical recurrence. Scores of greater than or equal to 2 indicate endoscopic recurrence, and patients with a score of 4 are expected to have disease recurrence within 4 years. Evaluation of the neoterminal ileum in the postoperative period allows for optimization of medical management and can prevent disease recurrence and the need for additional resections.

THERAPEUTIC ENDOSCOPY IN INFLAMMATORY BOWEL DISEASE

Transmural inflammation is a hallmark of CD and can often result in intestinal strictures, which occur in approximately 25% to 40% of patients with CD and in 10% of those specifically with Crohn colitis.[60] Strictures typically are identified either endoscopically or by radiographic studies, which have the added benefit of being able to identify concomitant abscess or fistula.[61,62] The most common location for stricture in CD is the terminal ileum in patients who have not undergone prior surgery or the neoterminal ileum just proximal to the site of prior ileocolic anastomosis in patients who have undergone prior resection.[63] Traditionally, strictures have been treated with surgical resection or strictureplasty, but, more recently, endoscopic balloon dilation (EBD) has been used with increasing frequency to help avoid surgery. Gustavsson and colleagues[62] reported a series of 776 EBDs for CD (80% of which were for anastomotic strictures), in which 52% required no further or 1 additional dilation only at 5-year follow-up. Generally, EBD is best suited for straight, short ($\leq$4 cm) strictures with minimal inflammation and without an adjacent fistula.[64] Symptomatic relief is achieved in greater than 70% of patients, and the perforation rate is approximately 3%.[65,66]

Colonic strictures generally are well tolerated, especially in the proximal colon where the stool is more liquid and, thus, typically present at a later stage. Patients may complain of a change in stool caliber, diarrhea or constipation, or abdominal pain. If a colonic stricture is seen endoscopically in the setting of suspected UC, and the stricture can be traversed, it is imperative to intubate the terminal ileum and obtain biopsies to rule out underlying CD. Colonic strictures in the setting of IBD typically are considered malignant until proven otherwise and should be biopsied in multiple quadrants when encountered.[67,68] EBD has become the preferred treatment in

Table 3	
Rutgeerts scale in assessment of postoperative Crohn disease	
Endoscopic remission	i0 = no lesions
	i1 = <5 aphthous lesions
Endoscopic recurrence	i2 = >5 aphthous lesions with normal intervening mucosa
	i3 = diffuse aphthous ileitis with diffusely inflamed mucosa
	i4 = diffuse inflammation with large ulcers/nodes/narrowing

Data from Rutgeerts P, Geboes K, Vantrappen G, Beyls J, Kerremans R, Hiele M. Predictability of the postoperative course of Crohn's disease. Gastroenterology. 1990;99(4):956-963.

most instances of ileal pouch strictures, with 87% of patients being able to retain a functional pouch.[69]

After exclusion of malignancy via endoscopic biopsies, colonic strictures can be treated with EBD using a pediatric colonoscope or enteroscope and a through-the-scope EBD. Pre-endoscopy imaging can help to estimate the diameter and length of the stricture. Performing the procedure under fluoroscopic guidance can be helpful as well, because injection of contrast via a biliary catheter placed though the biopsy channel of the endoscope can help to delineate the length of the stricture. Otherwise, the diameter of the scope can be used as a visual aid during endoscopic visualization of the stricture to help estimate the diameter of the stricture and aid in selection of the size of the balloon dilator to be used. Typically, balloons of 18 mm to 20 mm are used in the colon and balloons of 12 mm to 15 mm are used in the SB. Inflation occurs by hydrostatic pressure at 1-mm intervals, with a duration varying from 20 seconds to 3 minutes at each interval. After dilation, the stricture should be assessed for any potential injury or perforation.[62]

Endoscopic stricturotomy is well established for upper gastrointestinal tract and biliary strictures. More recently, endoscopic stricturotomy has been evaluated as a possible treatment modality of colonic strictures in the setting of IBD. A study from the Cleveland Clinic evaluated 127 strictures in 85 treatments that were treated with an endoscopic needle knife. In this study, strictures averaged 1.5 cm in length, and all were able to be traversed by an endoscope after treatment. At 1-year follow-up, 84.5% remained surgery-free, although most required additional endoscopic treatments. Adverse events occurred in less than 4% of procedures.[70]

Although no specific antifibrotic agents exist for stricturing CD, attempts have been made to directly inject medications into strictures endoscopically. Results of long-acting corticosteroid injection have been mixed. A randomized trial by East and colleagues[71] did not find a reduction in time to redilation of strictures after endoscopic injection of triamcinolone versus placebo; in fact, results trended toward favoring placebo. An Italian study of pediatric CD patients, however, found endoscopic corticosteroid steroid injection to statistically reduce the need for redilation and the time to subsequent surgery after EBD.[72] Due to lack of convincing data, intralesional steroid injection is not recommended at this time. Likewise, attempts have been made to heal inflammatory strictures in CD by directly injecting infliximab directly into the lesions. Studies thus far have been small but show promising results.[73–75]

Balloon-dilated strictures often recur and require multiple treatments. In this scenario, various types of self-expanding or balloon-expanded endoscopic stents have been used in an attempt to maintain patency of dilated strictures with promising results. Unfortunately, these stents are not designed to be left in place long term for benign disease (such as IBD), and therefore, if metal stents are used, they should be covered. Due to concern for possible stent migration, it is recommended that these stents be removed by 4 weeks. Several studies have investigated the use of biodegradable stents, initially developed for esophageal strictures and made from various synthetic polymers, for the treatment of strictures of both the small intestine and colon.[76–78] No currently available endoscopic stents are designed specifically for stricturing disease in IBD.[70]

Fistulizing disease can occur as a long-term complication of IBD, or it can occur after surgery with an anastomosis. A fistula by definition has a primary opening along the gastrointestinal tract and a secondary opening at other parts of bowel, other organs, or skin. Fistulae traditionally have been treated surgically or with medications, but endoscopic treatments have been developed in more recent years. Following the principles of surgical fistulotomy, endoscopic fistulotomy can be used to drain short, superficial fistulas (<3-cm long and <2-mm thick). This technique consists of traversing the tract with a soft tipped guide wire and opening the tract with a needle knife. For larger fistulas, a guide wire can be passed and used to introduce a seton.[70,79]

The introduction of over-the-scope clips has resulted in attempts to endoscopically close the primary opening of a fistula in an effort to reduce drainage and possibly prevent abscess formation. This technique seems to be more effective in closing fistulas from anastomotic leaks, and the efficacy of clipping CD-associated fistulae has been found to be low.[70,80]

SUMMARY

Flexible endoscopy is an essential tool for the diagnosis, staging, observation, and treatment of IBD. Frequent endoscopic assessment and use of standardized scoring systems allow for monitoring of treatment effect with a goal of achieving and maintaining mucosal healing. Biopsies allow endoscopists to evaluate histologic disease activity and screen for dysplastic changes. New technologies allow for better evaluation of the mucosa to find disease that may not be easily seen by the naked eye. Furthermore, endoscopic technologies allow for diagnostic and therapeutic endoscopy for IBD patients, such as stricture dilation and treatment of fistulas and absceses.

REFERENCES

1. Chutkan RK, Scherl E, Waye JD. Colonoscopy in inflammatory bowel disease. Gastrointest Endosc Clin N Am 2002;12(3):463–83, viii.
2. Pera A, Bellando P, Caldera D, et al. Colonoscopy in inflammatory bowel disease. Diagnostic accuracy and proposal of an endoscopic score. Gastroenterology 1987;92(1):181–5.
3. Peyrin-Biroulet L, Loftus EV Jr, Tremaine WJ, et al. Perianal Crohn's disease findings other than fistulas in a population-based cohort. Inflamm Bowel Dis 2012; 18(1):43–8.
4. Silverberg MS, Satsangi J, Ahmad T, et al. Toward an integrated clinical, molecular and serological classification of inflammatory bowel disease: report of a Working Party of the 2005 Montreal World Congress of Gastroenterology. Can J Gastroenterol 2005;19(Suppl A):5A–36A.
5. Mitselos IV, Christodoulou DK, Katsanos KH, et al. The role of small bowel capsule endoscopy and ileocolonoscopy in patients with nonspecific but suggestive symptoms of Crohn's disease. Eur J Gastroenterol Hepatol 2016;28(8): 882–9.
6. Annese V, Daperno M, Rutter MD, et al. European evidence based consensus for endoscopy in inflammatory bowel disease. J Crohns Colitis 2013;7(12): 982–1018.
7. Oberhuber G, Hirsch M, Stolte M. High incidence of upper gastrointestinal tract involvement in Crohn's disease. Virchows Arch 1998;432(1):49–52.
8. IBD Working Group of the European Society for Paediatric Gastroenterology, Hepatology, and Nutrition. Inflammatory bowel disease in children and adolescents: recommendations for diagnosis–the Porto criteria. J Pediatr Gastroenterol Nutr 2005;41(1):1–7.
9. Colombel JF, Rutgeerts P, Reinisch W, et al. Early mucosal healing with infliximab is associated with improved long-term clinical outcomes in ulcerative colitis. Gastroenterology 2011;141(4):1194–201.

10. Rutgeerts P, Diamond RH, Bala M, et al. Scheduled maintenance treatment with infliximab is superior to episodic treatment for the healing of mucosal ulceration associated with Crohn's disease. Gastrointest Endosc 2006;63(3):433–42 [quiz: 464].

11. Dave M, Loftus EV Jr. Mucosal healing in inflammatory bowel disease-a true paradigm of success? Gastroenterol Hepatol (N Y) 2012;8(1):29–38.

12. D'Haens GR, Fedorak R, Lemann M, et al. Endpoints for clinical trials evaluating disease modification and structural damage in adults with Crohn's disease. Inflamm Bowel Dis 2009;15(10):1599–604.

13. Schroeder KW, Tremaine WJ, Ilstrup DM. Coated oral 5-aminosalicylic therapy for mildly to moderately active ulcerative colitis. A randomized study. N Engl J Med 1987;317(26):1625–9.

14. Travis SP, Schnell D, Krzeski P, et al. Developing an instrument to assess the endoscopic severity of ulcerative colitis: the Ulcerative Colitis Endoscopic Index of Severity (UCEIS). Gut 2012;61(4):535–42.

15. Mohammed Vashist N, Samaan M, Mosli MH, et al. Endoscopic scoring indices for evaluation of disease activity in ulcerative colitis. Cochrane Database Syst Rev 2018;1:CD011450.

16. Mary JY, Modigliani R. Development and validation of an endoscopic index of the severity for Crohn's disease: a prospective multicentre study. Groupe d'Etudes Therapeutiques des Affections Inflammatoires du Tube Digestif (GETAID). Gut 1989;30(7):983–9.

17. Daperno M, D'Haens G, Van Assche G, et al. Development and validation of a new, simplified endoscopic activity score for Crohn's disease: the SES-CD. Gastrointest Endosc 2004;60(4):505–12.

18. Folsch UR, Nitschmann S. New therapeutic option for M. Crohn : SONIC study (study of biologic and immunomodulator naive patients in Crohn's disease). Internist (Berl) 2010;51(9):1202–4 [in German].

19. Kulaylat MN, Dayton MT. Ulcerative colitis and cancer. J Surg Oncol 2010;101(8): 706–12.

20. Wan J, Wang X, Yang Z, et al. Systematic review with meta-analysis: chromoendoscopy versus white light endoscopy in detection of dysplasia in patients with inflammatory bowel disease. J Dig Dis 2019;20(4):206–14.

21. Eaden JA, Abrams KR, Mayberry JF. The risk of colorectal cancer in ulcerative colitis: a meta-analysis. Gut 2001;48(4):526–35.

22. Laine L, Kaltenbach T, Barkun A, et al. SCENIC international consensus statement on surveillance and management of dysplasia in inflammatory bowel disease. Gastrointest Endosc 2015;81(3):489–501 e426.

23. Itzkowitz SH, Present DH. Crohn's, Colitis Foundation of America Colon Cancer in IBDSG. Consensus conference: Colorectal cancer screening and surveillance in inflammatory bowel disease. Inflamm Bowel Dis 2005;11(3):314–21.

24. Karlen P, Kornfeld D, Brostrom O, et al. Is colonoscopic surveillance reducing colorectal cancer mortality in ulcerative colitis? A population based case control study. Gut 1998;42(5):711–4.

25. Rutter MD, Saunders BP, Wilkinson KH, et al. Thirty-year analysis of a colonoscopic surveillance program for neoplasia in ulcerative colitis. Gastroenterology 2006;130(4):1030–8.

26. Lindberg J, Stenling R, Palmqvist R, et al. Efficiency of colorectal cancer surveillance in patients with ulcerative colitis: 26 years' experience in a patient cohort from a defined population area. Scand J Gastroenterol 2005;40(9):1076–80.

27. Galanopoulos M, Tsoukali E, Gkeros F, et al. Screening and surveillance methods for dysplasia in inflammatory bowel disease patients: where do we stand? World J Gastrointest Endosc 2018;10(10):250–8.

28. American Society for Gastrointestinal Endoscopy Standards of Practice Committee, Shergill AK, Lightdale JR, Bruining DH, et al. The role of endoscopy in inflammatory bowel disease. Gastrointest Endosc 2015;81(5):1101–21.e1-13.

29. Riddell RH, Goldman H, Ransohoff DF, et al. Dysplasia in inflammatory bowel disease: standardized classification with provisional clinical applications. Hum Pathol 1983;14(11):931–68.

30. van den Broek FJ, Stokkers PC, Reitsma JB, et al. Random biopsies taken during colonoscopic surveillance of patients with longstanding ulcerative colitis: low yield and absence of clinical consequences. Am J Gastroenterol 2014;109(5):715–22.

31. Watanabe T, Ajioka Y, Mitsuyama K, et al. Comparison of targeted vs random biopsies for surveillance of ulcerative Colitis-associated colorectal cancer. Gastroenterology 2016;151(6):1122–30.

32. Van Assche G, Dignass A, Bokemeyer B, et al. Second European evidence-based consensus on the diagnosis and management of ulcerative colitis part 3: special situations. J Crohns Colitis 2013;7(1):1–33.

33. Kiesslich R, Fritsch J, Holtmann M, et al. Methylene blue-aided chromoendoscopy for the detection of intraepithelial neoplasia and colon cancer in ulcerative colitis. Gastroenterology 2003;124(4):880–8.

34. Kudo S, Tamura S, Nakajima T, et al. Diagnosis of colorectal tumorous lesions by magnifying endoscopy. Gastrointest Endosc 1996;44(1):8–14.

35. Carballal S, Maisterra S, Lopez-Serrano A, et al. Real-life chromoendoscopy for neoplasia detection and characterisation in long-standing IBD. Gut 2018;67(1):70–8.

36. Ohmiya N, Horiguchi N, Tahara T, et al. Usefulness of confocal laser endomicroscopy to diagnose ulcerative colitis-associated neoplasia. Dig Endosc 2017;29(5):626–33.

37. De Palma GD, Colavita I, Zambrano G, et al. Detection of colonic dysplasia in patients with ulcerative colitis using a targeted fluorescent peptide and confocal laser endomicroscopy: A pilot study. PLoS One 2017;12(6):e0180509.

38. Karstensen JG, Saftoiu A, Brynskov J, et al. Confocal laser endomicroscopy in ulcerative colitis: a longitudinal study of endomicroscopic changes and response to medical therapy (with videos). Gastrointest Endosc 2016;84(2):279–86.e1.

39. Olivera P, Spinelli A, Gower-Rousseau C, et al. Surgical rates in the era of biological therapy: up, down or unchanged? Curr Opin Gastroenterol 2017;33(4):246–53.

40. Shen B. The evaluation of postoperative patients with ulcerative colitis. Gastrointest Endosc Clin N Am 2016;26(4):669–77.

41. Steinhart AH, Ben-Bassat O. Pouchitis: a practical guide. Frontline Gastroenterol 2013;4(3):198–204.

42. Ben-Bassat O, Tyler AD, Xu W, et al. Ileal pouch symptoms do not correlate with inflammation of the pouch. Clin Gastroenterol Hepatol 2014;12(5):831–7.e2.

43. Sandborn WJ, Tremaine WJ, Batts KP, et al. Pouchitis after ileal pouch-anal anastomosis: a Pouchitis Disease Activity Index. Mayo Clin Proc 1994;69(5):409–15.

44. Shen B, Achkar JP, Connor JT, et al. Modified pouchitis disease activity index: a simplified approach to the diagnosis of pouchitis. Dis Colon Rectum 2003;46(6):748–53.

45. Heuschen UA, Allemeyer EH, Hinz U, et al. Diagnosing pouchitis: comparative validation of two scoring systems in routine follow-up. Dis Colon Rectum 2002; 45(6):776–86 [discussion: 786–8].

46. Okita Y, Araki T, Kawamura M, et al. Clinical features and management of afferent limb syndrome after ileal pouch-anal anastomosis for ulcerative colitis. Surg Today 2016;46(10):1159–65.

47. Elder K, Lopez R, Kiran RP, et al. Endoscopic features associated with ileal pouch failure. Inflamm Bowel Dis 2013;19(6):1202–9.

48. Wu XR, Wong RCK, Shen B. Endoscopic needle-knife therapy for ileal pouch sinus: a novel approach for the surgical adverse event (with video). Gastrointest Endosc 2013;78(6):875–85.

49. Kochhar GS, Shen B. Endoscopic treatment of leak at the tip of the "J" ileal pouch. Endosc Int Open 2017;5(1):E64–6.

50. Rottoli M, Di Simone MP, Vallicelli C, et al. Endoluminal-assisted therapy as treatment for anastomotic leak after ileal pouch-anal anastomosis: a pilot study. Tech Coloproctol 2018;22(3):223–9.

51. Sherman J, Greenstein AJ, Greenstein AJ. Ileal j pouch complications and surgical solutions: a review. Inflamm Bowel Dis 2014;20(9):1678–85.

52. Francone TD, Champagne B. Considerations and complications in patients undergoing ileal pouch anal anastomosis. Surg Clin North Am 2013;93(1):107–43.

53. Kariv R, Remzi FH, Lian L, et al. Preoperative colorectal neoplasia increases risk for pouch neoplasia in patients with restorative proctocolectomy. Gastroenterology 2010;139(3):806–12, 812.e1-2.

54. Mark-Christensen A, Erichsen R, Brandsborg S, et al. Long-term risk of cancer following ileal pouch-anal anastomosis for ulcerative Colitis. J Crohns Colitis 2018;12(1):57–62.

55. Samaan MA, Forsyth K, Segal JP, et al. Current practices in ileal pouch surveillance for patients with ulcerative Colitis: a multinational, retrospective cohort study. J Crohns Colitis 2019;13(6):735–43.

56. Gu J, Remzi FH, Lian L, et al. Practice pattern of ileal pouch surveillance in academic medical centers in the United States. Gastroenterol Rep (Oxf) 2016;4(2): 119–24.

57. McLaughlin SD, Clark SK, Tekkis PP, et al. Review article: restorative proctocolectomy, indications, management of complications and follow-up–a guide for gastroenterologists. Aliment Pharmacol Ther 2008;27(10):895–909.

58. Hashash JG, Regueiro M. A Practical Approach to Preventing Postoperative Recurrence in Crohn's Disease. Cur Gastroenterol Rep 2016;18(5):25.

59. Rutgeerts P, Geboes K, Vantrappen G, et al. Predictability of the postoperative course of Crohn's disease. Gastroenterology 1990;99(4):956–63.

60. Rieder F, Zimmermann EM, Remzi FH, et al. Crohn's disease complicated by strictures: a systematic review. Gut 2013;62(7):1072–84.

61. Spiceland CM, Lodhia N. Endoscopy in inflammatory bowel disease: Role in diagnosis, management, and treatment. World J Gastroenterol 2018;24(35): 4014–20.

62. Gustavsson A, Magnuson A, Blomberg B, et al. Endoscopic dilation is an efficacious and safe treatment of intestinal strictures in Crohn's disease. Aliment Pharmacol Ther 2012;36(2):151–8.

63. Cosnes J, Cattan S, Blain A, et al. Long-term evolution of disease behavior of Crohn's disease. Inflamm Bowel Dis 2002;8(4):244–50.

64. Chen M, Shen B. Endoscopic therapy in Crohn's disease: principle, preparation, and technique. Inflamm Bowel Dis 2015;21(9):2222–40.

65. Navaneethan U, Lourdusamy V, Njei B, et al. Endoscopic balloon dilation in the management of strictures in Crohn's disease: a systematic review and meta-analysis of non-randomized trials. Surg Endosc 2016;30(12):5434–43.
66. Morar PS, Faiz O, Warusavitarne J, et al. Systematic review with meta-analysis: endoscopic balloon dilatation for Crohn's disease strictures. Aliment Pharmacol Ther 2015;42(10):1137–48.
67. Rutter MD, Saunders BP, Wilkinson KH, et al. Cancer surveillance in longstanding ulcerative colitis: endoscopic appearances help predict cancer risk. Gut 2004; 53(12):1813–6.
68. Fumery M, Pineton de Chambrun G, Stefanescu C, et al. Detection of dysplasia or cancer in 3.5% of patients with inflammatory bowel disease and colonic strictures. Clin Gastroenterol Hepatol 2015;13(10):1770–5.
69. Sunada K, Shinozaki S, Nagayama M, et al. Long-term outcomes in patients with small intestinal strictures secondary to Crohn's disease after double-balloon endoscopy-assisted Balloon Dilation. Inflamm Bowel Dis 2016;22(2):380–6.
70. Shen B, Kochhar G, Navaneethan U, et al. Role of interventional inflammatory bowel disease in the era of biologic therapy: a position statement from the Global Interventional IBD Group. Gastrointest Endosc 2019;89(2):215–37.
71. East JE, Brooker JC, Rutter MD, et al. A pilot study of intrastricture steroid versus placebo injection after balloon dilatation of Crohn's strictures. Clin Gastroenterol Hepatol 2007;5(9):1065–9.
72. Di Nardo G, Oliva S, Passariello M, et al. Intralesional steroid injection after endoscopic balloon dilation in pediatric Crohn's disease with stricture: a prospective, randomized, double-blind, controlled trial. Gastrointest Endosc 2010;72(6): 1201–8.
73. Hendel J, Karstensen JG, Vilmann P. Serial intralesional injections of infliximab in small bowel Crohn's strictures are feasible and might lower inflammation. United European Gastroenterol J 2014;2(5):406–12.
74. Swaminath A, Lichtiger S. Dilation of colonic strictures by intralesional injection of infliximab in patients with Crohn's colitis. Inflamm Bowel Dis 2008;14(2):213–6.
75. Chen M, Shen B. Endoscopic therapy for Kock pouch strictures in patients with inflammatory bowel disease. Gastrointest Endosc 2014;80(2):353–9.
76. Rejchrt S, Kopacova M, Brozik J, et al. Biodegradable stents for the treatment of benign stenoses of the small and large intestines. Endoscopy 2011;43(10): 911–7.
77. Rodrigues C, Oliveira A, Santos L, et al. Biodegradable stent for the treatment of a colonic stricture in Crohn's disease. World J Gastrointest Endosc 2013;5(5): 265–9.
78. Karstensen JG, Vilmann P, Hendel J. Successful endoscopic treatment of a 12-cm small-bowel Crohn stricture with a custom-made biodegradable stent. Endoscopy 2014;46(Suppl 1 UCTN):E227–8.
79. Kochhar G, Shen B. Endoscopic fistulotomy in inflammatory bowel disease (with video). Gastrointest Endosc 2018;88(1):87–94.
80. Prosst RL, Joos AK. Short-term outcomes of a novel endoscopic clipping device for closure of the internal opening in 100 anorectal fistulas. Tech Coloproctol 2016;20(11):753–8.

Preoperative Considerations in Inflammatory Bowel Disease

Nicholas P. McKenna, MD[a], Amy L. Lightner, MD[b],*

KEYWORDS

- Crohn's disease • Ulcerative colitis • Preoperative medications • Corticosteroids
- Biologics • Enteral nutrition

KEY POINTS

- The effect of biologic therapy on adverse postoperative outcomes remains controversial. In the setting of multiple risk factors in CD, or when performing an IPAA, it may be best to divert the anastomosis to prevent intra-abdominal sepsis.
- Corticosteroids are associated with adverse postoperative outcomes. All attempts should be made to wean the dose of corticosteroids prior to surgical intervention, and patients on high dose corticosteroids should have their intestinal anastomoses diverted.
- The use of preoperative nutritional optimization is best done with enteral versus parenteral nutrition, and has shown the greatest benefit in Crohn's patients. Prospective randomized trials are needed to define the optimal nutritional formula and duration.
- Timing of surgery in both UC and CD can be difficult. Prolonged waiting in a failing patient will lead to worse outcomes.

INTRODUCTION

Between 15% and 25% of patients with ulcerative colitis (UC)[1,2] and 60% of patients with Crohn's disease (CD)[3] will require a resection for medically refractory disease or dysplasia during their lifetime. With the risk of perioperative morbidity and mortality high, it is critical to optimize these patients preoperatively to ensure optimal postoperative outcomes. In an era of ever-increasing pharmaceutical options for the treatment of inflammatory bowel disease (IBD), patients seem to be presenting to surgery later and often sicker. The advent of new medical therapies also makes the decision of when to proceed to surgery versus attempt another class of biologic or

Disclosure: N.P. McKenna has no conflicts of interest. A.L. Lightner is a consultant for Takeda. There were no sources of funding for this research work. The disclosed conflicts of interest did not affect our investigation.
[a] Department of Surgery, Mayo Clinic, 200 1st Street Southwest, Rochester, MN 55905, USA;
[b] Digestive Diseases Institute, Cleveland Clinic, 9500 Euclid Avenue, Cleveland, OH 44195, USA
* Corresponding author.
E-mail address: lightna@ccf.org

escalate to combination therapy more challenging. In this article, we review the latest literature on the influence of preoperative immunosuppressive therapy and its influence on operative decision making and perioperative outcomes, the role of preoperative enteral nutrition in optimizing a patient for surgery, and how to decide when to pivot from ongoing medical management to an operation in patients with IBD.

MEDICATIONS
Biologics

Anti-tumor necrosis factors
Anti-tumor necrosis factor (anti-TNF) agents (infliximab, adalimubmab, and certolizumab) were approved for the treatment of CD in 1998 and UC in 2005. The anti-TNF agents induce mucosal healing, achieve corticosteroid sparing remission, and improve overall quality of life in both CD and UC.[4,5] However, perioperative anti-TNF agents have been associated with increased postoperative complications, including anastomotic leak and increased use of proximal intestinal diversion, both of which are associated with increased cost and decreased quality of life.[6–12] Controversy surrounds the decisions of when to hold or discontinue anti-TNF therapy preoperatively to minimize adverse postoperative outcomes, whether serum levels are relevant to postoperative outcomes and should be checked before surgery, and whether diversion of an anastomosis should be performed following exposure to anti-TNF therapy. These decisions have different implications for CD and UC, and are therefore discussed separately.

Ulcerative colitis Some studies have implicated anti-TNF agents as a risk factor for pelvic sepsis and major morbidity after ileal pouch anal anastomosis (IPAA)[8,13,14]; others have reported no increased risk in pelvic sepsis following exposure to anti-TNF agents.[11,15] Owing to the retrospective nature of these studies and the varying degrees of disease severity in the patients included, it is difficult to determine whether increased complications are a direct result of anti-TNF agents, a surrogate marker of disease severity, or both. In addition, the window from dose of an anti-TNF to operation has varied from 2 to 16 weeks, making it difficult to compare studies side by side. However, it is worth noting that the timing of the last dose has not been found to be associated with a change in outcome.[14,16] Regardless of whether anti-TNF agents play a direct role in pelvic sepsis, surgeons have responded by increased use of a modified 3-stage IPAA as compared with the prebiologic era, when a traditional 2-stage IPAA was used more frequently. This has been demonstrated in a study using the Nationwide Inpatient Sample with an increased proportion of subtotal colectomies performed after 2005.[17] This seems prudent given the impaired function associated with pelvic sepsis and the likely relationship between preoperative biologic exposure and pelvic sepsis.[18]

Crohn's disease Owing to the heterogeneity of operations performed for CD and the varying use of proximal diversion, the literature with respect to anti-TNFs impact on anastomotic leak is even more controversial.[7,19–23] Meta-analyses have largely come to the conclusion that preoperative anti-TNF exposure increases complications,[9,24] but one found no difference.[25] The most recent prospective study of anti-TNF agents before ileocolic resection in CD did find that anti-TNF agents increased morbidity, and that this persisted after they performed a propensity-weighted analysis to account for varying disease severity and likelihood of receiving anti-TNF agents preoperatively.[6]

Lau and colleagues[10] found that, as serum levels of anti-TNF agents increased, the risk of infectious complications, including intra-abdominal sepsis, also increased for

CD. Interestingly, 45% of patients on preoperative anti-TNF agents did not have detectable serum levels. They also found that detectable levels of anti-TNF agents increased complications, lending credence to the theory that anti-TNF agents are themselves deleterious, and that it is not simply an association between disease severity and increased likelihood of being exposed. Conversely, another study of 214 patients with CD who underwent an ileocecal resection collected serum drug levels on every patient within 48 hours of surgery, and found no correlation of serum drug levels and postoperative complications. Currently, it is still unclear if the biologic itself is responsible for postoperative complications.[26]

Vedolizumab
Vedolizumab is less well studied than the anti-TNF agents because it was only approved by the US Food and Drug Administration in 2014. There are few existing studies on vedolizumab, and these are further limited by small sample sizes, even when combining patients with UC and CD.

Ulcerative colitis Studies have reported mixed results for UC and vedolizumab.[27–29] Two meta-analyses provide the most robust data comparing vedolizumab with both no biologic therapy and to anti-TNFs.[30,31] Law and colleagues[30] combined patients undergoing surgery for both UC and CD, and found no increased risk in the vedolizumab-exposed cohort. Yung and colleagues[31] separated patients with UC from those with CD, but they also did not find a significant increased risk of infection. The inherent limitation to both these meta-analyses is the inclusion of all infectious complications and the inclusion of operations in which an anastomotic leak is not possible (ie, subtotal colectomy stage of UC treatment).

Crohn's disease A meta-analysis of 140 patients showed similar complication rates for vedolizumab in comparison with anti-TNF agents.[31] A single-center retrospective study of only patients with CD found an increased risk of postoperative surgical site infection (SSI) in patients exposed to vedolizumab compared with anti-TNF agents and to no biologic therapy.[32] A 2018 study used propensity score matching to better balance the groups, and SSI rates were similar for vedolizumab and anti-TNF agents.[33]

Ustekinumab
Crohn's disease Two studies have reported similar rates of complications between anti-TNF agents and ustekinumab.[34,35] Another study using case matching showed no difference in outcomes between ustekinumab and vedolizumab.[36]

Biologics summary
The impact of biologic therapy remains controversial. Regardless of whether the biologic itself is deleterious or simply a surrogate marker of disease severity, careful attention should be paid to these patients intraoperatively when deciding whether to divert an anastomosis and postoperatively when recovering. Ideally, the last dose of an anti-TNF agent or ustekinumab would be at least 4 weeks before surgery, and the last dose of vedolizumab would be 4 to 8 weeks before surgery,[37,38] with a plan to restart, when necessary, 4 weeks after surgery to maintain an evert 8-week dosing regimen and prevent antibody formation.

Corticosteroids
Corticosteroids have a well-established detrimental effect on anastomotic healing, with increased rates of intra-abdominal sepsis shown in patients undergoing surgery for both UC[39,40] and CD.[41,42] However, pelvic sepsis can sometimes be limited by using 2- and 3-stage approaches to UC and CD.[43]

Ulcerative colitis

Studies on IPAA formation in a 2-stage manner demonstrated increased risk of pelvic sepsis for patients on corticosteroids preoperatively, with the highest risk in those on ≥40 mg prednisone.[39] Other studies have shown an increased risk of pelvic sepsis with as little as 20 mg of prednisone and possibly lower.[44–46] Based on this evidence, the ECCO guidelines recommend delayed IPAA formation in patients who cannot be weaned to less than 20 mg per day for more than 6 weeks before surgery.[47]

Crohn's disease

Corticosteroids have been associated with an increased rate of intra-abdominal sepsis after ileocolic resection in patients with CD in numerous studies and in a meta-analysis.[41,42,48] When a stoma is used, the risk of sepsis is similar to those not on steroids.[6] Recent studies have shown that steroid use is strongly associated with stoma formation.[49,50]

Two papers have recently demonstrated an increased risk of sepsis after ileocolic resection with either dual therapy with a steroid and a biologic[51] or triple therapy with a corticosteroid, a biologic, and an immunomodulator.[50] This is an important finding because therapy for CD is becoming increasingly multimodal.[52–54]

Operation selection and intestinal diversion

Ulcerative colitis Although the American Society of Colon and Rectal Surgeon guidelines do not directly advise an operative approach based on patient medication profile,[55] it is reasonable to perform total abdominal colectomy with end ileostomy when patients are on preoperative high-dose steroids, thus performing pouch formation at a subsequent surgery when steroids are no longer needed.

The question of omission of temporary diversion at the time of total proctocolectomy with IPAA has been studied extensively, with conflicting results as to whether it is safe or not.[56–59] Most studies are retrospective in nature, with 1 randomized trial from 1992.[60] This randomized trial did not find a difference in pelvic sepsis based on the presence or absence of a diverting loop ileostomy. However, it only included 45 patients and took place before the biologic era. They also specifically excluded all patients on preoperative corticosteroids. A meta-analysis of studies comparing no diversion with diversion at time of IPAA found an increased risk of anastomotic leak and concluded that omission of an ileostomy is only potentially reasonable in those patients not taking corticosteroids and should only be considered in select cases.[58] Modified 2-stage procedures were shown to be safe in select patients,[61,62] but the 3-staged approach is considered the best choice for high-risk patients.[63] There is also geographic variation in approaches to these patients, and a consensus is difficult to achieve.[64]

Crohn's disease There is increased use of diversion in patients with CD on corticosteroids.[50] A National Surgery Quality Improvement Program study found a reduced risk of leak requiring reoperation with a loop ileostomy in patients undergoing open ileocolic resection, but they did not perform a CD-specific analysis.[49] Currently, there are few data to help the surgeon decide between an ileocolic anastomosis with loop ileostomy and an end ileostomy with long Hartmann's pouch.

NUTRITION
Ulcerative Colitis

Operation choice

Much of the attention on nutrition in IBD has been focused on CD, but the rate of malnutrition at surgery is also increasing in patients with UC. This increase has coincided with the advent of biologic therapies.[65] Patients who fail to respond to multiple biologics slowly worsen from a nutritional perspective before undergoing surgery, which can impact the choice of operation.[63,66] Initial total abdominal colectomy with end ileostomy allows the removal of the chronically inflamed, diseased colon, and for subsequent optimization of nutritional status before pursuing an IPAA.

Enteral versus parenteral nutrition

Many advocate for delaying surgery until the patient's nutrition can be improved. In 1 case series of 42 patients who were suffering from moderate to severe UC flares, those fed by supplemental enteral nutrition (EN) had a greater increase in serum albumin than those treated by total parenteral nutrition (TPN) alone.[67] Another series of 17 patients treated with EN demonstrated increased prealbumin after treatment for a mean of 12 days.[68]

Preoperative TPN has been studied extensively in patients with IBD before surgery with mixed results,[69] but only 1 study has looked exclusively at patients with UC. This study compared 56 patients who received preoperative TPN with 179 who did not and found no benefit to preoperative TPN.[70] However, patients receiving TPN were more malnourished and had worse disease severity, so it is possible that preoperative TPN contributes to outcomes being equal, because outcomes would be expected to be worse in patients with higher rates of malnutrition and increased disease severity. Given the significant increase in morbidity secondary to central line complications, routine TPN is not warranted preoperatively, except perhaps for the sickest of patients who also have a contraindication to EN.

Crohn's Disease

Operation choice

CD is traditionally thought of as a disease of wasting and malnutrition. It has been shown in pediatric patients that surgical intervention significantly improves nutritional status, with increased growth seen after surgical intervention for CD.[71,72] Therefore, the choice of operation in pediatric patients is a decision of timing to prevent growth stunting at critical ages of development.

Moreover, in malnourished adult patients, the operative choice is more about staging to prevent complications and optimize patients preoperatively. Both malnutrition and weight loss are associated with increased rates of intra-abdominal septic complications and overall postoperative complications in CD.[41,73–75] Because anastomotic leak is the most feared complication after intestinal resection, anastomosis and proximal intestinal diversion or an end ileostomy with a long Hartmann's stump is advised in malnourished patients to minimize this risk. Once the diseased intestine is removed, the patient's nutritional status can then be optimized to allow optimized conditions at the time of restoration of intestinal continuity.

Enteral nutrition versus total parenteral nutrition

EN for 3 months before surgery has been associated with improved albumin levels and decreased C-reactive protein levels in patients scheduled for intestinal resection for intra-abdominal fistulizing disease. Supplemental EN was protective against postoperative intra-abdominal septic complications at 3 months postoperatively.[76–78]

A recent meta-analysis examining the role of TPN for CD identified a trend toward reduced overall complications in patients whom received preoperative TPN.[79] However, only 1 of the included studies had taken place in the era of biologic treatment, and analysis was performed on the outcome of overall complications as opposed to intra-abdominal sepsis, so the results must be interpreted with caution. The first study of preoperative TPN in the biologic era included 15 patients on preoperative TPN who received between 18 and 90 days of TPN. All patients experienced CD remission defined as a Crohn's Disease Activity Index of less than 150 and a significant increase in albumin was noted. No patients experienced a 30-day postoperative complication, but 4 of the 15 patients experienced central line-associated thromboses preoperatively.[80]

Another study included 55 patients on preoperative TPN, and found similar rates of infectious and noninfectious complications compared with those without TPN. On multivariable analysis, receipt of TPN for greater than 60 days preoperatively was protective against noninfectious complications, but was not a significantly protective lfactor for infectious complications.[81]

Nutrition Summary

Malnutrition is a common problem in patients with IBD who require surgery. EN is favored over TPN when preoperative nutrition optimization is being considered. The optimal formulation of EN and the duration of treatment remain unknown.

CLINICAL DETERIORATION DURING MEDICAL THERAPY
Ulcerative Colitis

Many patients with UC can be successfully managed with medical therapy in the outpatient setting. However, a proportion of patients will suffer disease flares that require inpatient medical therapy with high-dose corticosteroids and possibly biologic agents. Several scoring systems exist to predict which hospitalized patients with UC will require surgery including the Travis score[82] and the Ho score.[83] Both have been shown to identify patients at high risk of being corticosteroid resistant, while the Travis score also identifies a high-risk patient group likely to be resistant to cyclosporine or infliximab as well. They are both also associated with increased odds of surgery in the same independent validation data set.[84]

More recently, it has been shown that early surgery is associated with reduced morbidity and decreased costs.[85,86] Multidisciplinary care with early consideration of colectomy is therefore indicated.[87] Starting the conversation about surgery on the day of admission may be useful to reduce patient anxiety and facilitate improved dialogue before the conversation becomes more time sensitive.

Crohn's Disease

Corticosteroids are the primary treatment for a CD flare and serve as a temporary bridge until biologics or immunomodulators can be initiated, escalated, or changed.[88] However, some patients with CD will fail medical salvage therapy and require semi-urgent or emergent surgery. Nonelective surgery is associated with a 3-fold increase in mortality,[89] and high rates of infectious complications are also seen in this setting.[90]

Unlike UC, no difference in postoperative complications has been demonstrated in patients with CD based on how long they were admitted preoperatively.[90] Patients who present with a localized abscess are typically candidates for interventional drainage, intravenous antibiotics, and hospital discharge with surgery scheduled in an elective manner.[91] Between percutaneous drainage and definitive operation, nutrition can be optimized and inflammation can be better controlled with medications, which may allow for a laparoscopic operation.[92]

SUMMARY

- The effect of biologic therapy on adverse postoperative outcomes remains controversial. In the setting of multiple risk factors in CD, or when performing

an IPAA, it may be best to divert the anastomosis to prevent intra-abdominal sepsis.
- Corticosteroids are associated with adverse postoperative outcomes. All attempts should be made to wean the dose of corticosteroids before surgical intervention, and patients on high-dose corticosteroids should have their intestinal anastomoses diverted.
- The use of preoperative nutritional optimization is best done with enteral versus parenteral nutrition, and has shown the greatest benefit in patients with CD. Prospective randomized trials are needed to define the optimal nutritional formula and duration.
- Timing of surgery in UC and CD can be difficult. Prolonged waiting in a failing patient will lead to worse outcomes.

REFERENCES

1. Langholz E, Munkholm P, Davidsen M, et al. Course of ulcerative colitis: analysis of changes in disease activity over years. Gastroenterology 1994;107(1):3–11.
2. Parragi L, Fournier N, Zeitz J, et al. Colectomy rates in ulcerative colitis are low and decreasing: 10-year follow-up data from the Swiss IBD Cohort Study. J Crohns Colitis 2018;12(7):811–8.
3. Frolkis AD, Dykeman J, Negron ME, et al. Risk of surgery for inflammatory bowel diseases has decreased over time: a systematic review and meta-analysis of population-based studies. Gastroenterology 2013;145(5):996–1006.
4. Cholapranee A, Hazlewood GS, Kaplan GG, et al. Systematic review with meta-analysis: comparative efficacy of biologics for induction and maintenance of mucosal healing in Crohn's disease and ulcerative colitis controlled trials. Aliment Pharmacol Ther 2017;45(10):1291–302.
5. Vogelaar L, Spijker AV, van der Woude CJ. The impact of biologics on health-related quality of life in patients with inflammatory bowel disease. Clin Exp Gastroenterol 2009;2:101–9.
6. Brouquet A, Maggiori L, Zerbib P, et al. Anti-TNF therapy is associated with an increased risk of postoperative morbidity after surgery for ileocolonic crohn disease: results of a prospective nationwide cohort. Ann Surg 2018;267(2):221–8.
7. Appau KA, Fazio VW, Shen B, et al. Use of infliximab within 3 months of ileocolonic resection is associated with adverse postoperative outcomes in Crohn's patients. J Gastrointest Surg 2008;12(10):1738–44.
8. Selvasekar CR, Cima RR, Larson DW, et al. Effect of infliximab on short-term complications in patients undergoing operation for chronic ulcerative colitis. J Am Coll Surg 2007;204(5):956–62 [discussion: 962–3].
9. Narula N, Charleton D, Marshall JK. Meta-analysis: peri-operative anti-TNFalpha treatment and post-operative complications in patients with inflammatory bowel disease. Aliment Pharmacol Ther 2013;37(11):1057–64.
10. Lau C, Dubinsky M, Melmed G, et al. The impact of preoperative serum anti-TNFalpha therapy levels on early postoperative outcomes in inflammatory bowel disease surgery. Ann Surg 2015;261(3):487–96.
11. Billioud V, Ford AC, Tedesco ED, et al. Preoperative use of anti-TNF therapy and postoperative complications in inflammatory bowel diseases: a meta-analysis. J Crohns Colitis 2013;7(11):853–67.
12. Eshuis EJ, Al Saady RL, Stokkers PC, et al. Previous infliximab therapy and postoperative complications after proctocolectomy with ileum pouch anal anastomosis. J Crohns Colitis 2013;7(2):142–9.

13. Gu J, Remzi FH, Shen B, et al. Operative strategy modifies risk of pouch-related outcomes in patients with ulcerative colitis on preoperative anti-tumor necrosis factor-alpha therapy. Dis Colon Rectum 2013;56(11):1243–52.

14. Kulaylat AS, Kulaylat AN, Schaefer EW, et al. Association of preoperative anti-tumor necrosis factor therapy with adverse postoperative outcomes in patients undergoing abdominal surgery for ulcerative colitis. JAMA Surg 2017;152(8): e171538.

15. Norgard BM, Nielsen J, Qvist N, et al. Pre-operative use of anti-TNF-alpha agents and the risk of post-operative complications in patients with ulcerative colitis - a nationwide cohort study. Aliment Pharmacol Ther 2012;35(11):1301–9.

16. Zittan E, Milgrom R, Ma GW, et al. Preoperative anti-tumor necrosis factor therapy in patients with ulcerative colitis is not associated with an increased risk of infectious and noninfectious complications after ileal pouch-anal anastomosis. Inflamm Bowel Dis 2016;22(10):2442–7.

17. Geltzeiler CB, Lu KC, Diggs BS, et al. Initial surgical management of ulcerative colitis in the biologic era. Dis Colon Rectum 2014;57(12):1358–63.

18. Kiely JM, Fazio VW, Remzi FH, et al. Pelvic sepsis after IPAA adversely affects function of the pouch and quality of life. Dis Colon Rectum 2012;55(4):387–92.

19. Canedo J, Lee SH, Pinto R, et al. Surgical resection in Crohn's disease: is immunosuppressive medication associated with higher postoperative infection rates? Colorectal Dis 2011;13(11):1294–8.

20. Colombel JF, Loftus EV Jr, Tremaine WJ, et al. Early postoperative complications are not increased in patients with Crohn's disease treated perioperatively with infliximab or immunosuppressive therapy. Am J Gastroenterol 2004;99(5):878–83.

21. Marchal L, D'Haens G, Van Assche G, et al. The risk of post-operative complications associated with infliximab therapy for Crohn's disease: a controlled cohort study. Aliment Pharmacol Ther 2004;19(7):749–54.

22. Myrelid P, Marti-Gallostra M, Ashraf S, et al. Complications in surgery for Crohn's disease after preoperative antitumour necrosis factor therapy. Br J Surg 2014; 101(5):539–45.

23. Kasparek MS, Bruckmeier A, Beigel F, et al. Infliximab does not affect postoperative complication rates in Crohn's patients undergoing abdominal surgery. Inflamm Bowel Dis 2012;18(7):1207–13.

24. Kopylov U, Ben-Horin S, Zmora O, et al. Anti-tumor necrosis factor and postoperative complications in Crohn's disease: systematic review and meta-analysis. Inflamm Bowel Dis 2012;18(12):2404–13.

25. Rosenfeld G, Qian H, Bressler B. The risks of post-operative complications following pre-operative infliximab therapy for Crohn's disease in patients undergoing abdominal surgery: a systematic review and meta-analysis. J Crohns Colitis 2013;7(11):868–77.

26. Fumery M, Seksik P, Auzolle C, et al. Postoperative complications after ileocecal resection in Crohn's disease: a prospective study from the REMIND Group. Am J Gastroenterol 2017;112(2):337–45.

27. Ferrante M, de Buck van Overstraeten A, Schils N, et al. Perioperative use of vedolizumab is not associated with postoperative infectious complications in patients with ulcerative colitis undergoing colectomy. J Crohns Colitis 2017; 11(11):1353–61.

28. Lightner AL, McKenna NP, Moncrief S, et al. Surgical outcomes in vedolizumab-treated patients with ulcerative colitis. Inflamm Bowel Dis 2017;23(12):2197–201.

29. Yamada A, Komaki Y, Patel N, et al. Risk of postoperative complications among inflammatory bowel disease patients treated preoperatively with vedolizumab. Am J Gastroenterol 2017;112(9):1423–9.

30. Law CCY, Narula A, Lightner AL, et al. Systematic review and meta-analysis: preoperative vedolizumab treatment and postoperative complications in patients with inflammatory bowel disease. J Crohns Colitis 2018;12(5):538–45.

31. Yung DE, Horesh N, Lightner AL, et al. Systematic review and meta-analysis: vedolizumab and postoperative complications in inflammatory bowel disease. Inflamm Bowel Dis 2018;24(11):2327–38.

32. Lightner AL, McKenna NP, Tse CS, et al. Postoperative outcomes in vedolizumab-treated Crohn's disease patients undergoing major abdominal operations. Aliment Pharmacol Ther 2018;47(5):573–80.

33. Park KT, Sceats L, Dehghan M, et al. Risk of post-operative surgical site infections after vedolizumab vs anti-tumour necrosis factor therapy: a propensity score matching analysis in inflammatory bowel disease. Aliment Pharmacol Ther 2018;48(3):340–6.

34. Shim HH, Ma C, Kotze PG, et al. Preoperative ustekinumab treatment is not associated with increased postoperative complications in Crohn's disease: a Canadian Multi-Centre Observational Cohort Study. J Can Assoc Gastroenterol 2018;1(3):115–23.

35. Lightner AL, McKenna NP, Tse CS, et al. Postoperative outcomes in ustekinumab-treated patients undergoing abdominal operations for Crohn's disease. J Crohns Colitis 2018;12(4):402–7.

36. Novello M, Stocchi L, Holubar S, et al. Surgical outcomes of patients treated with ustekinumab vs. vedolizumab in inflammatory bowel disease: a matched case analysis. Int J Colorectal Dis 2019;34(3):451–7.

37. Lightner AL. Perioperative management of biologic and immunosuppressive medications in patients with Crohn's disease. Dis Colon Rectum 2018;61(4):428–31.

38. Lightner AL, Shen B. Perioperative use of immunosuppressive medications in patients with Crohn's disease in the new "biological era". Gastroenterol Rep (Oxf) 2017;5(3):165–77.

39. Heuschen UA, Hinz U, Allemeyer EH, et al. Risk factors for ileoanal J pouch-related septic complications in ulcerative colitis and familial adenomatous polyposis. Ann Surg 2002;235(2):207–16.

40. Lake JP, Firoozmand E, Kang JC, et al. Effect of high-dose steroids on anastomotic complications after proctocolectomy with ileal pouch-anal anastomosis. J Gastrointest Surg 2004;8(5):547–51.

41. Alves A, Panis Y, Bouhnik Y, et al. Risk factors for intra-abdominal septic complications after a first ileocecal resection for Crohn's disease: a multivariate analysis in 161 consecutive patients. Dis Colon Rectum 2007;50(3):331–6.

42. Tzivanakis A, Singh JC, Guy RJ, et al. Influence of risk factors on the safety of ileocolic anastomosis in Crohn's disease surgery. Dis Colon Rectum 2012;55(5):558–62.

43. McKenna NP, Glasgow AE, Cima RR, et al. Risk factors for organ space infection after ileal pouch anal anastomosis for chronic ulcerative colitis: an ACS NSQIP analysis. Am J Surg 2018;216(5):900–5.

44. Ferrante M, D'Hoore A, Vermeire S, et al. Corticosteroids but not infliximab increase short-term postoperative infectious complications in patients with ulcerative colitis. Inflamm Bowel Dis 2009;15(7):1062–70.

45. Aberra FN, Lewis JD, Hass D, et al. Corticosteroids and immunomodulators: postoperative infectious complication risk in inflammatory bowel disease patients. Gastroenterology 2003;125(2):320–7.

46. Sahami S, Bartels SA, D'Hoore A, et al. A multicentre evaluation of risk factors for anastomotic leakage after restorative proctocolectomy with ileal pouch-anal anastomosis for inflammatory bowel disease. J Crohns Colitis 2016;10(7):773–8.

47. Oresland T, Bemelman WA, Sampietro GM, et al. European evidence based consensus on surgery for ulcerative colitis. J Crohns Colitis 2015;9(1):4–25.

48. Huang W, Tang Y, Nong L, et al. Risk factors for postoperative intra-abdominal septic complications after surgery in Crohn's disease: a meta-analysis of observational studies. J Crohns Colitis 2015;9(3):293–301.

49. Hawkins AT, Dharmarajan S, Wells KK, et al. Does diverting loop ileostomy improve outcomes following open ileo-colic anastomoses? A nationwide analysis. J Gastrointest Surg 2016;20(10):1738–43.

50. McKenna NP, Habermann EB, Glasgow AE, et al. Intra-abdominal sepsis after ileocolic resection in Crohn's disease: the role of combination immunosuppression. Dis Colon Rectum 2018;61(12):1393–402.

51. Serradori T, Germain A, Scherrer ML, et al. The effect of immune therapy on surgical site infection following Crohn's disease resection. Br J Surg 2013;100(8): 1089–93.

52. Sebastian S, Black C, Pugliese D, et al. The role of multimodal treatment in Crohn's disease patients with perianal fistula: a multicentre retrospective cohort study. Aliment Pharmacol Ther 2018;48(9):941–50.

53. Colombel JF, Sandborn WJ, Reinisch W, et al. Infliximab, azathioprine, or combination therapy for Crohn's disease. N Engl J Med 2010;362(15):1383–95.

54. Sokol H, Seksik P, Carrat F, et al. Usefulness of co-treatment with immunomodulators in patients with inflammatory bowel disease treated with scheduled infliximab maintenance therapy. Gut 2010;59(10):1363–8.

55. Ross H, Steele SR, Varma M, et al. Practice parameters for the surgical treatment of ulcerative colitis. Dis Colon Rectum 2014;57(1):5–22.

56. Lavryk OA, Hull TL, Duraes LC, et al. Outcomes of ileal pouch-anal anastomosis without primary diverting loop ileostomy if postoperative sepsis develops. Tech Coloproctol 2018;22(1):37–44.

57. Sahami S, Buskens CJ, Fadok TY, et al. Defunctioning ileostomy is not associated with reduced leakage in proctocolectomy and ileal pouch anastomosis surgeries for IBD. J Crohns Colitis 2016;10(7):779–85.

58. Weston-Petrides GK, Lovegrove RE, Tilney HS, et al. Comparison of outcomes after restorative proctocolectomy with or without defunctioning ileostomy. Arch Surg 2008;143(4):406–12.

59. Mark-Christensen A, Erichsen R, Brandsborg S, et al. Pouch failures following ileal pouch-anal anastomosis for ulcerative colitis. Colorectal Dis 2018;20(1): 44–52.

60. Grobler SP, Hosie KB, Keighley MR. Randomized trial of loop ileostomy in restorative proctocolectomy. Br J Surg 1992;79(9):903–6.

61. Samples J, Evans K, Chaumont N, et al. Variant two-stage ileal pouch-anal anastomosis: an innovative and effective alternative to standard resection in ulcerative colitis. J Am Coll Surg 2017;224(4):557–63.

62. Zittan E, Wong-Chong N, Ma GW, et al. Modified two-stage ileal pouch-anal anastomosis results in lower rate of anastomotic leak compared with traditional two-stage surgery for ulcerative colitis. J Crohns Colitis 2016;10(7):766–72.

63. Mege D, Figueiredo MN, Manceau G, et al. Three-stage laparoscopic ileal pouch-anal anastomosis is the best approach for high-risk patients with inflammatory bowel disease: an analysis of 185 consecutive patients. J Crohns Colitis 2016; 10(8):898–904.

64. Richardson D, deMontbrun S, Johnson PM. Surgical management of ulcerative colitis: a comparison of Canadian and American colorectal surgeons. Can J Surg 2011;54(4):257–62.

65. Hatch QM, Ratnaparkhi R, Althans A, et al. Is modern medical management changing ultimate patient outcomes in inflammatory bowel disease? J Gastrointest Surg 2016;20(11):1867–73.

66. Bikhchandani J, Polites SF, Wagie AE, et al. National trends of 3- versus 2-stage restorative proctocolectomy for chronic ulcerative colitis. Dis Colon Rectum 2015; 58(2):199–204.

67. Gonzalez-Huix F, Fernandez-Banares F, Esteve-Comas M, et al. Enteral versus parenteral nutrition as adjunct therapy in acute ulcerative colitis. Am J Gastroenterol 1993;88(2):227–32.

68. Klaassen J, Zapata R, Mella JG, et al. [Enteral nutrition in severe ulcerative colitis. Digestive tolerance and nutritional efficiency]. Rev Med Chil 1998;126(8): 899–904.

69. Schwartz E. Perioperative parenteral nutrition in adults with inflammatory bowel disease: a review of the literature. Nutr Clin Pract 2016;31(2):159–70.

70. Salinas H, Dursun A, Konstantinidis I, et al. Does preoperative total parenteral nutrition in patients with ulcerative colitis produce better outcomes? Int J Colorectal Dis 2012;27(11):1479–83.

71. Fahy AS, Potter DD, Ravi A, et al. Colectomy in refractory Crohn's colitis improves nutrition and reduces steroid use. J Pediatr Surg 2017;52(11):1769–75.

72. Singh Ranger G, Lamparelli MJ, Aldridge A, et al. Surgery results in significant improvement in growth in children with Crohn's disease refractory to medical therapy. Pediatr Surg Int 2006;22(4):347–52.

73. Lindor KD, Fleming CR, Ilstrup DM. Preoperative nutritional status and other factors that influence surgical outcome in patients with Crohn's disease. Mayo Clin Proc 1985;60(6):393–6.

74. Yamamoto T, Allan RN, Keighley MR. Risk factors for intra-abdominal sepsis after surgery in Crohn's disease. Dis Colon Rectum 2000;43(8):1141–5.

75. Iesalnieks I, Kilger A, Glass H, et al. Intraabdominal septic complications following bowel resection for Crohn's disease: detrimental influence on long-term outcome. Int J Colorectal Dis 2008;23(12):1167–74.

76. Li G, Ren J, Wang G, et al. Preoperative exclusive enteral nutrition reduces the postoperative septic complications of fistulizing Crohn's disease. Eur J Clin Nutr 2014;68(4):441–6.

77. Li Y, Zuo L, Zhu W, et al. Role of exclusive enteral nutrition in the preoperative optimization of patients with Crohn's disease following immunosuppressive therapy. Medicine (Baltimore) 2015;94(5):e478.

78. Heerasing N, Thompson B, Hendy P, et al. Exclusive enteral nutrition provides an effective bridge to safer interval elective surgery for adults with Crohn's disease. Aliment Pharmacol Ther 2017;45(5):660–9.

79. Brennan GT, Ha I, Hogan C, et al. Does preoperative enteral or parenteral nutrition reduce postoperative complications in Crohn's disease patients: a meta-analysis. Eur J Gastroenterol Hepatol 2018;30(9):997–1002.

80. Jacobson S. Early postoperative complications in patients with Crohn's disease given and not given preoperative total parenteral nutrition. Scand J Gastroenterol 2012;47(2):170–7.

81. Ayoub F, Kamel AY, Ouni A, et al. Pre-operative total parenteral nutrition improves post-operative outcomes in a subset of Crohn's disease patients undergoing major abdominal surgery. Gastroenterol Rep (Oxf) 2018;7(2):107–14.

82. Travis SP, Farrant JM, Ricketts C, et al. Predicting outcome in severe ulcerative colitis. Gut 1996;38(6):905–10.

83. Ho GT, Mowat C, Goddard CJ, et al. Predicting the outcome of severe ulcerative colitis: development of a novel risk score to aid early selection of patients for second-line medical therapy or surgery. Aliment Pharmacol Ther 2004;19(10): 1079–87.

84. Lynch RW, Churchhouse AM, Protheroe A, et al. Predicting outcome in acute severe ulcerative colitis: comparison of the Travis and Ho scores using UK IBD audit data. Aliment Pharmacol Ther 2016;43(11):1132–41.

85. Coakley BA, Telem D, Nguyen S, et al. Prolonged preoperative hospitalization correlates with worse outcomes after colectomy for acute fulminant ulcerative colitis. Surgery 2013;153(2):242–8.

86. Leeds IL, Truta B, Parian AM, et al. Early surgical intervention for acute ulcerative colitis is associated with improved postoperative outcomes. J Gastrointest Surg 2017;21(10):1675–82.

87. Seah D, De Cruz P. Review article: the practical management of acute severe ulcerative colitis. Aliment Pharmacol Ther 2016;43(4):482–513.

88. Lichtenstein GR, Loftus EV, Isaacs KL, et al. ACG clinical guideline: management of Crohn's disease in adults. Am J Gastroenterol 2018;113(4):481–517.

89. Singh S, Al-Darmaki A, Frolkis AD, et al. Postoperative mortality among patients with inflammatory bowel diseases: a systematic review and meta-analysis of population-based studies. Gastroenterology 2015;149(4):928–37.

90. Ananthakrishnan AN, McGinley EL. Weekend hospitalisations and post-operative complications following urgent surgery for ulcerative colitis and Crohn's disease. Aliment Pharmacol Ther 2013;37(9):895–904.

91. Berg DF, Bahadursingh AM, Kaminski DL, et al. Acute surgical emergencies in inflammatory bowel disease. Am J Surg 2002;184(1):45–51.

92. Fleshman JW. Pyogenic complications of Crohn's disease, evaluation, and management. J Gastrointest Surg 2008;12(12):2160–3.

Postoperative Considerations in Inflammatory Bowel Disease

Lea Lowenfeld, MD, Kyle G. Cologne, MD*

KEYWORDS

- Postoperative complications • Inflammatory bowel disease • Colorectal surgery

KEY POINTS

- The care of patients with inflammatory bowel disease (IBD) requires coordination of medical and surgical treatments. However, there are limited data to suggest that preoperative medical treatment increases the risk of postoperative complications or that medical treatment should be held postoperatively to decrease the risk of postoperative complications.
- Patients should be monitored closely for postoperative complications, specifically abdominal sepsis or venothromboembolism (VTE), which are increased in patients with IBD. Routine extended VTE prophylaxis may be considered postoperatively in patients with IBD.
- Postoperative recurrence of Crohn's disease can be detected endoscopically or clinically, and those at high risk of recurrence should consider early initiation or resumption of medical therapy.

INTRODUCTION

Treatment of inflammatory bowel disease (IBD), including Crohn's diseases (CD) and ulcerative colitis (UC), is often multidimensional, requiring both medical and surgical therapies at different times throughout the course of the disease. Both medical and surgical treatments may be used in the acute setting, during a flare, or in a more elective maintenance role. These treatments should be planned as complementary and synergistic. Gastroenterologists and colorectal surgeons should collaborate to create a cohesive treatment plan, arranging the sequence and timing of various treatments. The previous Nicholas P. McKenna and Amy L. Lightner's article, "Preoperative Considerations in Inflammatory Bowel Disease," in this issue discussed the preoperative considerations in IBD. This article reviews the anticipated postoperative recovery

Surgery, Division of Colorectal Surgery, University of Southern California Keck School of Medicine, 1441 Eastlake Avenue, Suite 7418, Los Angeles, CA 90033, USA
* Corresponding author.
E-mail address: kyle.cologne@med.usc.edu

Surg Clin N Am 99 (2019) 1095–1109
https://doi.org/10.1016/j.suc.2019.08.003
0039-6109/19/© 2019 Elsevier Inc. All rights reserved.

surgical.theclinics.com

after surgical treatment of IBD, possible postoperative complications, and considerations of timing surgery with medical therapy.

POSTOPERATIVE CONSIDERATIONS
Stoma Issues

One of the most common areas of postoperative complications surrounds the topic of stomas (ileostomy versus colostomy, temporary versus permanent). These issues, in part, can be averted, starting in the preoperative period. Discussing the lifestyle changes associated with ostomy and pouch creation with patients preemptively can help patients understand the surgery, manage postoperative expectations, and alleviate some of the patient's anxiety and resistance to surgery.

Ostomy creation is commonly performed in IBD surgery as a method of diverting the stool proximal to a new anastomosis, in the situation where an anastomosis cannot be safely performed, or when severe left-sided/perianal disease makes a restorative procedure unlikely to give acceptable bowel function. Even if temporary, ostomy creation is often dreaded by patients more than any complication because of the external alteration of their body image. Patients may receive medical information from their physicians and wound care stoma nurses, empowering self-care; and there are also support groups in person or on the Internet.[1–4] Preoperative stoma education has been associated with fewer peristomal complications, such as pouching difficulty and a variety of other problems.[2] Support groups offer aid for patients who have or will have stomas, their caregivers, and their family and friends, and are often helpful for new ostomates. A well-functioning stoma allows a much better quality of life than a poorly functioning anorectum. With this in mind, the surgeon should be familiar with several stoma-related complications and how to manage them.

Superficial stomal complications include leakage, skin irritation, difficulty maintaining a seal, retraction, ischemia, and mucocutaneous separation.[5] These nuisances can often be managed with appropriate preoperative skin marking (including skin folds and location of belt lines) as well as skilled stoma care. When education about proper appliance placement is not enough, there are numerous products on the market for the care of ostomies, including different shaped appliances (eg, convex wafer), powders or ointments to protect the skin around the ostomy, adhesive glues to provide a strong seal between the appliance and the skin, and belts or binders to provide additional support.

Specific to IBD, pyoderma gangrenosum (PG) is an extraintestinal manifestation of IBD, which develops most commonly on the lower extremities, but can also develop around the stoma sites. Parastomal pyoderma gangrenosum (PPG) can occur around any type of stoma and is a factor in approximately 15% of all pyoderma cases. This condition occurs in only 0.6% of all stomas created, but has been reported to occur in 2% to 5% of patients who have had stoma surgery for IBD.[6,7] Surgical treatment of the underlying disease, colitis, or perianal lesions can lead to improvement of PG.[8,9] However, stoma relocation, excision of ulcers, and skin grafting have been largely unsuccessful[10–13] and have high rates of recurrent disease. Wound and stoma care is crucial for the treatment of PPG; in addition, Funayama and colleagues[14] demonstrated the importance of early recognition and treatment with corticosteroids to promote healing of peristomal PG.

Overall, the risk of readmission after colorectal surgery is increased in patients with IBD.[15] Ileostomy creation has been identified as a major risk factor driving these readmission rates,[16–18] specifically due to the risk of dehydration and acute kidney injury.[19–22] The biggest risk factors associated with dehydration include older age, hypertension, the requirement of diuretics before initial discharge, and shortened length of stay.[19,21,23] Inflammatory and infectious pathology may also contribute to the risk of readmission; *Clostridium difficile* infection is a potential cause of high-output ileostomy or pouch and should be considered in refractory cases.[24,25] Initiatives involving preoperative and predischarge education and outpatient follow-up have been advocated to reduce the risk of readmission and prevent acute kidney injury without causing harm or increasing costs but with variable success in reducing the rate of readmission.[22,26,27] Scheduled early postoperative phone calls or office visits can also allow for early intervention in high-risk patients and prevent a readmission.

The lifestyle changes after surgery to create a pouch and after surgery resulting in short bowel syndrome are discussed in detail Jennifer A. Leinicke's article, "Ileal Pouch Complications," and Matthew A. Fuglestad and Jon S. Thompson's article, "Inflammatory Bowel Disease and Short Bowel Syndrome," elsewhere in this issue.

PATIENT-RELATED FACTORS AND DECISION MAKING

Postoperative complications are common in patients with IBD and may be attributable to the underlying condition, the associated malnutrition, or the treatment, specifically the use of immunomodulators or corticosteroids. These and the overall health of the patient may predispose to infectious complications (such as anastomotic leak, stump blowout, and pouch sepsis). Thus, appropriate decision making should be used in these patients with more severe disease, considering multistaged procedures (eg, 3-stage versus 2-stage proctocolectomy and an ileoanal pouch), as well as liberal use of proximal diverting stomas or end stomas to avoid a high-risk anastomoses or avoid an anastomosis altogether.

Older age and lower albumin level have been shown to be associated with an increased risk of postoperative complications. However, conflicting results have been reported with the use of medical therapies. It is well established that corticosteroid use preoperatively results in higher infectious-related complications.[28–30] Although some have found a higher rate of postoperative complications in patients treated with anti-tumor necrosis factor (TNF) therapy,[31] others have found no difference in postoperative complications in patients who received biologics within 2 or 3 months of surgery compared with patients who received biologics more than 2 or 3 months before surgery[32] or never received biologics.[33,34] Lau and colleagues[35] looked specifically at the serum level of anti-TNFα drugs and showed that increasing levels of preoperative serum anti-TNF levels were associated with increased risk of postoperative complications in CD but not in UC. Canedo and colleagues[36] showed no difference in intraoperative or postoperative complications in patients who had been exposed to infliximab, steroids or other immunosuppressive agents, or no medication, and Yamada and colleagues[37] showed that patients treated with nonbiologic therapy, anti-TNF agents, or vidolizumab had similar rates of postoperative infection.

Infection

Infection after surgery may present as superficial skin infection or deep/organ-space infection. The reported incidence of surgical site infections in patients with IBD range from 6.9% to 31.4%.[38–42] In the United States, postoperative infection rates are reported at approximately 15%, with similar incidences reported for patients with UC and CD.[43] Risk factors associated with postoperative infection are numerous and include patient demographics (age >60 years, Medicare insurance, insurance enrollment <24 months before surgery); comorbidities (such as anemia, cirrhosis, diabetes, chronic obstructive pulmonary disease, deep vein thrombosis [DVT], or rheumatoid arthritis); and IBD-related variables (previous postoperative infection, bacterial or *Clostridium difficile* infection, or $\geq$2 previous IBD-related hospitalizations). Notably, steroid use within 14 days of surgery is one of the biggest risk factors. There are also certain surgery-related risk factors (such as preoperative stay $\geq$4 days, intraoperative blood transfusion, open surgery, and ostomy creation).[43] Although most of these risk factors are nonmodifiable or procedure related, they raise awareness of the high risk of postoperative infection in patients with IBD.

This section focuses on the risk of intraabdominal sepsis; specifically, intraabdominal sepsis after colorectal surgery in IBD due to intraperitoneal abscess or anastomotic leak. McKenna and colleagues[44] examined patients with CD who underwent ileocolonic resection and found an overall incidence of intraabdominal sepsis of 8%, diagnosed at a median of 9 days after surgery, and nearly 2-thirds of patients were diagnosed after discharge from the hospital. Patients with intraabdominal infections were at increased risk of other complications, such as surgical site infection, urinary tract infection, pneumonia, partial small bowel obstruction or ileus, readmission, and increased total length of hospital stay.

Risk factors for postoperative intraabdominal sepsis after intestinal resection in CD included treatment with steroids,[45] biological agents,[46–48] positive histologic margins,[49] and repeat resections.[50,51] In the era of combination medical therapy and multiple repeat surgeries, McKenna and colleagues[44] showed that triple immunosuppression, but not any individual single or double agent immunosuppression, was associated with an increased risk of intraabdominal sepsis, and the risk of intraabdominal sepsis was increased with each additional intestinal resection. The group also showed that patients at highest risk of intraabdominal sepsis were those who were on triple immunosuppression and had undergone a previous intestinal resection (22%). This was greater than the risk for either factor alone (patients on triple immunosuppression [15%], patients with previous resection [11%]), and patients with neither of these risk factors (5%).[44] Special consideration should be given to performing a temporary diversion or forego an anastomosis in patients with the highest risk.

Patients with CD have a reported risk of anastomotic leak of 1.2% to 16.7%, which is associated with significantly increased morbidity, mortality, length of hospital stay, and total costs.[52] Anastomotic leaks most commonly present with abdominal pain and fevers, diagnosed at a mean of 9.8 days after surgery. Management of anastomotic leaks depends on the timing of presentation and degree of fecal contamination and may include bowel rest and antibiotics, percutaneous drainage, repeat bowel resection and anastomosis, fecal diversion with or without primary repair, and resection with end stoma formation.

Johnston and colleagues[51] showed that repeat intestinal resection is associated with an increased risk of anastomotic leak, with a 5% leak rate in patients with no previous intestinal resection and 17% leak rate in patients with a history of previous intestinal resection. Furthermore, they showed that increasing the number of previous intestinal resections further increased the risk; 13% leak rate in patients with 1 previous intestinal resection and 23% leak rate in patients with 2 or more previous intestinal resections.[51] Again, these data suggest that patients undergoing repeat resection are at particularly high risk of anastomotic leak and that efforts should be made to correct any modifiable risk factors. Again, special consideration should be given to the liberal use of fecal diversion in those patients with multiple risk factors.

Studies looking at the outcomes of different anastomotic configurations after intestinal resection for patients with CD have shown a reduced anastomotic leak rate after a stapled side-to-side anastomosis compared with a hand-sewn end-to-end anastomosis.[53–56] In a meta-analysis of these studies, Simillis and colleagues[57] found that end-to-end anastomoses were associated with an increased anastomotic leak rate, whereas side-to-side anastomoses were associated with a significant reduction in the anastomotic leak rate, overall postoperative complications, complications other than anastomotic leak, and length of hospital stay. They hypothesized that the decreased risk of leak may be due to lower intraoperative septic contamination, reduced tissue manipulation, less overall inflammation, or a more favorable anastomosis configuration—a wider diameter resulting in lower intraluminal pressure and reduced proximal ischemia. However, these findings have not been uniformly reproduced; some studies have shown no difference in complication rates, leak rates, or reoperation rates.[58] The authors prefer a stapled isoperistaltic resection in ileocolonic resections to allow ease of future ileocolonoscopy. The authors prefer to use a circular stapler or hand sew colo-rectal or colo-colonic anastomosis, respectively. Additional data on anastomotic construction types are presented later in this article.

RECTAL STUMP BLOWOUT

Operations without an anastomosis, such as subtotal colectomy in severe UC and CD, carry a risk of enteric leak at the rectal stump. Techniques purported to minimize the risk of rectal stump blowout, including oversewing the staple line or inserting a tube into the rectum to decompress the stump, have limited evidence. Another technique often described includes bringing the tip of the stump up and securing it above the fascia (with or without skin closure; eg, as a mucous fistula). In the event of a blowout, the stump can decompress via a skin fistula. The authors do not prefer this approach, because it does carry a small risk of necrotizing soft tissue infection if not discovered early. If a poor quality stump is anticipated, wide drainage (via intraabdominal and transrectal routes) can be sufficient to locally control fecal contamination and allow for healing. Although these drains can be uncomfortable, when left for 5 to 7 days, the subsequent stump blowout rate is low in the author's experience.

POUCH-RELATED COMPLICATIONS/SEPSIS

Restorative proctocolectomy and ileal pouch–anal anastomosis have become the standard surgical therapy for UC, with low morbidity, acceptable functional outcome, and high rates of patient satisfaction. Pouch-related septic complications related to anastomotic leak, abscess, and fistula have been reported to occur in 6% to 37% of patients.[59–61] Patients with pelvic sepsis had a higher rate of anastomotic leak, wound infection, fistula formation, and postoperative hemorrhage, and had higher rates of incontinence and seepage.[62] Patients with pelvic sepsis also experienced a higher rate of pouch failure compared with patients without pelvic sepsis (19% versus 4%); pelvic sepsis may result in defunctionalization of the pouch or necessitate pouch excision. Pouch leaks can be managed much in the same way that any low-pelvic anastomosis leaks are handled. Imaging can help determine if the source of a leak is low (eg, coloanal) or high (eg, tip of the J or transverse staple line). Drainage can be performed at the bedside or under radiologic guidance; on the other hand, drainage and diversion necessitate a return to the operating room.

If sepsis is controlled early with adequate directed interventions, often the long-term sequelae of pouch dysfunction and pouch failure can be avoided. Currently, novel techniques are being developed to increase the chance of pouch salvage.[63] Additional discussion of pouch complications is included in Jennifer A. Leinicke's article, "Ileal Pouch Complications," elsewhere in this issue.

Venothromboembolism

Vascular complications including both arterial thromboembolism and venous thromboembolism are more common in patients with IBD than in the general population and occur at a younger index age.[64–66] Reports of venous vascular complications include DVT, pulmonary emboli (PE),[67,68] portal vein thrombosis,[68] pseudotumor cerebri,[69] cerebral venous sinus thrombosis,[70,71] Budd Chiari syndrome,[72] and retinal vein thrombosis.[72] VTE events are now considered as extra-intestinal manifestations of IBD[64,73,74] and occur at a similar rate as other extraintestinal manifestations.

All patients are known to be at increased risk of VTE during hospitalization and postoperatively, presumably due to decreased mobility and an increased inflammatory response. Patients with IBD have a chronic immune-mediated inflammatory condition, which contributes to a hypercoagulable state and increased risk of VTE. Most of the studies looking at postoperative VTE use data from the American College of Surgeons (ACS) National Surgical Quality Improvement Program (NSQIP) to study the postoperative incidence of VTE in patients with IBD,[75–77] the risk factors associated with increased risk of VTE in patients with IBD,[76] and the indications for extended postoperative VTE prophylaxis.[78,79]

Overall, the 30-day rate of postoperative VTE in patients with IBD was approximately 2.5%.[76–78] Waellert and colleagues[76] found that VTE events occurred in 2.3% of patients with IBD who underwent colorectal procedures, with a higher rate in patients with UC (3.3%) compared with patients with CD (1.4%). Wilson and colleagues[77] also demonstrated a significantly higher risk of VTE in patients with UC undergoing colon resection (2.74%) compared with patients who underwent colonic resection for CD (1.21%), diverticulitis (1.41%), colorectal cancer (1.74%), or a benign neoplasm (1.10%).

McKenna and colleagues,[75,80] looking individually at CD and UC, showed that the risk of VTE was more closely associated with the type of operation (emergent extensive abdominal operations, including subtotal colectomy and total proctocolectomy), rather than the underlying disease. Obesity, American Society of Anesthesiologists (ASA) class III/IV, increased age, and preoperative systemic inflammatory response syndrome were all associated with increased risk of VTE.[77] Malnutrition, functional status, bleeding disorders, hematocrit less than 37%, steroid use, emergency surgery, and anesthesia time were identified as potentially modifiable risk factors that were associated with VTE.[76] Benlice and colleagues[79] developed a nomogram, with points accrued for age, hypertension requiring medications, ASA classification, bleeding disorder, transfusion, steroid use, days in the hospital before surgery, and surgical approach (laparoscopic versus open) and operative time.

VTE occurred at a mean of 10.8 days postoperatively but ranged from events at postoperative day 0 to postoperative day 30 in studies that evaluated 30-day morbidity and mortality.[79] Benlice and colleagues[79] showed that the 30-day VTE rate was 2.5%, with a postdischarge VTE rate of 1.0%; and 41% of VTE events were diagnosed after discharge. Studies looking at 90-day VTE rates showed a higher VTE rate (3.3%–4.3%) within 90 days after surgery.[81,82] Almost a third (29%) of VTEs occur within 7 days after surgery and most patients (64%–70%) developed a VTE within the first 30 days after discharge; nevertheless, the risk of VTE continues with 22% of VTEs occurring within 30 to 60 days and 14% within 60 to 90 days.[81,82]

Patients with IBD who experienced a VTE postoperatively also had a higher risk of other complications (41% versus 18%), a longer length of hospitalization (18.8 days versus 8.9 days), and an increased mortality rate (4% versus 0.9%).[76] Complications rates of bleeding, both superficial and deep incisional surgical site infections, sepsis, pneumonia, urinary tract infection, myocardial infarction, acute renal failure, and death were increased in patients with VTE. However, it is not clear whether the VTE event increases the risk of complication or if the complication increases the risk of VTE. Despite the significant risk of VTE and the associated morbidity and mortality, Brady and colleagues[81] found that only 0.6% of patients undergoing surgery for IBD received prophylactic anticoagulation on discharge from the hospital; furthermore, they also found that 21% of patients on anticoagulation had a VTE event.

Previous studies have described a particularly increased risk of portomesenteric venous thrombosis (PMVT) following total colectomy and proctocolectomy.[83–89] PMVT is believed to occur due to manipulation of the mesentery intraoperatively.[75,87,90] The NSQIP database includes PMVT within the category DVT; and Brady and colleagues,[81] using an insurance-based database, showed that 30% of postoperative VTEs are PMVT. Prophylaxis regimens to prevent postoperative PMVT have been shown to have varying success.[91–93] Therefore, it is possible that extended postoperative VTE prophylaxis will have no effect on the risk of postoperative PMVT.

Nearly all of these studies conclude with a call for extended postoperative prophylactic anticoagulation in the way that is recommended after colorectal surgery for cancer. Gross and colleagues[78] specifically compared patients with IBD who underwent colorectal surgery with patients with colorectal cancer who underwent colorectal surgery and showed an increased rate of VTE in patients with IBD (2.7% versus 2.1%). Approximately one-third of VTE events occurred after discharge from the hospital in each group (38% in patients with IBD, 35% in patients with colorectal cancer), with similar overall rates of postdischarge VTE (1.1% in patients with IBD, 0.7% in patients with colorectal cancer). Both groups carry a persistent risk of developing VTE during the 30-day postoperative period, and both having a median VTE occurrence at 9 days postoperatively.

This direct comparison by Gross and colleagues supports the proposal that postdischarge VTE prophylaxis recommendations for patients with IBD undergoing major abdominal surgery should be similar to the recommendations issued for 4 weeks of postoperative out-of-hospital VTE prophylaxis after surgery for colorectal cancer.[78,94,95] However, additional evidence has called into question the cost-effectiveness of long-term VTE prophylaxis, which requires predicted DVT rates of greater than 3%.[96] Therefore, the appropriate patients to treat, after which specific operations, and types of VTE that may be prevented require additional research. Current Clinical Practice Guidelines by The American Society of Colon and Rectal Surgeons recommend consideration for 4 weeks of extended duration prophylaxis in patients with IBD, but this is a weak recommendation based on low-quality evidence.[97]

RECURRENCE OF CROHN'S DISEASE

Nearly half of patients with CD require surgery at some point in their lives, and, although the rate of major abdominal surgery has decreased in the last 4 decades, the rate of surgical recurrence has increased, suggesting that surgery is reserved for more severe and complicated disease. Postoperative recurrence may be diagnosed based on histologic, endoscopic, clinical, and surgical features and often evolves in a sequential manner with endoscopic recurrence noted before the onset of symptomatic clinical recurrence.

Endoscopic recurrence occurs in up to 80% to 90% of postoperative patients within 5 years.[98–101] Risk factors include low preoperative albumin level, high perioperative inflammation, and history of previous intestinal resection.[102–107] Clinical recurrence, defined as the presence of IBD-related symptoms in the Crohn's Disease Activity Index, is observed in 28% to 50% of postoperative patients within 5 years.[98]

Because most recurrences occur at the proximal site of the anastomosis, the role of anastomotic configuration has been investigated as an influencing factor. However, there is great heterogeneity in the literature regarding the method (stapled versus hand-sewn) and configuration (isoperistaltic versus antiperistaltic, end-to-end versus side-to-side) without convincing evidence of a single superior technique.[53–55,57,108,109] The Kono-S anastomosis, which was first developed in Japan as an antimesenteric functional end-to-end hand-sewn anastomosis, has shown promise as a novel technique to limit disease recurrence.[110–112]

RESUMPTION OF MEDICAL THERAPY

Perioperative medication management in patients with IBD varies depending on the clinical situation of the patient and the type of surgery performed. Patients with UC undergoing proctocolectomy will no longer require immunosuppressant therapy, simplifying the postoperative medication management. In patients with IBD who require ongoing medical therapy, management will not differ between patients undergoing gastrointestinal surgery and patients undergoing nongastrointestinal surgeries; however, the nature of the surgical procedure (elective versus emergent, total proctocolectomy with end ileostomy versus total proctocolectomy with J pouch, or laparoscopic versus open surgery) may have a significant implication on the perioperative risk.

Early use of medical therapy, within 2 to 8 weeks after surgery, is effective in reducing the risk of endoscopic or clinical recurrence. Conversely, endoscopically guided therapy, in which treatment is only initiated after establishment of endoscopic recurrence, avoids the unnecessary overtreatment of low-risk patients, but may allow for permanent intestinal damage that cannot be reversed by delaying the initiation of medical therapy.

The current American Gastroenterological Association (AGA) guidelines are based on limited, low-quality evidence comparing these approaches and indirect evidence drawn from nonoperative treatment.[113]

- "The benefit of routine early postoperative prophylaxis over endoscopically guided therapy in decreasing the risk of recurrence of CD is uncertain.
- Anti-TNF monotherapy and thiopurine monotherapy probably result in the largest reductions in disease recurrence. Antibiotic monotherapy probably reduces the risk of recurrence, but the effect was not as strong. Thiopurines combined with antibiotics may reduce the risk of recurrence. There is an unclear benefit with the use of 5-aminosalicylates, probiotics, or budesonide.
- Routine endoscopic monitoring 6-12 months after surgical resection is probably superior to no endoscopic monitoring regardless of early postoperative management.
- Anti-TNF monotherapy or thiopurine monotherapy probably reduces the risk of recurrence in patients with asymptomatic endoscopic recurrence."

Ultimately, the guidelines recommend using anti-TNF therapy or thiopurines for postoperative prophylaxis. However, the AGA acknowledges that "patients, particularly those at lower risk of recurrence, who place a higher value on avoiding the small risks of pharmacologic prophylaxis and a lower value on the potential risk of early disease recurrence, may reasonably select endoscopically-guided pharmacological treatment over routine prophylaxis".[114]

The AGA strongly recommends routine endoscopy at 6 to 12 months after surgical resection in patients who choose to forego early postoperative prophylaxis but also weakly offers the same recommendation for patients who are treated with routine prophylaxis. Currently, biomarkers, such as fecal calprotectin, are being studied as predictors of recurrence but are not yet recommended for routine clinical use.

SUMMARY

IBD surgery is fraught with potential complications. Patients in general are high risk and often have comorbid conditions, such as malnutrition/weight loss, anemia, and chronic use of immunosuppressive medication. Surgical planning should avoid high-risk anastomoses or stage high-risk procedures. A high index of suspicion is required to appropriately diagnose, prevent, and treat the potential complications outlined in this article. Finally, the more complicated cases may require referral to specialized centers who are equipped to deal with these scenarios in a multidisciplinary fashion.

REFERENCES

1. Pittman J, Nichols T, Rawl SM. Evaluation of web-based ostomy patient support resources. J Wound Ostomy Continence Nurs 2017;44(6):550–6.
2. Stokes AL, Tice S, Follett S, et al. Institution of a preoperative stoma education group class decreases rate of peristomal complications in new stoma patients. J Wound Ostomy Continence Nurs 2017;44(4):363–7.
3. O'Connor G. Teaching stoma-management skills: the importance of self-care. Br J Nurs 2005;14(6):320–4.
4. Metcalf C. Stoma care: empowering patients through teaching practical skills. Br J Nurs 1999;8(9):593–600.
5. Ratliff CR. Early peristomal skin complications reported by WOC nurses. J Wound Ostomy Continence Nurs 2010;37(5):505–10.
6. Greenstein AJ, Janowitz HD, Sachar DB. The extra-intestinal complications of Crohn's disease and ulcerative colitis: a study of 700 patients. Medicine (Baltimore) 1976;55(5):401–12.
7. Sloan WP Jr, Bargen JA, Gage RP. Life histories of patients with chronic ulcerative colitis: a review of 2,000 cases. Gastroenterology 1950;16(1):25–38.
8. Tjandra JJ, Hughes LE. Parastomal pyoderma gangrenosum in inflammatory bowel disease. Dis Colon Rectum 1994;37(9):938–42.
9. Talansky AL, Meyers S, Greenstein AJ, et al. Does intestinal resection heal the pyoderma gangrenosum of inflammatory bowel disease? J Clin Gastroenterol 1983;5(3):207–10.
10. Hughes AP, Jackson JM, Callen JP. Clinical features and treatment of peristomal pyoderma gangrenosum. JAMA 2000;284(12):1546–8.
11. Cairns BA, Herbst CA, Sartor BR, et al. Peristomal pyoderma gangrenosum and inflammatory bowel disease. Arch Surg 1994;129(7):769–72.
12. Sheldon DG, Sawchuk LL, Kozarek RA, et al. Twenty cases of peristomal pyoderma gangrenosum: diagnostic implications and management. Arch Surg 2000;135(5):564–8 [discussion: 568–9].
13. Kiran RP, O'Brien-Ermlich B, Achkar JP, et al. Management of peristomal pyoderma gangrenosum. Dis Colon Rectum 2005;48(7):1397–403.
14. Funayama Y, Kumagai E, Takahashi K, et al. Early diagnosis and early corticosteroid administration improves healing of peristomal pyoderma gangrenosum in inflammatory bowel disease. Dis Colon Rectum 2009;52(2):311–4.

15. Bliss LA, Maguire LH, Chau Z, et al. Readmission after resections of the colon and rectum: predictors of a costly and common outcome. Dis Colon Rectum 2015;58(12):1164–73.

16. Damle RN, Cherng NB, Flahive JM, et al. Clinical and financial impact of hospital readmissions after colorectal resection: predictors, outcomes, and costs. Dis Colon Rectum 2014;57(12):1421–9.

17. Kulaylat AN, Dillon PW, Hollenbeak CS, et al. Determinants of 30-d readmission after colectomy. J Surg Res 2015;193(2):528–35.

18. Orcutt ST, Li LT, Balentine CJ, et al. Ninety-day readmission after colorectal cancer surgery in a Veterans Affairs cohort. J Surg Res 2016;201(2):370–7.

19. Messaris E, Sehgal R, Deiling S, et al. Dehydration is the most common indication for readmission after diverting ileostomy creation. Dis Colon Rectum 2012; 55(2):175–80.

20. Hayden DM, Pinzon MC, Francescatti AB, et al. Hospital readmission for fluid and electrolyte abnormalities following ileostomy construction: preventable or unpredictable? J Gastrointest Surg 2013;17(2):298–303.

21. Paquette IM, Solan P, Rafferty JF, et al. Readmission for dehydration or renal failure after ileostomy creation. Dis Colon Rectum 2013;56(8):974–9.

22. Nagle D, Pare T, Keenan E, et al. Ileostomy pathway virtually eliminates readmissions for dehydration in new ostomates. Dis Colon Rectum 2012;55(12): 1266–72.

23. Chen SY, Stem M, Cerullo M, et al. Predicting the risk of readmission from dehydration after ileostomy formation: the dehydration readmission after ileostomy prediction score. Dis Colon Rectum 2018;61(12):1410–7.

24. Navaneethan U, Giannella RA. Thinking beyond the colon-small bowel involvement in *Clostridium difficile* infection. Gut Pathog 2009;1(1):7.

25. Mann SD, Pitt J, Springall RG, et al. *Clostridium difficile* infection–an unusual cause of refractory pouchitis: report of a case. Dis Colon Rectum 2003;46(2):267–70.

26. Hardiman KM, Reames CD, McLeod MC, et al. Patient autonomy-centered self-care checklist reduces hospital readmissions after ileostomy creation. Surgery 2016;160(5):1302–8.

27. Grahn SW, Lowry AC, Osborne MC, et al. System-wide improvement for transitions after ileostomy surgery: can intensive monitoring of protocol compliance decrease readmissions? A randomized trial. Dis Colon Rectum 2019;62(3):363–70.

28. Furst MB, Stromberg BV, Blatchford GJ, et al. Colonic anastomoses: bursting strength after corticosteroid treatment. Dis Colon Rectum 1994;37(1):12–5.

29. Ehrlich HP, Hunt TK. Effects of cortisone and vitamin A on wound healing. Ann Surg 1968;167(3):324–8.

30. Aszodi A, Ponsky JL. Effects of corticosteroid on the healing bowel anastomosis. Am Surg 1984;50(10):546–8.

31. Appau KA, Fazio VW, Shen B, et al. Use of infliximab within 3 months of ileocolonic resection is associated with adverse postoperative outcomes in Crohn's patients. J Gastrointest Surg 2008;12(10):1738–44.

32. Myrelid P, Marti-Gallostra M, Ashraf S, et al. Complications in surgery for Crohn's disease after preoperative antitumour necrosis factor therapy. Br J Surg 2014; 101(5):539–45.

33. Kasparek MS, Bruckmeier A, Beigel F, et al. Infliximab does not affect postoperative complication rates in Crohn's patients undergoing abdominal surgery. Inflamm Bowel Dis 2012;18(7):1207–13.

34. Krane MK, Allaix ME, Zoccali M, et al. Preoperative infliximab therapy does not increase morbidity and mortality after laparoscopic resection for inflammatory bowel disease. Dis Colon Rectum 2013;56(4):449–57.

35. Lau C, Dubinsky M, Melmed G, et al. The impact of preoperative serum anti-TNFalpha therapy levels on early postoperative outcomes in inflammatory bowel disease surgery. Ann Surg 2015;261(3):487–96.

36. Canedo J, Lee SH, Pinto R, et al. Surgical resection in Crohn's disease: is immunosuppressive medication associated with higher postoperative infection rates? Colorectal Dis 2011;13(11):1294–8.

37. Yamada A, Komaki Y, Patel N, et al. Risk of postoperative complications among inflammatory bowel disease patients treated preoperatively with vedolizumab. Am J Gastroenterol 2017;112(9):1423–9.

38. Uchino M, Ikeuchi H, Matsuoka H, et al. Surgical site infection and validity of staged surgical procedure in emergent/urgent surgery for ulcerative colitis. Int Surg 2013;98(1):24–32.

39. Maeda K, Nagahara H, Shibutani M, et al. A preoperative low nutritional prognostic index correlates with the incidence of incisional surgical site infections after bowel resection in patients with Crohn's disease. Surg Today 2015;45(11):1366–72.

40. Guo K, Ren J, Li G, et al. Risk factors of surgical site infections in patients with Crohn's disease complicated with gastrointestinal fistula. Int J Colorectal Dis 2017;32(5):635–43.

41. Lightner AL, Raffals LE, Mathis KL, et al. Postoperative outcomes in vedolizumab-treated patients undergoing abdominal operations for inflammatory bowel disease. J Crohns Colitis 2017;11(2):185–90.

42. Bhakta A, Tafen M, Glotzer O, et al. Increased incidence of surgical site infection in IBD patients. Dis Colon Rectum 2016;59(4):316–22.

43. Liang H, Jiang B, Manne S, et al. Risk factors for postoperative infection after gastrointestinal surgery among adult patients with inflammatory bowel disease: findings from a large observational US cohort study. JGH Open 2018;2(5):182–90.

44. McKenna NP, Habermann EB, Glasgow AE, et al. Intra-abdominal sepsis after ileocolic resection in Crohn's disease: the role of combination immunosuppression. Dis Colon Rectum 2018;61(12):1393–402.

45. Alves A, Panis Y, Bouhnik Y, et al. Risk factors for intra-abdominal septic complications after a first ileocecal resection for Crohn's disease: a multivariate analysis in 161 consecutive patients. Dis Colon Rectum 2007;50(3):331–6.

46. Brouquet A, Maggiori L, Zerbib P, et al. Anti-TNF therapy is associated with an increased risk of postoperative morbidity after surgery for ileocolonic Crohn disease: results of a prospective nationwide cohort. Ann Surg 2018;267(2):221–8.

47. Jouvin I, Lefevre JH, Creavin B, et al. Postoperative morbidity risks following ileocolic resection for Crohn's disease treated with anti-TNF alpha therapy: a retrospective study of 360 patients. Inflamm Bowel Dis 2018;24(2):422–32.

48. Billioud V, Ford AC, Tedesco ED, et al. Preoperative use of anti-TNF therapy and postoperative complications in inflammatory bowel diseases: a meta-analysis. J Crohns Colitis 2013;7(11):853–67.

49. Shental O, Tulchinsky H, Greenberg R, et al. Positive histological inflammatory margins are associated with increased risk for intra-abdominal septic complications in patients undergoing ileocolic resection for Crohn's disease. Dis Colon Rectum 2012;55(11):1125–30.

50. Yamamoto T, Spinelli A, Suzuki Y, et al. Risk factors for complications after ileocolonic resection for Crohn's disease with a major focus on the impact of

preoperative immunosuppressive and biologic therapy: a retrospective international multicentre study. United Eur Gastroenterol J 2016;4(6):784–93.

51. Johnston WF, Stafford C, Francone TD, et al. What is the risk of anastomotic leak after repeat intestinal resection in patients with Crohn's disease? Dis Colon Rectum 2017;60(12):1299–306.

52. Post S, Betzler M, von Ditfurth B, et al. Risks of intestinal anastomoses in Crohn's disease. Ann Surg 1991;213(1):37–42.

53. Yamamoto T, Bain IM, Mylonakis E, et al. Stapled functional end-to-end anastomosis versus sutured end-to-end anastomosis after ileocolonic resection in Crohn disease. Scand J Gastroenterol 1999;34(7):708–13.

54. Munoz-Juarez M, Yamamoto T, Wolff BG, et al. Wide-lumen stapled anastomosis vs. conventional end-to-end anastomosis in the treatment of Crohn's disease. Dis Colon Rectum 2001;44(1):20–5 [discussion: 25–6].

55. Hashemi M, Novell JR, Lewis AA. Side-to-side stapled anastomosis may delay recurrence in Crohn's disease. Dis Colon Rectum 1998;41(10):1293–6.

56. Resegotti A, Astegiano M, Farina EC, et al. Side-to-side stapled anastomosis strongly reduces anastomotic leak rates in Crohn's disease surgery. Dis Colon Rectum 2005;48(3):464–8.

57. Simillis C, Purkayastha S, Yamamoto T, et al. A meta-analysis comparing conventional end-to-end anastomosis vs. other anastomotic configurations after resection in Crohn's disease. Dis Colon Rectum 2007;50(10):1674–87.

58. McLeod RS, Wolff BG, Ross S, et al. Recurrence of Crohn's disease after ileocolic resection is not affected by anastomotic type: results of a multicenter, randomized, controlled trial. Dis Colon Rectum 2009;52(5):919–27.

59. Reissman P, Piccirillo M, Ulrich A, et al. Functional results of the double-stapled ileoanal reservoir. J Am Coll Surg 1995;181(5):444–50.

60. Mikkola K, Luukkonen P, Jarvinen HJ. Long-term results of restorative proctocolectomy for ulcerative colitis. Int J Colorectal Dis 1995;10(1):10–4.

61. Lim M, Sagar P, Abdulgader A, et al. The impact of preoperative immunomodulation on pouch-related septic complications after ileal pouch-anal anastomosis. Dis Colon Rectum 2007;50(7):943–51.

62. Kiely JM, Fazio VW, Remzi FH, et al. Pelvic sepsis after IPAA adversely affects function of the pouch and quality of life. Dis Colon Rectum 2012;55(4):387–92.

63. Worley GHT, Segal JP, Warusavitarne J, et al. Management of early pouch-related septic complications in ulcerative colitis: a systematic review. Colorectal Dis 2018;20(8):O181–9.

64. Miehsler W, Reinisch W, Valic E, et al. Is inflammatory bowel disease an independent and disease specific risk factor for thromboembolism? Gut 2004; 53(4):542–8.

65. Grip O, Svensson PJ, Lindgren S. Inflammatory bowel disease promotes venous thrombosis earlier in life. Scand J Gastroenterol 2000;35(6):619–23.

66. Levy PJ, Tabares AH, Olin JW. Lower extremity arterial occlusions in young patients with Crohn's colitis and premature atherosclerosis: report of six cases. Am J Gastroenterol 1997;92(3):494–7.

67. Srirajaskanthan R, Winter M, Muller AF. Venous thrombosis in inflammatory bowel disease. Eur J Gastroenterol Hepatol 2005;17(7):697–700.

68. Ha C, Magowan S, Accortt NA, et al. Risk of arterial thrombotic events in inflammatory bowel disease. Am J Gastroenterol 2009;104(6):1445–51.

69. Levine JB, Lukawski-Trubish D. Extraintestinal considerations in inflammatory bowel disease. Gastroenterol Clin North Am 1995;24(3):633–46.

70. Umit H, et al. Cerebral sinus thrombosis in patients with inflammatory bowel disease: a case report. World J Gastroenterol 2005;11(34):5404–7.
71. Tsujikawa T, Urabe M, Bamba H, et al. Haemorrhagic cerebral sinus thrombosis associated with ulcerative colitis: a case report of successful treatment by anticoagulant therapy. J Gastroenterol Hepatol 2000;15(6):688–92.
72. Koutroubakis IE. Therapy insight: vascular complications in patients with inflammatory bowel disease. Nat Clin Pract Gastroenterol Hepatol 2005;2(6):266–72.
73. Koutroubakis IE, Sfiridaki A, Tsiolakidou G, et al. Genetic risk factors in patients with inflammatory bowel disease and vascular complications: case-control study. Inflamm Bowel Dis 2007;13(4):410–5.
74. Tan VP, Chung A, Yan BP, et al. Venous and arterial disease in inflammatory bowel disease. J Gastroenterol Hepatol 2013;28(7):1095–113.
75. McKenna NP, Behm KT, Ubl DS, et al. Analysis of postoperative venous thromboembolism in patients with chronic ulcerative colitis: is it the disease or the operation? Dis Colon Rectum 2017;60(7):714–22.
76. Wallaert JB, De Martino RR, Marsicovetere PS, et al. Venous thromboembolism after surgery for inflammatory bowel disease: are there modifiable risk factors? Data from ACS NSQIP. Dis Colon Rectum 2012;55(11):1138–44.
77. Wilson MZ, Connelly TM, Tinsley A, et al. Ulcerative colitis is associated with an increased risk of venous thromboembolism in the postoperative period: the results of a matched cohort analysis. Ann Surg 2015;261(6):1160–6.
78. Gross ME, Vogler SA, Mone MC, et al. The importance of extended postoperative venous thromboembolism prophylaxis in IBD: a National Surgical Quality Improvement Program analysis. Dis Colon Rectum 2014;57(4):482–9.
79. Benlice C, Holubar SD, Gorgun E, et al. Extended venous thromboembolism prophylaxis after elective surgery for IBD patients: nomogram-based risk assessment and prediction from nationwide cohort. Dis Colon Rectum 2018; 61(10):1170–9.
80. McKenna NP, Bews KA, Behm KT, et al. Do patients with Inflammatory bowel disease have a higher postoperative risk of venous thromboembolism or do they undergo more high-risk operations? Ann Surg 2018. https://doi.org/10. 1097/SLA.0000000000003017.
81. Brady MT, Patts GJ, Rosen A, et al. Postoperative venous thromboembolism in patients undergoing abdominal surgery for IBD: a common but rarely addressed problem. Dis Colon Rectum 2017;60(1):61–7.
82. Ali F, Al-Kindi SG, Blank JJ, et al. Elevated venous thromboembolism risk following colectomy for IBD is equal to those for colorectal cancer for ninety days after surgery. Dis Colon Rectum 2018;61(3):375–81.
83. Robinson KA, O'Donnell ME, Pearson D, et al. Portomesenteric venous thrombosis following major colon and rectal surgery: incidence and risk factors. Surg Endosc 2015;29(5):1071–9.
84. Allaix ME, Krane MK, Zoccali M, et al. Postoperative portomesenteric venous thrombosis: lessons learned from 1,069 consecutive laparoscopic colorectal resections. World J Surg 2014;38(4):976–84.
85. Gorgun E, Sapci I, Onder A, et al. Factors associated with portomesenteric venous thrombosis after total colectomy with ileorectal anastomosis or end ileostomy. Am J Surg 2018;215(1):62–5.
86. Gu J, Stocchi L, Gorgun E, et al. Risk factors associated with portomesenteric venous thrombosis in patients undergoing restorative proctocolectomy for medically refractory ulcerative colitis. Colorectal Dis 2016;18(4):393–9.

87. Remzi FH, Fazio VW, Oncel M, et al. Portal vein thrombi after restorative procto-colectomy. Surgery 2002;132(4):655–61 [discussion: 661–2].
88. Millan M, Hull TL, Hammel J, et al. Portal vein thrombi after restorative proctoco-lectomy: serious complication without long-term sequelae. Dis Colon Rectum 2007;50(10):1540–4.
89. Baker ME, Remzi F, Einstein D, et al. CT depiction of portal vein thrombi after creation of ileal pouch-anal anastomosis. Radiology 2003;227(1):73–9.
90. Goitein D, Matter I, Raziel A, et al. Portomesenteric thrombosis following laparo-scopic bariatric surgery: incidence, patterns of clinical presentation, and etiol-ogy in a bariatric patient population. JAMA Surg 2013;148(4):340–6.
91. Qi X, Bai M, Guo X, et al. Pharmacologic prophylaxis of portal venous system thrombosis after splenectomy: a meta-analysis. Gastroenterol Res Pract 2014; 2014:292689.
92. Kawanaka H, Akahoshi T, Kinjo N, et al. Impact of antithrombin III concentrates on portal vein thrombosis after splenectomy in patients with liver cirrhosis and hypersplenism. Ann Surg 2010;251(1):76–83.
93. Lai W, Lu SC, Li GY, et al. Anticoagulation therapy prevents portal-splenic vein thrombosis after splenectomy with gastroesophageal devascularization. World J Gastroenterol 2012;18(26):3443–50.
94. Merkow RP, Bilimoria KY, McCarter MD, et al. Post-discharge venous thrombo-embolism after cancer surgery: extending the case for extended prophylaxis. Ann Surg 2011;254(1):131–7.
95. Rasmussen MS, Jorgensen LN, Wille-Jørgensen P, et al. Prolonged prophylaxis with dalteparin to prevent late thromboembolic complications in patients under-going major abdominal surgery: a multicenter randomized open-label study. J Thromb Haemost 2006;4(11):2384–90.
96. Leeds IL, Canner JK, DiBrito SR, et al. Justifying total costs of extended veno-thromboembolism prophylaxis after colorectal cancer surgery. J Gastrointest Surg 2019. https://doi.org/10.1007/s11605-019-04206-z.
97. Fleming F, Gaertner W, Ternent CA, et al. The American Society of Colon and Rectal Surgeons Clinical Practice Guideline for the Prevention of Venous Throm-boembolic Disease in Colorectal Surgery. Dis Colon Rectum 2018;61(1):14–20.
98. Buisson A, Chevaux JB, Allen PB, et al. Review article: the natural history of postoperative Crohn's disease recurrence. Aliment Pharmacol Ther 2012; 35(6):625–33.
99. Tytgat GN, Mulder CJ, Brummelkamp WH. Endoscopic lesions in Crohn's dis-ease early after ileocecal resection. Endoscopy 1988;20(5):260–2.
100. Olaison G, Smedh K, Sjodahl R. Natural course of Crohn's disease after ileocolic resection: endoscopically visualised ileal ulcers preceding symptoms. Gut 1992;33(3):331–5.
101. Rutgeerts P, Geboes K, Vantrappen G, et al. Natural history of recurrent Crohn's disease at the ileocolonic anastomosis after curative surgery. Gut 1984;25(6): 665–72.
102. Ikeda A, Miyoshi N, Fujino S, et al. A novel predictive nomogram for early endo-scopic recurrence after intestinal resection for Crohn's disease. Digestion 2019. https://doi.org/10.1159/000495981.
103. Toh JWT, Wang N, Young CJ, et al. Major abdominal and perianal surgery in Crohn's Disease: long-term follow-up of Australian patients with Crohn's disease. Dis Colon Rectum 2018;61(1):67–76.

104. Simillis C, Yamamoto T, Reese GE, et al. A meta-analysis comparing incidence of recurrence and indication for reoperation after surgery for perforating versus nonperforating Crohn's disease. Am J Gastroenterol 2008;103(1):196–205.
105. Lautenbach E, Berlin JA, Lichtenstein GR. Risk factors for early postoperative recurrence of Crohn's disease. Gastroenterology 1998;115(2):259–67.
106. Han YM, Kim JW, Koh SJ, et al. Patients with perianal Crohn's disease have poor disease outcomes after primary bowel resection. J Gastroenterol Hepatol 2016; 31(8):1436–42.
107. Reese GE, Nanidis T, Borysiewicz C, et al. The effect of smoking after surgery for Crohn's disease: a meta-analysis of observational studies. Int J Colorectal Dis 2008;23(12):1213–21.
108. Caprilli R, Corrao G, Taddei G, et al. Prognostic factors for postoperative recurrence of Crohn's disease. Gruppo Italiano per lo Studio del Colon e del Retto (GISC). Dis Colon Rectum 1996;39(3):335–41.
109. Ikeuchi H, Kusunoki M, Yamamura T. Long-term results of stapled and hand-sewn anastomoses in patients with Crohn's disease. Dig Surg 2000;17(5):493–6.
110. Kono T, Ashida T, Ebisawa Y, et al. A new antimesenteric functional end-to-end handsewn anastomosis: surgical prevention of anastomotic recurrence in Crohn's disease. Dis Colon Rectum 2011;54(5):586–92.
111. Kono T, Fichera A, Maeda K, et al. Kono-S anastomosis for surgical prophylaxis of anastomotic recurrence in Crohn's disease: an international multicenter study. J Gastrointest Surg 2016;20(4):783–90.
112. Shimada N, Ohge H, Kono T, et al. Surgical recurrence at anastomotic site after bowel resection in Crohn's disease: comparison of Kono-S and end-to-end anastomosis. J Gastrointest Surg 2019;23(2):312–9.
113. Regueiro M, Velayos F, Greer JB, et al. American Gastroenterological Association Institute technical review on the management of Crohn's disease after surgical resection. Gastroenterology 2017;152(1):277–95.e3.
114. Nguyen GC, Loftus EV Jr, Hirano I, et al. American Gastroenterological Association Institute guideline on the management of Crohn's disease after surgical resection. Gastroenterology 2017;152(1):271–5.

Surgical Management of Dysplasia and Cancer in Inflammatory Bowel Disease

James Ansell, MD[a], Fabian Grass, MD[a], Amit Merchea, MD[b],*

KEYWORDS

- Crohn • Ulcerative colitis • Cancer • Dysplasia

KEY POINTS

- Patients with inflammatory bowel disease (IBD) and high-grade dysplasia, multifocal low-grade dysplasia and nonadenoma dysplasia-associated mass or lesion, high-grade or invasive cancer should undergo total proctocolectomy.
- Segmental resection in IBD–colorectal cancer (CRC) has a limited role because of the risk of developing secondary malignancies in other areas of colon.
- Ileal pouch anal anastomosis (IPAA) surgery for ulcerative colitis restores intestinal continuity and is associated with a very small risk of pouch neoplasia. High-risk patients with a history of dysplasia or CRC before IPAA should undergo pouchoscopy with biopsy every 1 to 3 years.
- IPAA surgery should not be considered in patients with a history of pelvic radiation, and indications for pouch excision include biopsy-confirmed high-grade dysplasia or synchronous cancer.

INTRODUCTION

Chronic inflammatory bowel disease (IBD) is characterized by recurrent episodes of mucosal inflammation, which can lead to an increased risk of dysplasia and cancer.[1] It is nearly a century since Crohn and Rosenberg[2] published their data linking IBD with colorectal cancer (CRC). A 2001 meta-analysis reported the overall IBD-CRC risk was 3 per 1000 per year and 2%, 8% and 18% in the first, second, and third decades after diagnosis, respectively.[3] More than a decade later, this risk has decreased to 1.69 per 1000 per year, possibly because of improved early detection and surveillance, earlier

Disclosure: The authors declare no relationship with a commercial company that has a direct financial interest in subject matter or materials discussed in the article or with a company making a competing product.
[a] Division of Colon and Rectal Surgery, Mayo Clinic, 200 First Street Southwest, Rochester, MN 55905, USA; [b] Division of Colon and Rectal Surgery, Mayo Clinic, 4500 San Pablo Road South, Jacksonville, FL 32224, USA
* Corresponding author.
E-mail address: Merchea.Amit@mayo.edu

surgical intervention in medically refractory disease, and the introduction of chemo-protective aminosalicytes.[4,5]

The overall incidence of IBD-CRC is 2.5%, but this varies based on the site of inflammation.[4,6] Colonic Crohn's disease (CD) is associated with CRC (relative risk, 4.5 [1.3–14.9]), but ileal CD is not (relative risk, 1.1 [0.8–1.5]).[4,6] The cumulative risk of CRC in CD at 10, 20, and 30 years after diagnosis is 2.9%, 5.6%, and 8.3%, respectively.

The cause and presentation of IBD-CRC differs from that of sporadic CRC. Sporadic disease is linked to the predictable adenoma-carcinoma sequence, but IBD-CRC is driven by cellular damage from chronic inflammation and does not follow in such an orderly fashion.[7,8] IBD-CRC tends to present at a younger age compared with sporadic disease (mean, 40–50 years vs 60 years)[9] and may arise in flat mucosa that is more difficult to visualize.[10]

Risk factors for IBD-CRC include a younger age at onset, duration greater than 8 years, extent of colitis, and the degree of endoscopic and histologic inflammation.[11,12] Other risks include primary sclerosing cholangitis (PSC) (odds ratio, 4.8; 95% confidence interval [CI], 3.6–6.4)[13] and a positive family history of CRC.[14]

Previous work by our group detailed the risk, pathogenesis, surveillance, and management of IBD dysplasia and CRC.[15] This article focuses on the surgical approach to IBD dysplasia and CRC.

COLORECTAL CANCER SCREENING

Current data on the survival benefit for screening in IBD are sparse, with a Cochrane Review failing to show a benefit,[16] so our review focuses on expert panel consensus.[12]

Most current guidelines recommend starting surveillance colonoscopy 6 to 10 years after the diagnosis of IBD, with surveillance colonoscopy every 1 to 2 years.[17–21] In the presence of coexisting PSC, patients should undergo colonoscopy followed by yearly surveillance.[17] Of note, PSC may be an indication for prophylactic colectomy, although the relative risk of IBD-CRC is lower in CD than in ulcerative colitis (UC).[22]

Surveillance technique normally involves 2 sets of 4-quadrant biopsies in each colon segment (right, transverse, left, rectosigmoid), producing more than 32 random biopsies, providing an 80% to 90% sensitivity for dysplasia.[23–25] Directed biopsies of polypoid lesions, masses, strictures, or irregular mucosa should also be performed.[23,26,27]

Recent research has shown that dysplasia may be better identified with advanced endoscopic imaging and targeted biopsies rather than random biopsies.[28–30]

Advanced Endoscopic Imaging

Chromoendoscopy (CE) uses a dye agent such as indigo carmine or methylene blue to enhance the detection of mucosal lesions.[30,31] This technique improves flat dysplastic lesion detection by 27%.[32,33] At present, most expert societies recommend the use of CE with targeted biopsies whenever the technology and expertise are available, particularly for high-risk patients.[33]

Digital or optical imaging technology, such as narrow band imaging (NBI; Olympus, Tokyo, Japan), uses specific light wavelengths that penetrate only the superficial mucosa to better delineate mucosal vasculature without the use of dyes,[34,35] but this has not been shown to provide a benefit in neoplasia detection rates.[36] Compared with chromoendoscopy, NBI is associated with a higher miss rate for neoplasia, and is not recommended for IBD surveillance.[35]

High-resolution endoscopy and endocytoscopy are emerging areas of interest for endoscopic surveillance, but have yet to show improved detection of neoplasia compared with conventional endoscopy.[37–43]

MANAGEMENT OF INFLAMMATORY BOWEL DISEASE–RELATED DYSPLASIA, CANCER, AND STRICTURES

Dysplasia can be microscopically classified into low-grade dysplasia (LGD), high-grade dysplasia (HGD), or indefinite for dysplasia depending on the degree of preservation or loss of cellular polarity reflected by nuclear stratification.[44] Dysplasia identified on random biopsies must be confirmed by 2 gastrointestinal pathologists. One of the most important determinants in managing patients with raised dysplastic lesions is whether the dysplasia is completely resectable.[44] If a lesion is nonresectable because of size, fixation, or adjacent dysplasia, it is referred to as a dysplasia-associated lesion or mass (DALM). DALMs can be further divided into adenomalike (polypoid) and nonadenomalike (nonpolypoid).[45]

Adenomalike DALMs tend to behave like sporadic adenomas and can be safely treated with polypectomy, tattoo, and continued surveillance,[46] a strategy associated with a low risk of progression to CRC (2.4% of patients after an average follow-up of 54 months).[47] However, if biopsy of the surrounding tissue identifies dysplasia, colectomy is recommended because of the high risk of associated CRC.[10,29,47]

Nonadenomalike DALMs can appear as velvety patches, plaques, irregular bumps and nodules, wartlike thickenings, stricturing lesions, or broad-based masses.[45] These flat DALMs are usually not amenable to endoscopic removal, and they have a 9-fold risk of developing cancer and a 12-fold risk of developing any advanced lesion,[48] so surgical resection is usually warranted.

Low-Grade Dysplasia

The management of unifocal, flat LGD in the setting of IBD remains controversial. Historically, the literature reports widely variable rates of progression to HGD, ranging from 0% to 53%.[10] Studies performed in the era of chromoendoscopy show that most patients with LGD do not progress to HGD over 3 to 4 years of follow-up.

Areas of LGD that are nonpolypoid, endoscopically invisible, 1 cm or larger, or preceded by indefinite dysplasia are at increased risk for progression and should be considered for colectomy.[20] Other considerations for colectomy include metachronous LGD after endoscopic removal and multifocal disease.[20]

High-Grade Dysplasia

In HGD the risk of harboring an underlying invasive malignancy can be greater than 40%.[49] Therefore, HGD has traditionally warranted surgical resection. However, there are emerging data suggesting that discrete areas of HGD can be safely removed via endoscopy, avoiding major surgery.[50,51] In 2015, the Surveillance for Colorectal Endoscopic Neoplasia Detection and Management in Inflammatory Bowel Disease Patients: International Consensus Recommendations (SCENIC) panel stated that, if dysplasia is not detected on follow-up, a decision regarding surveillance or colectomy can be individualized.[52] This statement is in contrast with the European Crohn's and Colitis Organization and The American Society for Gastrointestinal Endoscopy, which state that HGD without an associated endoscopically visible lesion is an indication for surgery.[21]

Strictures

Colonic strictures develop in 5% to 10% of patients with IBD and should be routinely biopsied because of an increased risk of CRC (hazard ratio, 18.8).[23,53,54] A negative biopsy may not completely rule out this risk because of sampling error and the more infiltrative nature of colitis-associated malignancies. All IBD strictures require surveillance and those that cannot be traversed and biopsied should be considered for surgical resection.[55]

SURGICAL OPTIONS

As with any cancer, when an IBD-CRC is found during screening or surveillance colonoscopy, preoperative staging is performed to inform appropriate treatment strategies.[56]

Ulcerative Colitis

In the elective setting, findings of IBD-CRC, a nonadenoma DALM, or HGD are almost uniformly accepted as indications for proctocolectomy with or without ileal pouch anal anastomosis (IPAA),[23] because 43% to 50% have associated malignancy at the time of colectomy.[49,57,58] The technical aspects of surgery for IBD-CRC mirror the approach to sporadic disease, and include high ligation of major colonic vessels and total mesorectal excision.[59]

In select cases, the rectum can be spared, and an ileorectal anastomosis can be performed. Although this surgery is usually less extensive, the risk of anastomotic leak is up to 13% in some studies.[60] A further issue is the cumulative risk of developing dysplasia in the retained rectum (5, 10, 15, 20 years is 7%, 9%, 20%, 25% respectively) and cancer (5, 10, 15, 20 years is 0%, 2%, 5%, 14% respectively).[61,62]

Segmental resection also has a limited role in UC because of the risk of developing secondary malignancies in other areas of colon.[10] Previous reports have shown that 12% to 55% of patients have an occult or synchronous cancer and 48% have synchronous dysplasia.[10,63,64]

Ileal Pouch Anal Anastomosis in Inflammatory Bowel Disease Colorectal Cancer

In 1978, Parks and Nicholls[65] published the technique of ileoanal pouch surgery in the *British Medical Journal.*[66] This technique is usually accomplished in either a 2-stage or 3-stage procedure. The ultimate result with IPAA involves forming a J-shaped pouch from the terminal ileum in order to replace the function of the rectum. The presence of UC-related dysplasia or cancer is not a contraindication to IPAA.

The most common method of creating an IPAA is a double-stapled technique with a distal rectal anastomosis, preserving the anal transition zone (ATZ)[66] (**Fig. 1**). This method leaves a cuff of residual columnar mucosa at the ATZ, which theoretically has the potential risk of future malignancy. The alternative method of IPAA creation involves performing a mucosectomy of the anal canal and a hand-sewn ileoanal anastomosis (**Fig. 2**). A double-stapled technique has better functional outcomes compared with a hand-sewn IPAA[67]; 2 randomized trials have shown reduced levels of nocturnal fecal incontinence with the double-stapled technique. Furthermore, occasional or frequent episodes of incontinence have been reported in 64% of hand-sewn groups compared with 38% of the stapled groups.[67–69]

With either technique, there is a small risk of subsequent dysplasia. A 2003 study of 289 patients undergoing a double-stapled IPAA found a 4.5% incidence of dysplasia in the residual ATZ at 10 years.[70] One 2011 review showed 43 known cases of dysplasia and cancer, including 30 patients with mucosectomy and 13 with a stapled

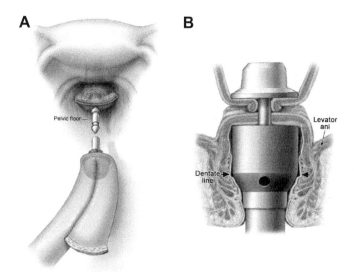

Fig. 1. Double-stapled technique for IPAA creation. (*A*) Intraabdominal view; (*B*) coronal anal of view IPAA creation with circular stapler. (Used with permission of Mayo Foundation for Medical Education and Research, all rights reserved.)

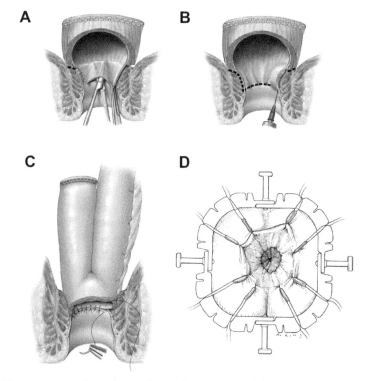

Fig. 2. Mucosectomy and hand-sewn ileoanal anastomosis. (*A*) Raising submucosal plain; (*B*) excision of mucosa; (*C*) suturing of pouch-anal anastomosis; (*D*) external view of hand-sewn pouch-anal anastomosis. (Used with permission of Mayo Foundation for Medical Education and Research, all rights reserved.)

anastomosis.[71] Another study of 1200 patients with IBD-related IPAA found that 1.83% developed pouch neoplasia, including 16 adenocarcinomas.[72] A similar review from Cleveland Clinic of 3202 patients reported that the cumulative incidences for pouch neoplasia at 5, 10, 15, and 20 years were 0.9%, 1.3%, 1.9%, and 4.2%.[10,73] Eleven (0.36%) patients developed adenocarcinoma of the anal canal or pouch.[73] The only independent risk factor for pouch neoplasia was a history of dysplasia or CRC before IPAA.[73]

Ileal Pouch Anal Anastomosis in Inflammatory Bowel Disease Colorectal Cancer and Radiation

Special consideration should be taken for patients with UC with locally advanced rectal cancer. Preoperative pelvic radiation can affect pouch-related sepsis and long-term pouch function.[74] Wu and colleagues[74] studied 63 IPAA patients with IBD-CRC and found that preoperative radiation was associated with chronic pouchitis. In the same study, pouch failure occurred in 13 patients after a median follow-up of 66.4 months.[74] The investigators showed a strong association between preoperative pelvic radiation and the risk for pouch failure ($P<.001$), but there was no correlation between pelvic radiation and pouch/anal transitional zone neoplasia, pouch stricture, pelvic abscess, and pouch fistula/sinus.[74]

Postoperative pelvic radiation after IPAA is even more significant and rarely allows acceptable pouch function. In 2012, Merchea and colleagues[75] published on 41 patients with UC and rectal cancer, which included 11 patients undergoing IPAA. Two patients had a failed pouch, 1 of which was secondary to radiation enteritis.[75] The conclusion of this study was that rectal cancer not requiring neoadjuvant chemoradiotherapy can safely undergo restorative proctocolectomy with good functional results.[75] Patients who require pelvic radiation or who have stage IV disease may be better served with proctocolectomy and end ileostomy.[75]

Crohn's Disease

Patients with CD and HGD, multifocal LGD, a nonadenoma DALM, or invasive cancer should undergo total proctocolectomy.[76] Approximately 40% of patients with CD undergoing segmental resection or subtotal colectomy develop metachronous cancers.[76] Approximately 44% of patients with known malignancy have multifocal disease in the final specimen and 40% have evidence of dysplasia remote from the cancer site.[76] In general, IPAA formation in the setting of CD is not recommended because it is associated with poor function and high failure rates. In highly selected patients who are not willing to have a permanent end ileostomy and have so-called rectal sparing with no active inflammation or dysplasia within the rectum, a total abdominal colectomy with ileorectal anastomosis can be considered as long as there is intense postoperative surveillance.

LONG-TERM OUTCOMES

As with sporadic CRC, in IBD-CRC the prognosis and survival depend on stage of disease and response to treatment. A study from the Mayo Clinic in 2006 comparing IBD-CRC (n = 290) and sporadic CRC (n = 290) over 20 years showed comparable 5-year survival (54% in IBD-CRC and 53% in sporadic CRC).[10,76] Several more recently published articles have also confirmed that IBD-associated CRCs have comparable rates of tumor recurrence and survival following postoperative chemotherapy with patients with CRC without IBD.[77] For metastatic disease, the situation may be different. Recent work from Memorial Sloan Kettering Cancer Center case matched 18 patients with metastatic IBD-CRC with sporadic cases. Median overall survival was significantly worse in the IBD-related group (15 months vs 34 months).[78]

SUMMARY

Patients with IBD are at an increased risk of cancer secondary to long-standing intestinal inflammation. Surgical options must take into account the significant risk of synchronous disease at other colonic sites. IPAA is a viable option for patients with UC but this should be restricted to early cancers that are unlikely to require preoperative or postoperative radiation treatment.

REFERENCES

1. Dulai PS, Sandborn WJ, Gupta S. Colorectal Cancer and Dysplasia in Inflammatory Bowel Disease: A Review of Disease Epidemiology, Pathophysiology, and Management. Cancer Prev Res (Phila) 2016;9(12):887–94.
2. Crohn BB, Rosenberg B. The sigmoidoscopic picture of chronic ulcerative colitis (nonspecific). Am J Med Sci 1925;170:220–7.
3. Eaden JA, Abrams KR, Mayberry JF. The risk of colorectal cancer in ulcerative colitis: a meta-analysis. Gut 2001;48:526–35.
4. Wang ZH, Fang JY. Colorectal Cancer in Inflammatory Bowel Disease: Epidemiology, Pathogenesis and Surveillance. Gastrointest Tumors 2014;1(3):146–54.
5. Castaño-Milla C, Chaparro M, Gisbert JP. Systematic review with meta-analysis: the declining risk of colorectal cancer in UC. Aliment Pharmacol Ther 2014;39(7):1001–2.
6. Canavan C, Abrams KR, Mayberry J. Meta-analysis: colorectal and small bowel cancer risk in patients with Crohn's disease. Aliment Pharmacol Ther 2006;23:1097–104.
7. Grivennikov SI. Inflammation and colorectal cancer: colitis-associated neoplasia. Semin Immunopathol 2012;35(2):229–44.
8. Fearon ER, Vogelstein B. A genetic model for colorectal Tumorigenesis. Cell 1990;61(5):759–67.
9. Munkholm P. Review article: the incidence and prevalence of colorectal cancer in inflammatory bowel disease. Aliment Pharmacol Ther 2003;18(Suppl 2):1–5.
10. Althumairi AA, Lazarev MG, Gearhart SL. Inflammatory bowel disease associated neoplasia: a surgeon's perspective. World J Gastroenterol 2016;22(3):961–73.
11. Kim ER, Chang DK. Colorectal cancer in inflammatory bowel disease: the risk, pathogenesis, prevention and diagnosis. World J Gastroenterol 2014;20(29):9872–81.
12. Mattar MC, Lough D, Pishvaian MJ, et al. Current management of inflammatory bowel disease and colorectal cancer. Gastrointest Cancer Res 2011;4(2):53–61.
13. Andersen NN, Jess T. Has the risk of colorectal cancer in inflammatory bowel disease decreased? World J Gastroenterol 2013;19(43):7561–8.
14. Askling J, Dickman PW, Karlén P, et al. Family history as a risk factor for colorectal cancer in inflammatory bowel disease. Gastroenterology 2001;120(6):1356–62.
15. Huang LC, Merchea A. Dysplasia and Cancer in Inflammatory Bowel Disease. Surg Clin North Am 2017;97(3):627–39.
16. Mpofu C, Watson AJM, Rhodes JM. Strategies for detecting colon cancer and/or dysplasia in patients with inflammatory bowel disease. Cochrane Database Syst Rev 2004;(2). John Wiley & Sons, Ltd, CD000279.
17. Guagnozzi D, Lucendo AJ. Colorectal cancer surveillance in patients with inflammatory bowel disease: What is new? World J Gastrointest Endosc 2012;4(4):108–16.

18. Itzkowitz SH, Present DH. Consensus conference: Colorectal cancer screening and surveillance in inflammatory bowel disease. Inflamm Bowel Dis 2005;11:314–21.

19. Bae SI, Kim YS. Colon cancer screening and surveillance in inflammatory bowel disease. Clin Endosc 2014;47(6):509–15.

20. Choi CH, Ignjatovic-Wilson A, Askari A, et al. Low-grade dysplasia in ulcerative colitis: risk factors for developing high-grade dysplasia or colorectal cancer. Am J Gastroenterol 2015;110(10):1461–71.

21. Huguet JM, Suárez P, Ferrer-Barceló L, et al. Endoscopic recommendations for colorectal cancer screening and surveillance in patients with inflammatory bowel disease: Review of general recommendations. World J Gastrointest Endosc 2017;9(6):255–62.

22. Broomé U, Löfberg R, Veress B, et al. Primary sclerosing cholangitis and ulcerative colitis: evidence for increased neoplastic potential. Hepatology 1995;22:1404–8.

23. Ross H, Steele SR, Varma M, et al. Practice Parameters for the Surgical Treatment of Ulcerative Colitis. Dis Colon Rectum 2014;57:5–22.

24. Awais D, Siegel CA, Higgins PD. Modelling dysplasia detection in ulcerative colitis: clinical implications of surveillance intensity. Gut 2009;58:1498–503.

25. Rubin CE, Haggitt RC, Burmer GC, et al. DNA aneuploidy in colonic biopsies predicts future development of dysplasia in ulcerative colitis. Gastroenterology 1992; 103:1611–20.

26. Blonski W, Kundu R, Lewis J, et al. Is dysplasia visible during surveillance colonoscopy in patients with ulcerative colitis? Scand J Gastroenterol 2008;43: 698–703.

27. Rubin DT, Rothe JA, Hetzel JT, et al. Are dysplasia and colorectal cancer endoscopically visible in patients with ulcerative colitis? Gastrointest Endosc 2007;65: 998–1004.

28. Watanabe T, Ajioka Y, Mitsuyama K, et al. Comparison of Targeted vs Random Biopsies for Surveillance of Ulcerative Colitis-Associated Colorectal Cancer. Gastroenterology 2016;151:1122–30.

29. Rutter MD, Saunders BP, Wilkinson KH, et al. Most dysplasia in ulcerative colitis is visible at colonoscopy. Gastrointest Endosc 2004;6:334–9.

30. Trivedi PJ, Braden B. Indications, stains and techniques in chromoendoscopy. QJM 2012;106(2):117–31.

31. Barkin JA, Sussman DA, Abreu MT. Chromoendoscopy and advanced imaging technologies for surveillance of patients with IBD. Gastroenterol Hepatol (N Y) 2012;8(12):796–802.

32. Subramanian V, Mannath J, Ragunath K, et al. Meta-analysis: the diagnostic yield of chromoendoscopy for detecting dysplasia in patients with colonic inflammatory bowel disease. Aliment Pharmacol Ther 2011;33(3):304–12.

33. Shukla R, Salem M, Hou JK. Use and barriers to chromoendoscopy for dysplasia surveillance in inflammatory bowel disease. World J Gastrointest Endosc 2017; 9(8):359–67.

34. Cho WY, Jang JY, Lee DH, Endoscopic Technology and Investigation Study Group. Recent Advances in Image-enhanced Endoscopy. Clin Endosc 2011; 44(2):65–75.

35. Pellisé M, López-Cerón M, Rodríguez de Miguel C, et al. Narrow-band imaging as an alternative to chromoendoscopy for the detection of dysplasia in long-standing inflammatory bowel disease: a prospective, randomized, crossover study. Gastrointest Endosc 2011;74(4):840–8.

36. Dekker E, van den Broek FJ, Reitsma JB, et al. Narrow-band imaging compared with conventional colonoscopy for the detection of dysplasia in patients with long-standing ulcerative colitis. Endoscopy 2007;39:216–21.
37. Galli J, Cammarota G, Rigante M, et al. High resolution magnifying endoscopy: a new diagnostic tool also for laryngeal examination? Acta Otorhinolaryngol Ital 2007;27(5):233–6.
38. Kiesslich R, Goetz M, Neurath MF. Confocal laser endomicroscopy for gastrointestinal diseases. Gastrointest Endosc Clin N Am 2008;18:451–66.
39. Kim ES. Role of Advanced Endoscopic Imaging Techniques in the Management of Inflammatory Bowel Disease. Clin Endosc 2017;50(5):424–8.
40. Beintaris I, Rutter M. Advanced imaging in colonoscopy: contemporary approach to dysplasia surveillance in inflammatory bowel disease. Frontline Gastroenterol 2016;7(4):308–15.
41. Günther U, Kusch D, Heller F, et al. Surveillance colonoscopy in patients with inflammatory bowel disease: comparison of random biopsy vs. targeted biopsy protocols. Int J Colorectal Dis 2011;26:667–72.
42. Freire P, Figueiredo P, Cardoso R. Surveillance in ulcerative colitis: is chromoendoscopy-guided endomicroscopy always better than conventional colonoscopy? A randomized trial. Inflamm Bowel Dis 2014;20:2038–45.
43. Wanders LK, Kuiper T, Kiesslich R. Limited applicability of chromoendoscopy-guided confocal laser endomicroscopy as daily-practice surveillance strategy in Crohn's disease. Gastrointest Endosc 2016;83:966–71.
44. Harpaz N, Polydorides AD. Colorectal Dysplasia in IBD. Arch Pathol Lab Med 2010;134:876–95.
45. Fogt F, Urbanski SJ, Sanders ME, et al. Distinction between dysplasia-associated lesion or mass (DALM) and adenoma in patients with ulcerative colitis. Hum Pathol 2000;31(3):288–91.
46. Quinn AM, Farraye FA, Naini BV, et al. Polypectomy is adequate treatment for adenoma-like dysplastic lesions (DALMs) in Crohn's disease. Inflamm Bowel Dis 2013;19(6):1186–93.
47. Wanders LK, Dekker E, Pullens B, et al. Cancer risk after resection of polypoid dysplasia in patients with longstanding ulcerative colitis: A Meta-analysis. Clin Gastroenterol Hepatol 2014;12:756–64.
48. Thomas T, Abrams KA, Robinson RJ, et al. Meta-analysis: cancer risk of low-grade dysplasia in chronic ulcerative colitis. Aliment Pharmacol Ther 2007;25:657–68.
49. Bernstein CN, Shanahan F, Weinstein WM. Are we telling patients the truth about surveillance colonoscopy in ulcerative colitis? Lancet 1994;343:71–4.
50. Blonski W, Kundu R, Furth EF, et al. High-grade dysplastic adenoma-like mass lesions are not an indication for colectomy in patients with ulcerative colitis. Scand J Gastroenterol 2008;43:817.
51. Smith LA, Baraza W, Tiffin N, et al. Endoscopic resection of adenoma-like mass in chronic ulcerative colitis using a combined endoscopic mucosal resection and cap assisted submucosal dissection technique. Inflamm Bowel Dis 2008;14:1380.
52. Laine L, Kaltenbach T, Barkun A, et al. SCENIC international consensus statement on surveillance and management of dysplasia in inflammatory bowel disease. Gastroenterology 2015;148(3):639–51.
53. Lashner BA, Turner BC, Bostwick DG, et al. Dysplasia and cancer complicating strictures in ulcerative coli- tis. Dig Dis Sci 1990;35:349–52.

54. Lovasz BD, Lakatos L, Golovics PA, et al. Risk of Colorectal Cancer in Crohn s Disease Patients with Colonic Involvement and Stenosing Disease in a Population-based Cohort from Hungary. J Gastrointestin Liver Dis 2013;22(3): 265–8.

55. Hwang JM, Varma MG. Surgery for inflammatory bowel disease. World J Gastro-enterol 2008;14(17):2678–90.

56. Wu JS. Rectal cancer staging. Clin Colon Rectal Surg 2007;20(3):148–57.

57. Blackstone MO, Riddell RH, Rogers BH, et al. Dysplasia- associated lesion or mass (Dalm) detected by colonoscopy in long-standing ulcerative colitis: an indication for colectomy. Gastroenterology 1981;80:366–74.

58. Riddell RH, Goldman H, Ransohoff DF. Dysplasia in inflammatory bowel disease: standardized classification with pro- visional clinical applications. Hum Pathol 1983;14:931–68.

59. Yao HW, Liu YH. Re-examination of the standardization of colon cancer surgery. Gastroenterol Rep (Oxf) 2013;1(2):113–8.

60. Segelman J, Mattsson I, Jung B, et al. Risk factors for anastomotic leakage following ileosigmoid or ileorectal anastomosis. Colorectal Dis 2018;20(4): 304–11.

61. Juviler A, Hyman N. Ulcerative colitis: the fate of the retained rectum. Clin Colon Rectal Surg 2004;17(1):29–34.

62. Scoglio D, Ahmed Ali U, Fichera A. Surgical treatment of ulcerative colitis: ileor-ectal vs ileal pouch-anal anastomosis. World J Gastroenterol 2014;20(37): 13211–8.

63. Beaugerie L, Svrcek M, Seksik P, et al. Risk of colorectal high-grade dysplasia and cancer in a prospective observational cohort of patients with inflammatory bowel disease. Gastroenterology 2013;145:166–75.

64. Jayaram H, Satsangi J, Chapman RW. Increased colorectal neoplasia in chronic ulcerative colitis complicated by primary sclerosing cholangitis: fact or fiction? Gut 2001;48:430–4.

65. Parks AG, Nicholls RJ. Proctocolectomy without ileostomy for ulcerative colitis. BMJ 1978;2:85–8.

66. Carne PW, Pemberton JH. Technical aspects of ileoanal pouch surgery. Clin Colon Rectal Surg 2004;17(1):35–41.

67. Deen KI, Williams JG, Grant EA, et al. Randomized trial to determine the optimum level of pouch-anal anastomosis in stapled restorative proctocolectomy. Dis Colon Rectum 1995;38(2):133–8.

68. Reilly WT, Pemberton JH, Wolff BG, et al. Randomized prospective trial comparing ileal pouch-anal anastomosis performed by excising the anal mucosa to ileal pouch-anal anastomosis performed by preserving the anal mucosa. Ann Surg 1997;225(6):666–76.

69. Hallgren TA, Fasth SB, Oresland TO, et al. Ileal pouch anal function after endoa-nal mucosectomy and handsewn ileoanal anastomosis compared with stapled anastomosis without mucosectomy. Eur J Surg 1995;161(12):915–21.

70. Remzi FH, Fazio VW, Delaney CP, et al. Dysplasia of the anal transitional zone after ileal pouch-anal anastomosis: results of prospective evaluation after a minimum of ten years. Dis Colon Rectum 2003;46(1):6–13.

71. Um JW, M'Koma AE. Pouch-related dysplasia and adenocarcinoma following restorative proctocolectomy for ulcerative colitis. Tech Coloproctol 2011; 15(1):7–16.

72. Derikx LA, Kievit W, Drenth JP, et al. Prior colorectal neoplasia is associated with increased risk of ileoanal pouch neoplasia in patients with inflammatory bowel disease. Gastroenterology 2014;146(1):119–28.
73. Kariv R, Remzi FH, Lian L, et al. Preoperative colorectal neoplasia increases risk for pouch neoplasia in patients with restorative proctocolectomy. Gastroenterology 2010;139:806–12.
74. Wu XR, Kiran RP, Remzi FH, et al. Preoperative pelvic radiation increases the risk for ileal pouch failure in patients with colitis-associated colorectal cancer. J Crohns Colitis 2013;7(10):e419–26.
75. Merchea A, Wolff BG, Dozois EJ, et al. Clinical features and oncologic outcomes in patients with rectal cancer and ulcerative colitis: a single-institution experience. Dis Colon Rectum 2012;55(8):881–5.
76. Delaunoit T, Limburg PJ, Goldberg RM, et al. Colorectal cancer prognosis among patients with inflammatory bowel disease. Clin Gastroenterol Hepatol 2006;4: 335–42.
77. Dugum M, Lin J, Lopez R, et al. Recurrence and survival rates of inflammatory bowel disease-associated colorectal cancer following postoperative chemotherapy: a comparative study. Gastroenterol Rep (Oxf) 2016;5(1):57–61.
78. Yaeger, Hersch J, Bates D, et al. Outcomes for matched patients with metastatic colitis-associated cancers versus sporadic colorectal cancer receiving chemotherapy. J Clin Oncol 2018;36(15S):e15534.

Elective Abdominal Surgery for Inflammatory Bowel Disease

Adina E. Feinberg, MDCM[a], Michael A. Valente, DO[b],*

KEYWORDS

- Elective surgery • Inflammatory bowel disease • Resection margins • Mesentery
- Strictureplasty • Ileal pouch–anal anastomosis

KEY POINTS

- Elective abdominal surgery for inflammatory bowel disease is common.
- Surgery for Crohn's disease is not curative, and treatment must be individualized to the disease process.
- Surgery for ulcerative colitis generally is curative but consideration of patient specific factors is important for staging of the procedure and determining whether ileal pouch–anal anastomosis is appropriate.

INTRODUCTION

Elective surgery for inflammatory bowel disease (IBD) is an essential part of the multimodal treatment. In Crohn's disease (CD), surgery is not curative and thus is usually indicated when a patient is refractory to medical therapy or for fibrostenosing or fistulizing disease–related complications. In ulcerative colitis (UC), surgery is curative, which influences the decision to undergo surgery. This article provides an overview of elective surgery in CD and UC.

CROHN'S DISEASE

Approximately 70% of patients with CD require surgery at some point during their lifetime.[1] Elective surgery may be undertaken for disease-associated complications, such as fibrostenotic stricture, dysplasia, or medically refractory disease. Patients who develop perforation and abscess initially may be managed with percutaneous drainage, but these patients often go on to require resection for control of ongoing

No disclosures.

[a] Department of General Surgery, Joseph Brant Hospital, 390 Brant Street, Suite 405, Burlington, Ontario L7R 4J4, Canada; [b] Department of Colorectal Surgery, Digestive Disease and Surgery Institute, Cleveland Clinic, 9500 Euclid Avenue, Desk A-30, Cleveland, OH 44195, USA
* Corresponding author.
E-mail address: valentm2@ccf.org

fistulas and sepsis.[2] Given that surgery for CD is not curative, any intervention should be considered in the context of these main goals:

- Control symptoms.
- Preserve bowel length.
- Maintain function.

The preoperative considerations in IBD surgery is covered detail in Nicholas P. McKenna and Amy L. Lightner's article, "Preoperative Considerations in Inflammatory Bowel Disease," in this issue. Preoperative assessment should include complete staging of disease to assist in surgical planning and minimize intraoperative surprises. The office evaluation should entail a thorough history of prior interventions to include a detailed review of any previous operative notes and pathology results and assessment of nutritional status as well as other risk factors for surgical complications, such as immunosuppression. Surgeons should maximize their understanding of the anatomic extent of disease using endoscopy and computed tomography or magnetic resonance enterography to complete this work-up. Preoperative meeting with an enterostomal therapist is essential to begin patient education and ensure appropriate location in the event that ostomy formation is required.

GENERAL PRINCIPLES
Surgical Approach

Laparoscopic techniques have been shown to be safe when feasible and are associated with decreased length of stay and incisional benefits.[3] In some cases, a minimally invasive approach may not be possible due to the nature of the disease or adhesions from prior procedures.

Extent of Resection

Conservative margins (2 cm) should be used with division where the bowel appears grossly normal because wider margins do not reduce the rate of recurrence.[4] Because CD involvement begins at the mesenteric border of the bowel, palpation along the mesenteric border is used to assess where the normal edge of bowel wall can be felt (**Fig. 1**).

Anastomosis

Although great controversy exists, there is no high-quality evidence to suggest that anastomotic technique (stapled vs hand-sewn) or configuration (end-to-end vs side-to-side) has an impact on disease recurrence. In the Canadian and American Surgical Crohn's Disease trial, patients undergoing surgery for ileocolic disease had no difference in endoscopic or symptomatic recurrence whether they were randomized to a stapled side-to-side anastomosis or a hand-sewn end-to-end anastomosis.[5] A recent prospective study found that patients undergoing ileocecal resection with an end-to-end anastomosis had lower health care utilization and better quality of life at 2 years than those with a side-to-side anastomosis,[6] but these results were limited by the nonrandomized nature of the study.

Recently, the Kono-S anastomosis (**Fig. 2**) has been shown in preliminary studies to have low surgical recurrence,[7] possibly due to the supporting column of the anastomosis, which is hypothetically more resistant to deformity from disease recurrence. It also is possible that the separation from the mesentery is protective. A randomized trial is under way and may provide further insights regarding the utility of the Kono-S anastomosis.

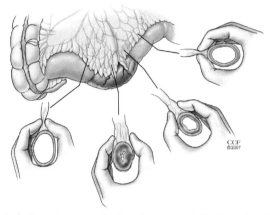

Fig. 1. Palpation technique to assess for involvement of CD. By palpating the mesenteric border, where the edge of the bowel becomes soft and normal can be felt. (Reprinted with permission, Cleveland Clinic Center for Medical Art & Photography © 1998–2019. All Rights Reserved.)

Internal Bypass

Internal bypass procedures generally should be avoided due to the risk of malignancy in bypassed segment over time.[8] In select situations, bypass may be the safest choice, such as in gastroduodenal disease that is not amenable to strictureplasty.

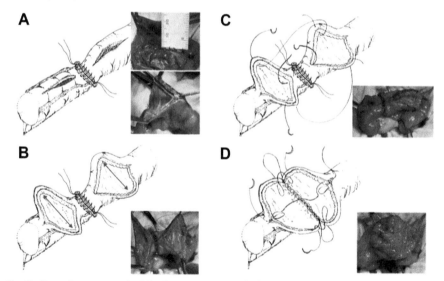

Fig. 2. Kono-S anastomosis. (*A*) after resection with closure of the 2 bowel ends, the ends of bowel are approximated to form the supporting column, and antimesenteric linear enterotomies are made on either side within 0.5 cm to 1 cm of the supporting column; (*B*) these enterotomies are joined in a transverse manner; (*C*) the posterior wall is approximated with interrupted or running suture; and (*D*) the anterior wall is closed in the same fashion. (Reprinted with permission from Springer Nature: Journal of Gastrointestinal Surgery, Kono-S Anastomosis for Surgical Prophylaxis of Anastomotic Recurrence in Crohn's Disease: an International Multicenter Study, Kono et al, 2015.)

Approach to the Mesentery

Proper respect and handling of the mesentery is necessary when operating on patients with CD. The diseased mesentery typically is thickened and difficult to control. Standard clamp-tie techniques and vessel sealing energy devices used to divide normal mesentery typically do not suffice. The vessels can retract within the adipose tissue, creating an enlarging hematoma and possibly ischemia. The authors prefer to use Kocher clamps to secure the mesentery before division with suture ligation (**Fig. 3**). Safe laparoscopic division of the mesentery can be done in appropriately selected patients,[9] but extreme caution should be used, and backup plans, including the use of endoloops and delivery into a minilaparotomy, should be prepared.

Because CD surgery does not require an oncologic lymphadenectomy and proximal division of the vessels can be hazardous, large mesenteric resections usually are avoided. Recent studies have shown, however, resection of the mesentery to be associated with lower rates of disease recurrence.[10] Further studies are necessary before adopting this more aggressive resection technique.

SPECIFIC ANATOMIC CONSIDERATIONS
Duodenal Disease

Duodenal CD most commonly presents with obstructive symptoms. Fistulas involving the duodenum usually are the result of adjacent small bowel or colonic disease with the duodenum as an innocent bystander, and fistulizing disease originating in the duodenum has not been reported.[11]

Malnutrition is common in patients with duodenal CD, so preoperative optimization with enteral feeding (when possible) is crucial.

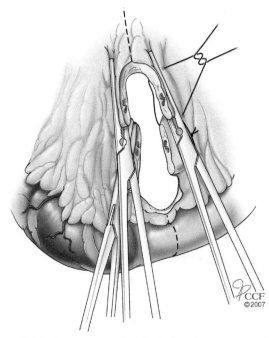

Fig. 3. Technique to divide the mesentery in CD. Kocher clamps are used to secure the mesentery and suture ligatures (U-stitch) are placed underneath to control hemostasis. (Reprinted with permission, Cleveland Clinic Center for Medical Art & Photography © 1998–2019. All Rights Reserved.)

Approaches to duodenal stricture include endoscopic dilatation, bypass, resection, or strictureplasty. Endoscopic dilatation is an attractive initial measure for short strictures but repeat procedures often are necessary.[12] When resection or strictureplasty is planned, complete kocherization and releasing the ligament of Treitz should be performed. The authors' preference is for Heineke-Mickulicz or Finney strictureplasties (discussed later) if they can be accomplished without undue tension.[13] (**Fig. 4**).

Lesions in the third or fourth portion of the duodenum may be best treated with resection and an end-to-end or end-to-side hand-sewn anastomosis. Gastroduodenal bypass is an appropriate option when strictureplasty or resection is not feasible in situations where the duodenum cannot be safely mobilized. An algorithm for the management of duodenal CD is presented in **Fig. 5**.

Small Bowel Disease

Documenting the bowel length, in particular the length of bowel that remains in situ, is necessary at every operation involving small bowel CD unless it is unsafe to do so due to adhesions. Patients with less than 200 cm of small bowel are at risk for short bowel syndrome and patients with less than 100 cm of small bowel almost certainly require parental nutrition.

Often multiple strictures are present and downstream lesions may not be obvious because there may be less prestenotic dilatation. An inflated urinary catheter balloon with approximately 8 mL of water or a 25-mm sphere made of surgical plastic (ie, Bakelite) may be used to identify all areas of problematic stricture (**Fig. 6**).[14] Any stricture resulting in a lumen greater than 20 mm should be addressed in some fashion.[15]

Strictureplasty

Resection of the diseased small bowel is preferred when disease is limited and there have not been significant prior bowel resections. Strictureplasty has an important role in complex disease where there is concern for development of short bowel syndrome. Strictureplasty is safe, with similar recurrence rates to resection procedures.[16] The overall rate of septic complications, including anastomotic leak, fistula, and abscess, is approximately 4%.[17] Although many of CD patients have subsequent operations, only 3% required further surgery for recurrence at sites of prior

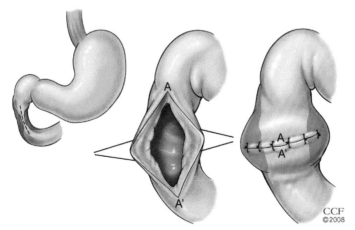

Fig. 4. Heineke-Mickulicz strictureplasty for duodenal strictures. (Reprinted with permission, Cleveland Clinic Center for Medical Art & Photography © 1998–2019. All Rights Reserved.)

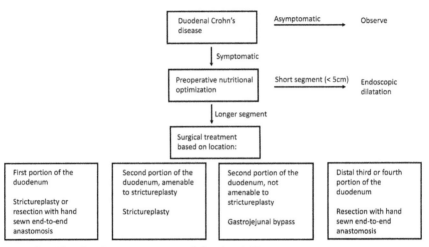

Fig. 5. Algorithm for the management of duodenal CD.

strictureplasties. Strictureplasty may be done in highly selected sites of active inflammation as well.[18]

Considerations for strictureplasty

- Multiple strictures with diffuse jejunoileal distribution[16]
- Prior significant bowel resection (>100 cm of small bowel previously resected)
- Existing short bowel syndrome with stricture(s)

Contraindications for strictureplasty

- Perforated bowel (peritonitis, abscess, fistula with phlegmonous features)
- Suspected malignancy
- Multiple strictures within short segment
- Stricture in close proximity to planned resection site
- Malnutrition with hypoalbuminemia (<2.0 g/dL)

Choice of strictureplasty

Short segment, less than 10 cm The Heineke-Mikulicz strictureplasty is the most straightforward anf commonly used technique.[19] A longitudinal incision is made along the length of the stricture and additional 1 cm to 2 cm of grossly healthy tissue on either side. The incision is then closed in a transverse fashion in either a 1 or

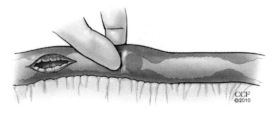

Fig. 6. Identification of significant strictures using a sphere. It may be hard to detect strictures by palpation alone; here, a calibration sphere of 20-mm to 25-mm diameter is used to identify tight areas that limit passage. (Reprinted with permission, Cleveland Clinic Center for Medical Art & Photography © 1998–2019. All Rights Reserved.)

2 layer technique with absorbable suture (**Fig. 7**). This can be modified to excise a fistula tract with the Judd procedure (**Fig. 8**). The Moskel-Walske-Neumayer modification can be done when there is a size mismatch with severely dilated bowel on 1 side (**Fig. 9**).

Intermediate segment, 10 cm to 20 cm Finney-type (**Fig. 10**) or Jabouley (**Fig. 11**) strictureplasties are preferred in this situation. Similar to the Heineke-Mickulicz technique, a longitudinal incision is made along the antimesenteric length of the stricture. The bowel is then folded on itself in a U-shaped configuration. A diverticulum can form and enlarge over time, leading to stasis and bacterial overgrowth. Therefore, this technique should be considered when a Heineke-Mickulicz strictureplasty cannot be done without undue tension.

Long segment, greater than 20 cm The side-to-side isoperistaltic strictureplasty (Michelassi)[20] (**Fig. 12**) can be used for any length of stricture. The bowel is divided halfway between the involved length and intestinal continuity is restored by anastomosing along the length of these segments. This technique should be reserved for patients at risk for short bowel syndrome with disease not amenable to simpler types of strictureplasty, due to significant risk of surgical recurrence.[21]

The authors selectively biopsy the strictureplasty site rather than a routine biopsy. There are thousands of reported strictureplasties, with rare case reports of malignancy occurring. The authors apply metallic clips to the mesentery when there are multiple strictureplasties to facilitate radiographic localization in the rare case of bleeding that is elucidated on angiography. The clips help to identify the bleeding strictureplasty, thereby helping to avoid the opening up of all strictureplasty sites.

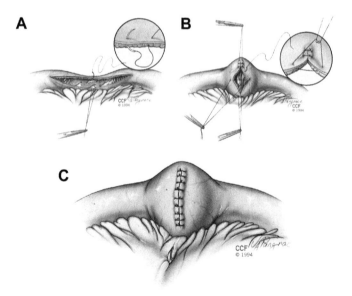

Fig. 7. Heineke-Mickulicz strictureplasty. (*A*) longitudinal incision should extend onto normal bowel for 1 cm to 2 cm in either direction; stay sutures are placed at the midpoint which will become the apices in the transverse closure; (*B*) closure is done transversely with interrupted or running sutures; and (*C*) final result after transverse closure. (Reprinted with permission, Cleveland Clinic Center for Medical Art & Photography © 1998–2019. All Rights Reserved.)

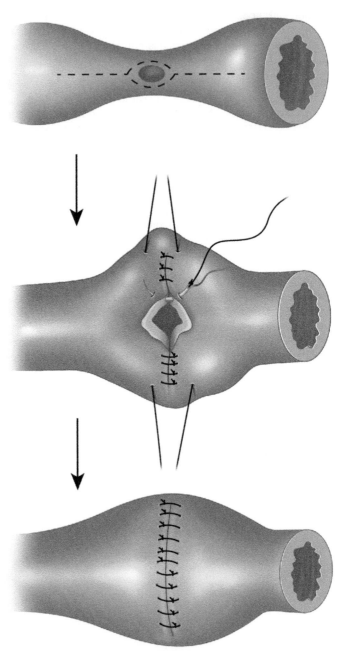

Fig. 8. Judd strictureplasty. (Top) The fistula tract is excised and the longitudinal incision is made. (Middle) This is closed in a transverse fashion. (Bottom) appearance after completion of the strictureplasty. (*From* Ambe R, Campbell L, Cagir B. A comprehensive review of strictureplasty techniques in Crohn's disease: types, indications, comparisons, and safety. J Gastrointest Surg. 2012 Jan;16(1):209-17. https://doi.org/10.1007/s11605-011-1651-2. Epub 2011 Sep 10.)

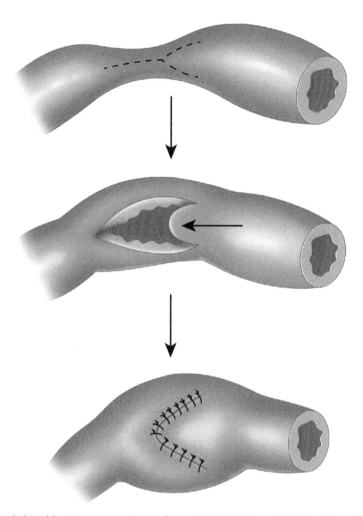

Fig. 9. Moskel-Walske-Neumayer strictureplasty. (Top) A 'Y' shaped incision is made to account for the size discrepancy. (Middle) This is closed in a 'V' fashion. (Bottom) Appearance after completion of the strictureplasty. (*From* Ambe R, Campbell L, Cagir B. A comprehensive review of strictureplasty techniques in Crohn's disease: types, indications, comparisons, and safety. J Gastrointest Surg. 2012 Jan;16(1):209-17. https://doi.org/10.1007/s11605-011-1651-2. Epub 2011 Sep 10.)

Ileocolic Disease

Ileocolic distribution is the most common presentation of CD. Surgery generally is indicated for disease-related complications or medically refractory disease. Surgery also is a viable alternative to biological therapy in a patient who has failed conventional therapy, and a recent randomized controlled trial showed similar quality of life outcomes between biologics and surgery.[22]

When present, fistulas are detected preoperatively in approximately 65% of cases,[23] so most patients should be placed in the lithotomy position in case a colonic procedure becomes necessary. For small bowel and colon fistulas that involve healthy, innocent bystander segments, wedge excision and primary repair are

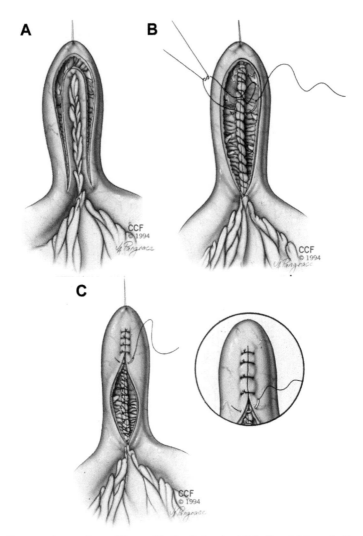

Fig. 10. Finney strictureplasty. (*A*) as with the Heinecke-Mickulicz strictureplasties, longitudinal incision should extend onto normal bowel for 1 cm to 2 cm; the bowel is then folded onto itself with a stay suture at the midpoint; (*B*) interrupted or running closure is used to create the back wall of the strictureplasty; and (*C*) closure of the front wall completes the Finney strictureplasty. (Reprinted with permission, Cleveland Clinic Center for Medical Art & Photography © 1998–2019. All Rights Reserved.)

appropriate rather than a second resection. In the finding of an ileosigmoid fistula, operative approach depends on its relationship to the mesentery. Fistulas located on the mesenteric side of the sigmoid often are not amenable to wedge excision, and a colectomy may be necessary.

Colorectal Disease

Surgical options for isolated Crohn's colitis include segmental colonic resection, total colectomy with ileorectal anastomosis, total proctocolectomy with end ileostomy,

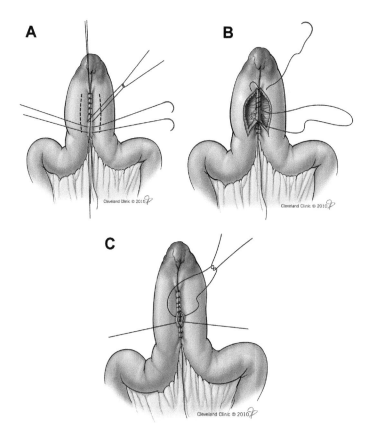

Fig. 11. Jaboulet strictureplasty. (*A*) the strictured area of bowel is folded over and a back row of sutures is placed to line up the area of strictureplasty; (*B*) separate enterotomies are created on either side and the back row of sutures is placed; and (*C*) closure of the front wall completes the Jaboulet strictureplasty. (Reprinted with permission, Cleveland Clinic Center for Medical Art & Photography © 1998–2019. All Rights Reserved.)

and, rarely, ileal pouch–anal anastomosis (IPAA). Strictureplasty is not recommended for colonic disease due to the possibility of malignancy.[24]

Segmental colectomy is certainly an option for segmental colonic disease but is associated with very high rates of disease recurrence, with more than 50% requiring repeat colonic resections.[25,26] Total colectomy with ileorectal anastomosis can maintain intestinal continuity and avoid a pelvic dissection, but 25% to 50% of patients progress to completion proctectomy.[25]

Perianal fistulous disease is discussed detail in Adam Truong's article, "Anorectal Crohn's Disease," in this issue. When total proctocolectomy is performed, the preference is for intersphincteric resection to minimize perineal wound complications. When a patient has severe perianal fistulous disease combined with colorectal disease then staged surgery, starting with diverting loop ileostomy may help to improve the integrity of the perineal skin before proctectomy. If severe perianal fistulous disease persists, then wider resection may be required and consideration for flap reconstruction is advised.

When the perianal disease is severe enough to require fecal diversion, the rate of sustained restoration of intestinal continuity is approximately 10%.[27] The presence

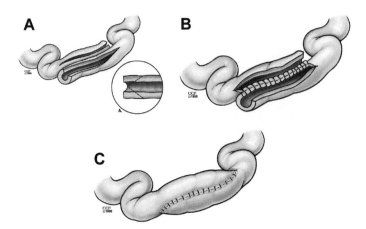

Fig. 12. Side-to-side isoperistaltic strictureplasty. (*A*) after the longitudinal incision is made over the extent of the stricture bowel, the bowel is divided at the midpoint and lined up side by side; (*A*) the edges of bowel can be trimmed to allow better approximation; (*B*) interrupted or running closure is used to create the back wall; and (*C*) closure of the front wall completes the side-to-side isoperistaltic strictureplasty. (Reprinted with permission, Cleveland Clinic Center for Medical Art & Photography © 1998–2019. All Rights Reserved.)

of proctitis decreases the likelihood that a patient will achieve stoma closure.[28] Patients should be given realistic expectations prior to diversion.

IPAA generally is not recommended for CD. In a well-informed and highly motivated patient, however, IPAA can be considered in the absence of small bowel and perianal disease.[29] IPAA in CD is associated with higher rates of complications and at least one-third of patients eventually have pouch failure.[25]

The presence of granulomas on pathology is associated with higher recurrence of CD and should be considered when making treatment decisions.[30]

Fecal Diversion

Proximal diversion may be prudent when there are multiple risk factors for anastomotic dehiscence. At the authors' center, the practice is usually to consider fecal diversion in patients with the following risk factors: long-term and/or high-dose steroid use, recent use of biologics, and malnutrition with hypoalbumenia (<2 g/dL). When proximal diversion entails a high jejunostomy, the patient requires intravenous hydration and likely total parenteral nutrition. The use of high ostomies is uncommon.

ULCERATIVE COLITIS

Approximately 15% of patients with UC proceed to surgery, making this patient population less likely to require surgery than patients with CD.[31] Surgery for UC is curative, and indications include patient preference, medically refractory disease, and dysplasia or carcinoma. Elective surgery in UC generally entails total proctocolectomy with either permanent end ileostomy or IPAA.

General Principles

There generally is no difference in the overall quality of life between patients who undergo IPAA versus permanent ileostomy because both groups report significant improvement[32] IPAA is associated with several short-term and long-term complications, described in Jennifer A. Leinicke's article, "Ileal Pouch Complications," elsewhere in this issue. Proper patient selection and informed decision making are essential to optimize outcomes with IPAA.

Special Considerations in Ileal Pouch–Anal Anastomosis

Patients with primary sclerosing cholangitis (PSC) pose a clinical dilemma. PSC both is a risk factor for chronic pouchitis[33] and may result in cirrhosis with portal hypertension leading to debilitating peristomal varices in patients with permanent ostomy.[34] The authors' preference is toward IPAA in these patients when no contraindication exists, given the difficulty of managing life-threatening bleeding when peristomal varices develop.

Indeterminate colitis on final pathology has similar pouch-related outcomes to UC[35,36] and, therefore, the authors do not change the surgical approach based on this factor alone.

Operative Approach

Ileal pouch

Open, laparoscopic, hybrid, robotic, and even transanal (*transanal* total mesorectal excision) approaches to IPAA have been utilized and shown to be safe. IPAA is typically performed in stages:

- Three-stage procedure: (1) total colectomy with end ileostomy and rectal stump, (2) proctectomy with IPAA and loop ileostomy, and (3) ileostomy takedown
- Two-stage procedure: (1) total proctocolectomy with IPAA and loop ileostomy and (2) ileostomy takedown
- One-stage procedure: total proctocolectomy with IPAA and no diversion

The authors tend to perform the 3-stage procedure in all patients who are hospitalized for refractory disease as well as outpatients who may be on biologicals or steroids. When a diagnosis is uncertain, this approach also allows additional pathologic information before committing to a pouch. It also may be used as a bridge to optimize patients for an eventual IPAA if, for example, weight loss is required. A 3-stage approach also is used for young women wishing to preserve fertility. The authors defer this decision to patients, however, because many would like to minimize their time with an ostomy and have resources available to help with pregnancy after IPAA.

For well patients with dysplasia or malignancy, the authors typically perform a 2-stage procedure. The authors do not favor constructing the IPAA without fecal diversion, given the long-term effects of pelvic sepsis on pouch function. In patients where a diverting loop ileostomy cannot be constructed without undue tension on the IPAA, the authors may omit diversion if all conditions are favorable.

One of the most challenging aspects of IPAA surgery is obtaining adequate length to perform a tension-free anastomosis. If obesity is a contributing factor, then staging the procedure and encouraging a weight loss program before pouch reconstruction are helpful. The following are intraoperative techniques to obtain maximal bowel length, in sequential order:

- Complete mobilization of the small bowel to the root of the mesentery
- Transverse incisions on the visceral peritoneum of the mesentery
- Careful division of select vascular arcades in the small bowel mesentery (**Fig. 13**)

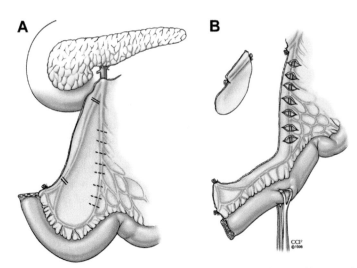

Fig. 13. Mesenteric lengthening procedures. (*A*) mesenteric slits enable stretch that can achieve some additional length and (*B*) division of branches of the superior mesenteric artery allow additional length with care not to devascularize the conduit. (Reprinted with permission, Cleveland Clinic Center for Medical Art & Photography © 1998–2019. All Rights Reserved.)

- Alternate pouch configurations, such as the S pouch, W pouch, and H pouch (**Fig. 14**)

Most IPAAs performed at the authors' institution are stapled J pouches, because they have been shown to have better pouch-related outcomes compared with hand-sewn S pouches.[33] This technique preserves the anal transition zone, which is important for pouch function.[37] When there is dysplasia of the rectum, then mucosectomy with hand-sewn anastomosis can be considered but does not eliminate the need for pouch surveillance.

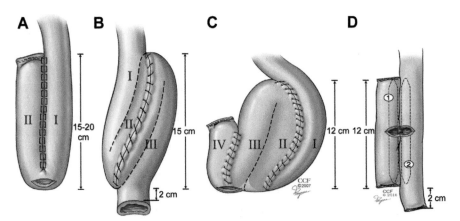

Fig. 14. Variations in ileal pouch configuration. (A) J-pouch (B) S-pouch (C) W-pouch (D) H-pouch. (Reprinted with permission, Cleveland Clinic Center for Medical Art & Photography © 1998–2019. All Rights Reserved.)

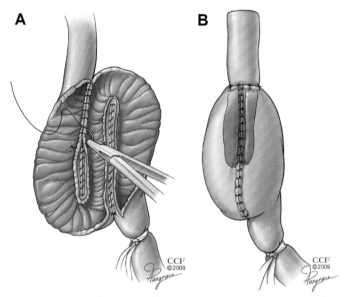

Fig. 15. Continent ileostomy. (*A*) the initial constructions begins in a similar fashion to the S pouch and (*B*) final configuration after creation of the continent valve. (Reprinted with permission, Cleveland Clinic Center for Medical Art & Photography © 1998–2019. All Rights Reserved.)

Continent ileostomy

The continent ileostomy, or Kock pouch (**Fig. 15**), was introduced in the 1960s as an alternative to the standard ileostomy and was later largely replaced by the IPAA. The pouch is constructed in a similar configuration to the S pouch but has modifications that create the continent nipple valve. Approximately 50 cm of small bowel are required to construct the pouch. Continent ileostomies are used when a patient is not a candidate for IPAA but desires to avoid wearing a stoma appliance.

Contraindications to a continent ileostomy include

- Obesity, which precludes passing the conduit through the abdominal wall
- Limitations in dexterity or cognitive impairment, which precludes self-intubation of the pouch
- CD involvement of the small bowel or prior significant small bowel resection
- Inability to access a surgeon who can manage complications of the pouch

Segmental resection

Total abdominal colectomy with ileorectal anastomosis was more commonly offered to patients with UC prior to the use of the IPAA. The procedure is rarely indicated, because there is an approximately 50% risk of future proctectomy,[38] and the risk of metachronous cancer in the rectal stump is 7% to 8%.[38,39]

SUMMARY

Elective surgery remains an important component in the multidisciplinary treatment of patients with IBD. There are numerous surgical approaches that can be considered in both CD and UC. Careful consideration of patient-specific details and shared decision making are necessary to select the appropriate operation. Multidisciplinary discussions are recommended in challenging cases.

REFERENCES

1. Bernell O, Lapidus A, Hellers G. Risk factors for surgery and postoperative recurrence in Crohn's disease. Ann Surg 2000;231(1):38–45.
2. Poritz LS, Koltun WA. Percutaneous drainage and ileocolectomy for spontaneous intraabdominal abscess in Crohn's disease. J Gastrointest Surg 2007;11(2):204–8.
3. Duepree HJ, Senagore AJ, Delaney CP, et al. Advantages of laparoscopic resection for ileocecal Crohn's disease. Dis Colon Rectum 2002;45(5):605–10.
4. Fazio VW, Marchetti F, Church M, et al. Effect of resection margins on the recurrence of Crohn's disease in the small bowel. A randomized controlled trial. Ann Surg 1996;224(4):563–71 [discussion: 571–3].
5. McLeod RS, Wolff BG, Ross S, et al, Investigators of the CAST Trial. Recurrence of Crohn's disease after ileocolic resection is not affected by anastomotic type: results of a multicenter, randomized, controlled trial. Dis Colon Rectum 2009; 52(5):919–27.
6. Gajendran M, Bauer AJ, Buchholz BM, et al. Ileocecal anastomosis type significantly influences long-term functional status, quality of life, and healthcare utilization in postoperative Crohn's disease patients independent of inflammation recurrence. Am J Gastroenterol 2018;113(4):576–83.
7. Kono T, Fichera A, Maeda K, et al. Kono-S anastomosis for surgical prophylaxis of anastomotic recurrence in Crohn's disease: an international multicenter study. J Gastrointest Surg 2016;20(4):783–90.
8. Greenstein AJ, Sachar D, Pucillo A, et al. Cancer in Crohn's disease after diversionary surgery. A report of seven carcinomas occurring in excluded bowel. Am J Surg 1978;135(1):86–90.
9. Bergamaschi R, Haughn C, Reed JF, et al. Laparoscopic intracorporeal ileocolic resection for Crohn's disease: is it safe? Dis Colon Rectum 2009;52(4):651–6.
10. Coffey CJ, Kiernan MG, Sahebally SM, et al. Inclusion of the mesentery in ileocolic resection for Crohn's disease is associated with reduced surgical recurrence. J Crohns Colitis 2018;12(10):1139–50.
11. Lightner AL. Duodenal Crohn's disease. Inflamm Bowel Dis 2018;24(3):546–51.
12. Matsui T, Hatakeyama S, Ikeda K, et al. Long-term outcome of endoscopic balloon dilation in obstructive gastroduodenal Crohn's disease. Endoscopy 1997;29(7):640–5.
13. Worsey MJ, Hull T, Ryland L, et al. Strictureplasty is an effective option in the operative management of duodenal Crohn's disease. Dis Colon Rectum 1999; 42(5):596–600.
14. García-Granero E, Esclápez P, García-Armengol J, et al. Simple technique for the intraoperative detection of Crohn's strictures with a calibration sphere. Dis Colon Rectum 2000;43(8):1168–70.
15. Alexander-Williams J, Haynes IG. Conservative operations for Crohn's disease of the small bowel. World J Surg 1985;9(6):945–51.
16. Dietz DW, Laureti S, Strong SA, et al. Safety and longterm efficacy of strictureplasty in 314 patients with obstructing small bowel Crohn's disease. J Am Coll Surg 2001;192(3):330–7 [discussion: 337–8].

17. Yamamoto T, Fazio VW, Tekkis PP. Safety and efficacy of strictureplasty for Crohn's disease: a systematic review and meta-analysis. Dis Colon Rectum 2007;50(11):1968–86.

18. Roy P, Kumar D. Strictureplasty for active Crohn's disease. Int J Colorectal Dis 2006;21(5):427–32.

19. Tichansky D, Cagir B, Yoo E, et al. Strictureplasty for Crohn's disease: meta-analysis. Dis Colon Rectum 2000;43(7):911–9.

20. Michelassi F. Side-to-side isoperistaltic strictureplasty for multiple Crohn's strictures. Dis Colon Rectum 1996;39(3):345–9.

21. Fazi M, Giudici F, Luceri C, et al. Long-term results and recurrence-related risk factors for Crohn disease in patients undergoing side-to-side isoperistaltic strictureplasty. JAMA Surg 2016;151(5):452–60.

22. Ponsioen CY, de Groof EJ, Eshuis EJ, et al. Laparoscopic ileocaecal resection versus infliximab for terminal ileitis in Crohn's disease: a randomised controlled, open-label, multicentre trial. Lancet Gastroenterol Hepatol 2017;2(11):785–92.

23. Melton GB, Stocchi L, Wick EC, et al. Contemporary surgical management for ileosigmoid fistulas in Crohn's disease. J Gastrointest Surg 2009;13(5):839–45.

24. Farraye FA, Odze RD, Eaden J, et al. AGA medical position statement on the diagnosis and management of colorectal neoplasia in inflammatory bowel disease. Gastroenterology 2010;138(2):738–45.

25. Lightner AL. Segmental resection versus total proctocolectomy for Crohn's Colitis: what is the best operation in the setting of medically refractory disease or dysplasia? Inflamm Bowel Dis 2018;24(3):532–8.

26. de Buck van Overstraeten A, Wolthuis AM, Vermeire S, et al. Intersphincteric proctectomy with end-colostomy for anorectal Crohn's disease results in early and severe proximal colonic recurrence. J Crohns Colitis 2013;7(6):e227–31.

27. Sauk J, Nguyen D, Yajnik V, et al. Natural history of perianal Crohn's disease after fecal diversion. Inflamm Bowel Dis 2014;20(12):2260–5.

28. Gu J, Valente MA, Remzi FH, et al. Factors affecting the fate of faecal diversion in patients with perianal Crohn's disease. Colorectal Dis 2015;17(1):66–72.

29. Le Q, Melmed G, Dubinsky M, et al. Surgical outcome of ileal pouch-anal anastomosis when used intentionally for well-defined Crohn's disease. Inflamm Bowel Dis 2013;19(1):30–6.

30. Li Y, Stocchi L, Liu X, et al. Presence of granulomas in mesenteric lymph nodes is associated with postoperative recurrence in Crohn's disease. Inflamm Bowel Dis 2015;21(11):2613–8.

31. Targownik LE, Singh H, Nugent Z, et al. The epidemiology of colectomy in ulcerative colitis: results from a population-based cohort. Am J Gastroenterol 2012; 107(8):1228–35.

32. Murphy PB, Khot Z, Vogt KN, et al. Quality of life after total proctocolectomy with ileostomy or IPAA: a systematic review. Dis Colon Rectum 2015;58(9):899–908.

33. Penna C, Dozois R, Tremaine W, et al. Pouchitis after ileal pouch-anal anastomosis for ulcerative colitis occurs with increased frequency in patients with associated primary sclerosing cholangitis. Gut 1996;38(2):234–9.

34. Khan F, Vessal S, Gordon-Williams R. Bleeding from peristomal varices: a complication of portal hypertension. BMJ Case Rep 2011;2011 [pii:bcr0820114598].

35. Manilich E, Remzi FH, Fazio VW, et al. Prognostic modeling of preoperative risk factors of pouch failure. Dis Colon Rectum 2012;55(4):393–9.

36. Jackson KL, Stocchi L, Duraes L, et al. Long-term outcomes in indeterminate colitis patients undergoing ileal pouch-anal anastomosis: function, quality of life, and complications. J Gastrointest Surg 2017;21(1):56–61.

37. Silvestri MT, Hurst RD, Rubin MA, et al. Chronic inflammatory changes in the anal transition zone after stapled ileal pouch-anal anastomosis: is mucosectomy a superior alternative? Surgery 2008;144(4):533–7 [discussion: 537–9].

38. da Luz Moreira A, Kiran RP, Lavery I. Clinical outcomes of ileorectal anastomosis for ulcerative colitis. Br J Surg 2010;97(1):65–9.

39. Uzzan M, Kirchgesner J, Oubaya N, et al. Risk of rectal neoplasia after colectomy and ileorectal anastomosis for ulcerative colitis. J Crohns Colitis 2017;11(8): 930–5.

Abdominal Emergencies in Inflammatory Bowel Disease

Robert N. Goldstone, MD[a], Randolph M. Steinhagen, MD[b],*

KEYWORDS

- Ulcerative colitis • Crohn's disease • Toxic colitis • Perforation • Abscess
- Stricture • Bowel obstruction • Hemorrhage

KEY POINTS

- Toxic colitis requires multidisciplinary management with early resuscitation, consideration of rescue therapy, and, if failure to improve, emergent total abdominal colectomy with end ileostomy.
- Intra-abdominal abscess formation is best managed with percutaneous drainage and antibiotic administration followed by elective resection when indicated.
- Intestinal obstruction from fibrostenotic Crohn's disease requires a multidisciplinary approach to guide treatment with medical therapy, endoscopic therapy, or surgery.
- Severe hemorrhage is rare in inflammatory bowel disease and requires emergent resuscitation, localization, and resection of the diseased segment.

INTRODUCTION

Ulcerative colitis (UC) and Crohn's disease (CD) are chronic inflammatory conditions of the gastrointestinal tract with both distinct and overlapping features that have a negative impact on quality of life.[1,2] Population studies have demonstrated that the prevalence of inflammatory bowel disease (IBD) in Western countries is approximately 0.5% of the population.[3,4] Because of this great disease burden, there has been a large focus on improvement of medical management. Despite this, the rates of operative intervention remain high, with 47% of patients with CD and 16% of patients with UC requiring resection within 10 years of diagnosis.[4,5] Rates of emergency surgery have remained unchanged or somewhat decreased.[6,7]

Given the broad spectrum of emergent presentations in IBD, a multidisciplinary team, including surgeons, gastroenterologists, radiologists, nutritional support services, and enterostomal therapists, is required for optimal patient care and decision

Disclosure Statement: The authors have nothing to disclose.
[a] Section of Colon and Rectal Surgery, Department of Surgery, Massachusetts General Hospital, 15 Parkman Street, WAC 4-460, Boston, MA 02114, USA; [b] Division of Colon and Rectal Surgery, Department of Surgery, Icahn School of Medicine at Mount Sinai, Box 1259, One Gustave L. Levy Place, New York, NY 10029, USA
* Corresponding author.
E-mail address: randolph.steinhagen@mountsinai.org

Surg Clin N Am 99 (2019) 1141–1150
https://doi.org/10.1016/j.suc.2019.08.007
surgical.theclinics.com

making.[8] Management of each emergency should be individualized based on patient age, disease type and duration, and patient goals of care.

TOXIC COLITIS

Toxic colitis, or fulminant colitis, is a potentially life-threatening condition that may occur in both UC or CD. The observed incidence of toxic colitis is approximately 10% in all patients with UC and studies have demonstrated that as many as 50% of all toxic colitis cases may be secondary to Crohn's colitis.[9–12] Despite differences in the underlying etiology of the disease, the work-up and management of the patient with toxic colitis in each disease process is the same.

Patients with toxic colitis present to the hospital with symptoms similar to a disease flare, including frequent bloody diarrhea, fever, and tachycardia. The most commonly used diagnostic criteria, as defined by Truelove and Witts,[13] include severe diarrhea (6 or more bloody bowel movements per day), temperature greater than 37.8°C, heart rate greater than 90 beats per minute, anemia (hemoglobin <10.5 g/dL), and an elevated erythrocyte sedimentation rate (<30 mm/h). Toxic megacolon, a rare and morbid variant of toxic colitis, includes these criteria together with radiographic imaging demonstrating dilation of the colon to at least 6 cm.

Any patient who presents with signs and symptoms concerning for toxic colitis should be admitted to the hospital for close monitoring and intensive medical therapy. On presentation, the patient should receive large-bore intravenous catheter placement to initiate sufficient fluid resuscitation in the setting of hypovolemia. All patients should undergo serial laboratory testing, including complete blood cell counts to assess for anemia and leukocytosis, and basic metabolic panels to assess for acute kidney injury and serum electrolyte imbalances, especially hypokalemia and hypomagnesemia, both of which may contribute toward colonic dilation and toxic megacolon.[14] Additional laboratory studies include liver function tests and serum albumin and prealbumin for nutritional assessment. An abdominal radiograph should be obtained to assess degree of small bowel or large bowel dilation and for the presence of free air.

Hepatitis B serology and tuberculin skin test or the interferon-gamma release assays also should be performed on admission to rule out latent TB in preparation for possible rescue therapy with biologic agents.[15] After initial emergent assessment, a multidisciplinary team composed of gastroenterologists, colorectal surgeons, nutritional support dieticians, and enterostomal therapists should coordinate goal-directed therapy.

Infectious colitis with organisms, such as Clostridium difficile and cytomegalovirus (CMV), must be excluded for all patients on admission b both of these entities have been identified to exacerbate the degree of colitis in IBD. Stool samples are cultured for Salmonella, Yersinia, and Shigella. C difficile infection may be tested by obtaining stool analysis for C difficile toxin, and, if positive, should be treated appropriately with oral vancomycin and possibly intravenous metronidazole therapy. Studies have demonstrated that C difficile infection in the setting of severe or toxic colitis is associated with increased morbidity and mortality.[14,16] CMV colitis, on the other hand, is definitively diagnosed by histology of ulcers biopsied during flexible sigmoidoscopy. Careful sigmoidoscopy with minimal insufflation is indicated within 24 hours of admission, but full colonoscopy should be avoided due to increased risk of bowel perforation. Treatment of CMV colitis requires IV ganciclovir followed by oral valganciclovir. Importantly, CMV infection has been identified in 25% to 36% of patients with steroid-refractory acute colitis.[17]

If any of these infections is present, antibiotic therapy or antiviral therapy, as previously discussed, is indicated. Empiric antibiotic coverage in the absence of demonstrated infection, however, has been investigated in several randomized controlled trials with agents, such as ciprofloxacin, metronidazole, and tobramycin, and has not been shown to increase rates of remission of toxic colitis or to avoid colectomy.[16,18–20]

Other important measures for optimal care in this acute setting include discontinuation and avoidance of opioids, anticholinergic agents, antidiarrheal agents, and nonsteroidal anti-inflammatory drugs, all of which may mask disease progression or exacerbate colonic dilation through impaired motility.[14,16] These patients also possess a 3-times to 6-times greater risk of venous thromboembolism than the general population and, thus, should be administered prophylactic subcutaneous low-molecular-weight heparin.[14,16]

Nutritional support for these patients is of great importance in their care. For all patients without concern for toxic megacolon or ileus, enteral nutrition should be provided and is preferred over parenteral nutrition. One prior study demonstrated that enteral nutrition is associated with fewer complications than parenteral nutrition (9% vs 35%, respectively).[21]

On diagnosis of toxic colitis, intensive medical therapy should be initiated, including serial abdominal examinations, laboratory studies, and abdominal radiograph. If a patient develops peritonitis on examination or evidence of free perforation on imaging, emergent exploration is warranted. In all other cases, however, medical management with steroids should be initiated. Intravenous methylprednisolone, 60 mg per day, in divided doses or hydrocortisone, 300 mg in divided doses, is the medication of choice.[22] Treatment with higher doses of intravenous corticosteroids have not been demonstrated to reduce colectomy rate and, thus, should not be considered.[23] If a patient responds to treatment with corticosteroids over the course of the next 3 days to 5 days, initiation of maintenance therapy and a steroid taper may be conducted. On the other hand, if a patient fails to improve with corticosteroid therapy, then care must transition to either rescue therapy or urgent colectomy.

Cyclosporine, a calcineurin inhibitor, was the first agent utilized for steroid refractory colitis. This medication was accepted among practitioners after a small randomized, double-blind, controlled trial where 9 of 11 patients who failed to improve after 7 days of corticosteroid treatment responded to cyclosporine therapy compared with 0 of 9 patients who received placebo[24]; 4 of the 9 placebo group patients underwent urgent colectomy and the remaining 5 patients received cyclosporine and improved. Since this initial study, there have been numerous observation and retrospective studies, along with a few randomized controlled trials, which evaluated immediate response, short-term response, and long-term response rates to cyclosporine therapy. Although the immediate response rates are encouraging, ranging from 64% to 82%, long-term response rates were significantly lower, ranging between 42% and 50%, with colectomy rates as high as 58%.[14,25] Some improvement in long-term remission has been observed in patients who were initiated on azathioprine and aminosalicylate maintenance therapy. For those who respond to this therapy, the response is generally rapid and occurs within the first 4 days. This medication should be stopped if no improvement is observed within 7 days.

Cyclosporine is associated with significant minor and major adverse effects, including hypertension, nephrotoxicity, opportunistic infections, neurotoxicity, and seizure. This extensive side-effect profile, along with the poor long-term response rate, has significantly limited the usage of this medication. Instead, infliximab has now emerged as the most widely used rescue therapy. One recent literature review demonstrated immediate response rates to infliximab as a rescue therapy agent range between 50% and 83%, with long-term response rates slightly lower at 50% to

63%.[14,25] These results are similar to those seen with cyclosporine therapy. Indeed, 2 randomized controlled trials (the Cyclosporine versus Infliximab and Comparison of Infliximab and Ciclosporin in Steroid Resistant Ulcerative Colitis trials) have been completed, both showing no difference in colectomy-free survival and similar rates of adverse events.[14,26–28] Despite the similarity in efficacy, infliximab remains the preferred agent due to its reduced toxicity, ease of administration, and ability to be continued for maintenance therapy.

Patients who clinically deteriorate within 24 hours to 72 hours of initiation of medical therapy or those who fail to respond to the previously discussed pharmacologic agents require emergent surgery. Surgical delay has been associated with increased postoperative morbidity.[29] Additionally, in patients who have developed a bowel perforation secondary to progression of disease, postoperative mortality rates increase from 2% to 8% up to 40%.[30,31] The surgical option of choice is total abdominal (subtotal) colectomy with creation of end ileostomy with or without mucous fistula. There is no role for segmental colectomy in the treatment of toxic colitis.

A total proctocolectomy should be avoided at this time because it is associated with greater postoperative morbidity and mortality due to increased operative time, risk of blood loss, pelvic sepsis, pelvic nerve damage, and small bowel obstruction.[8,10] Moreover, a subtotal colectomy allows for future reconstructive options with either an ileorectal anastomosis for patients with CD without rectal or perianal involvement or elective completion proctectomy with ileal pouch anal anastomosis for those with UC. Finally, for patients without a definitive diagnosis of either UC or CD, a subtotal colectomy may assist with establishing the correct diagnosis by pathologic examination of the resected colon and thus guide future interventions. The only rare time in which an emergent proctectomy may be necessary is if there is acute perforation of the rectum or exsanguinating hemorrhage. An algorithm for the management of toxic colitis for patients with inflammatory bowel disease is demonstrated in **Fig. 1**.

PERFORATION AND ABSCESS

Free perforation is a rare complication of both UC and CD, accounting for approximately 2% and 1% to 3% of cases, respectively.[8,32,33] Rates of perforation requiring

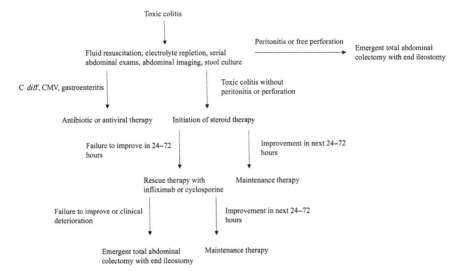

Fig. 1. Treatment algorithm for IBD patient with toxic colitis.

emergency colectomy that were previously reported are likely overestimates of the current situation due to improved IBD medical management. In patients with UC, perforation typically occurs in the setting of toxic megacolon but also may occur secondary to iatrogenic injury during surveillance colonoscopy.[8] Diagnosis of perforation in this setting may be delayed if the patient is on high-dose steroids or other immunosuppressants. In these settings, the appropriate management involves urgent resuscitation, administration of broad-spectrum antibiotics, and emergent surgical intervention. The procedure of choice for management of colonic perforation in UC remains a subtotal colectomy with creation of end ileostomy. This allows for a more rapid operation with less morbidity and mortality than a total proctocolectomy and preserves the option of future restorative intervention.

Although perforation in patients with UC is restricted to the colon and rectum, perforation in CD may occur throughout the gastrointestinal tract.[8] The location of bowel perforation in CD as well as management depends on the etiology and area of bowel affected by the disease. Small bowel perforation often occurs in the setting of a complete bowel obstruction from an inflammatory stricture. In this instance, the site of perforation usually is immediately proximal to the small bowel stricture and may be treated with emergent small bowel or ileocolic resection with primary anastomosis. Proximal diversion should be considered if patients are in critical condition, have large associated abscesses or fistulas, have had numerous prior resections, or are malnourished.[34–36] If the perforation occurs secondary to a colonic stricture causing large bowel obstruction, the site of perforation is typically the cecum. In this case, the operation of choice would be a subtotal colectomy, including removal of the segment with the stricture, with end ileostomy, with or without creation of a mucus fistula. For patients with focal diseased segments of Crohn's colitis with perforation at the site of the disease, consideration may be made for performing a segmental resection with primary anastomosis with or without proximal diversion versus Hartmann procedure. Segmental resection, however, is associated with earlier disease recurrence.[37]

Abscesses remain a far more common indication for surgery in CD than free perforation, accounting for 7% to 25% of operations performed.[38] CD is characterized by transmural inflammation of the bowel, which in turn may lead to focal microperforation and subsequent abscess formation. The most common location for abscesses to form is the right lower quadrant of the abdomen adjacent to the terminal ileum and cecum. These abscesses may be intraperitoneal, extraperitoneal, or intramesenteric. Diagnosis is typically made with either computed tomography (CT) or magnetic resonance imaging (MRI).

On initial presentation and diagnosis, patients should be administered intravenous antibiotics for coverage of all enteric gram-negative bacteria and anaerobes. If an abscess is well defined and less than 3 cm in diameter, medical therapy alone with antibiotics may prove successful. For larger, well-defined abscesses, percutaneous drainage should be performed and clinical improvement should be observed within 3 days to 5 days. If the patient fails to improve or drain output is minimal, repeat imaging should be performed to rule out malposition of the drain, fistulous communication with the bowel, or progression of disease with new abscess formation.

Percutaneous drainage resolves the acute infection in more than 90% of cases.[38–40] After that, 20% to 77% of patients go on to require elective bowel resection.[39–41] The decision to proceed with elective surgery is individualized based on disease location and presence or absence of appropriate medical therapy. Patients naïve to biologic therapy often can be initiated on medical therapy, such as infliximab, which may allow fistula closure and avoid surgery. An algorithm for the management of intra-abdominal abscesses in patients with IBD is depicted in **Fig. 2**.

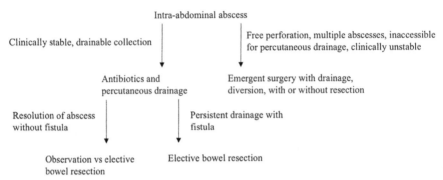

Fig. 2. Treatment algorithm for IBD patient with intra-abdominal abscess.

OBSTRUCTION

Although intestinal obstruction may occur in patients with UC, it is far more common in patients with CD and accounts for approximately 20% to 25% of operative interventions.[38,40] Obstruction in CD typically occurs intermittently over time secondary to acute inflammation during flares in regions of bowel fibrosis due to scarring from the chronic transmural disease process.[8] Diagnosis and determination of the etiology of obstruction typically are made with CT imaging. MRI may help in differentiating between a fibrotic stricture, inflammatory stricture, or mixed inflammatory and fibrotic stricture. The most common location for bowel obstruction in CD is the terminal ileum, although obstruction also may occur in the colon or rectum, with an incidence as low as 5% of cases.[42]

If the obstruction is thought to be secondary to an inflammatory stricture, patients typically improve with medical management with steroid therapy or initiation/alteration of biologic therapy. Approximately 75% of patients diagnosed with an intestinal stricture from CD go on to require either endoscopic dilation or surgical resection.[43]

The 2 primary procedures for the surgical management of small bowel obstruction in CD are bowel resection and strictureplasty. Typically, bowel resection with primary anastomosis is performed in the elective setting for inflammatory, fibrotic, or mixed strictures when limited bowel is involved. Strictureplasty, on the other hand, remains an option for patients with extensive fibrostenosing disease for which bowel resection is deemed inappropriate due to risk of short bowel syndrome. This procedure has been demonstrated to be durable and effective in long-term studies.[44] When performing a strictureplasty, it is important to obtain biopsy of the stricture to rule out an underlying malignancy.

Endoscopic approaches, including balloon dilation or stricturotomy, have also proved successful in management of primary intestinal strictures or anastomotic strictures in CD. For fibrotic strictures, endoscopic balloon dilation has a technical success rate of 89% to 92%, with 70% to 81% patients experiencing short-term relief of symptoms.[45,46] Long-term results are less impressive, with 73.5% of patients requiring a repeat dilation and 43% requiring surgical intervention within 2 years.[45] Endoscopic stricturotomy is an evolving, novel therapy for which only few short-term retrospective studies exist demonstrating its safety and efficacy compared with endoscopic balloon dilation or ileocolic resection.[47]

Large bowel strictures, especially in UC, should raise high concern for malignancy.[48] When forced to perform an emergent colectomy, oncologic principles should be followed. An algorithm for the management of large and small bowel obstruction for patients with IBD is demonstrated in **Fig. 3.**

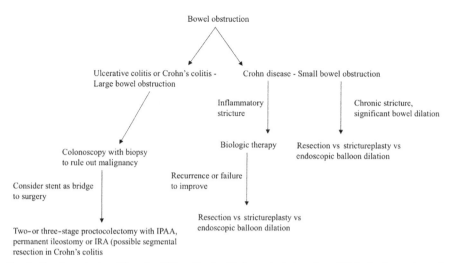

Fig. 3. Treatment algorithm for IBD patient with bowel obstruction. IPAA, ileal pouch anal anastomosis; IRA, ileorectal anastomosis.

BLEEDING

Severe intestinal hemorrhage is a rare occurrence in IBD, with reported incidence between 0% and 6%.[8] The underlying pathophysiology of the hemorrhage differs between UC and CD. In UC, the bleeding typically occurs in patients with pancolitis from diffuse areas of mucosal ulceration. In CD, however, the bleeding most often is a result of focal erosion into an intestinal vessel.[8]

Because of the low incidence of severe hemorrhage in IBD, a limited number of studies are available to guide management. The initial approach is similar to any patient with severe bleeding and includes large-bore intravenous access and aggressive resuscitation. A nasogastric tube should be inserted with gastric lavage to investigate for an upper gastrointestinal bleed, with 1 study reporting approximately 30% of patients with CD presenting with severe hemorrhage having a bleeding duodenal ulcer.[49] Surgery is indicated for patients who demonstrate continued hemorrhage despite resuscitation with 6+ units of packed red blood cells or have other indications for resection of diseased bowel.

In UC, the operation of choice is a total abdominal colectomy with creation of end ileostomy. A total proctocolectomy is contraindicated due to the emergent nature of the surgery, critical condition of the patient, and, thus, increased postoperative morbidity and mortality. After this operation, rectal bleeding may persist with rates of up to 12% but can be managed with nonoperative interventions, such as packing of the retained rectum or the administration of mixed saline-epinephrine enemas.[8,50,51]

For patients with CD, identification of the bleeding location is far more important than for UC because it may occur anywhere throughout the gastrointestinal tract. Endoscopy should be performed if blood is detected within bilious fluid aspirated with the nasogastric tube. Colonoscopy should also be performed if the patient is stable enough to tolerate this examination. Other studies that may aid in localization of the bleed are CT angiography or selective angiography, with reported identification rates of 40% to 45%.[49,52] Other proposed methods of localization include injection of isosulfan blue or methylene blue through an angiocatheter with provocative angiography in the operating room.[53,54] If the bleeding is identified in the small intestine, operative intervention with resection of the involved segment of intestine and primary anastomosis may be completed. If the bleeding occurs in the setting of Crohn's colitis, consideration should be made for performing a total abdominal colectomy with end ileostomy. A total abdominal colectomy with ileorectal anastomosis may be considered if the rectum is disease-free and the patient remains hemodynamically stable.

SUMMARY

Emergent surgery in IBD may be required as a result of a variety of conditions, including toxic colitis, perforation, abscess formation, bowel obstruction, or severe gastrointestinal hemorrhage. Each of these presentations requires multidisciplinary team management with ideal resuscitative approaches. Optimal care significantly reduces patient morbidity and mortality and improves patient outcomes.

REFERENCES

1. Ordas I, Eckmann L, Talamini M, et al. Ulcerative colitis. Lancet 2012;380: 1606–19.
2. Baumgart DC, Sandborn WJ. Crohn's disease. Lancet 2012;380:1590–605.
3. Molodecky NA, Soon IS, Rabi DM, et al. Increasing incidence and prevalence of the inflammatory bowel disease with time, based on systematic review. Gastroenterology 2012;142:46–54.e42.
4. Frolkis AD, Dykeman J, Negron ME, et al. Risk of surgery for inflammatory bowel diseases has decreased over time: a systematic review and Meta-analysis of population-based studies. Gastroenterology 2013;145:996–1006.
5. Justiniano CF, Aquina CT, Becerra AZ, et al. Postoperative mortality after nonelective surgery for inflammatory bowel disease patients in the era of biologics. Ann Surg 2019;269(4):686–91.
6. Ma C, Moran GW, Benchimol EI, et al. Surgical rates for Crohn's disease are decreasing: a population-based time trend analysis and validation study. Am J Gastroenterol 2017;112(12):1840–8.
7. Kaplan GG, Seow CH, Ghosh S, et al. Decreasing colectomy rates for ulcerative colitis: a population-based time trend study. Am J Gastroenterol 2012;107(12):1879–87.
8. Berg DF, Bahadursingh AM, Kaminski DL, et al. Acute surgical emergencies in inflammatory bowel disease. Am J Surg 2002;184(1):45–51.
9. Marion JF, Present DH. The modern medical management of acute. Severe ulcerative colitis. Eur J Gastroenterol Hepatol 1998;9:831–5.
10. Fazio VW. Toxic megacolon in ulcerative colitis and Crohn's colitis. In: Farmer RG, editor. Clinics in gastroenterology. Philadelphia: WB Saunders; 1980. p. 389–407.
11. Farmer RG, Easley KA, Rankin GBZ. Clinical patterns, natural history, and progression of ulcerative colitis. A long-term follow-up of 1116 patients. Dig Dis Sci 1993;38:1137–46.
12. Cima RR. Timing and indications for colectomy in chronic ulcerative colitis: surgical consideration. Dig Dis 2010;28:501–7.
13. Truelove SC, Witts LJ. Cortisone in ulcerative colitis; final report on a therapeutic trial. Br Med J 1955;2(4947):1041–8.
14. Gisbert JP, Chaparro M. Acute severe ulcerative colitis: state of the art treatment. Best Pract Res Clin Gastroenterol 2018;32-33:56–69.
15. Singh JA, Wells GA, Christensen R, et al. Adverse effects of biologics: a network meta-analysis and Cochrane overview. Cochrane Database Syst Rev 2011;(2):CD008794.

16. Harbord M, Eliakim R, Bettenworth D, et al. Third European evidence-based consensus on diagnosis and management of ulcerative colitis. Part 2: current management. J Crohns Colitis 2017;11(7):769–84.
17. Lawlor G, Moss AC. Cytomegalovirus in inflammatory bowel disease: pathogen or innocent bystander? Inflamm Bowel Dis 2010;16(9):1620–7.
18. Chapman RW, Selby WS, Jewell DP. Controlled trial of intravenous metronidazole as an adjunct to corticosteroids in severe ulcerative colitis. Gut 1986;27:1210–2.
19. Mantzaris GJ, Hatzis A, Kontogiannis P, et al. Intravenous tobramycin and metronidazole as an adjunct to corticosteroids in acute, severe ulcerative colitis. Am J Gastroenterol 1994;89:43–6.
20. Mantzaris GJ, Petraki K, Archavlis E, et al. A prospective randomized controlled trial of intravenous ciprofloxacin as an adjunct to corticosteroids in acute, severe ulcerative colitis. Scand J Gastroenterol 2001;36:971–4.
21. Gonzalez-Huix F, Fernandez-Banares F, Esteve-Comas M, et al. Enteral versus parenteral nutrition as adjunct therapy in acute ulcerative colitis. Am J Gastroenterol 1993;88:227–32.
22. Kornbluth A, Sachar DB, Practice parameters committee of the American College of Gastroenterology. Ulcerative colitis practice guidelines in adults: American College of Gastroenterology, Practice Parameters Committee. Am J Gastroenterol 2010;105(3):501–23.
23. Turner D, Walsh CM, Steinhart AH, et al. Response to corticosteroids in severe ulcerative colitis: a systematic review of the literature and a meta-regression. Clin Gastroenterol Hepatol 2007;5:103–10.
24. Lichtiger S, Present DH, Kornbluth A, et al. Cyclosporine in severe ulcerative colitis refractory to steroid therapy. N Engl J Med 1994;330(26):1841–5.
25. Seah D, De Cruz P. Review article: the practical management of acute severe ulcerative colitis. Aliment Pharmacol Ther 2016;43:482–513.
26. Laharie D, Bourreille A, Branche J, et al. Ciclosporin versus infliximab in patients with severe ulcerative colitis refractory to intravenous steroids: a parallel, open-label randomized controlled trial. Lancet 2012;380:1909–15.
27. Laharie D, Bourreille A, Branche J, et al. Long-term outcome of patients with steroid-refractory acute severe UC treated with ciclosporin or infliximab. Gut 2018;67:237–43.
28. Williams JG, Alam MF, Alrubaiy L, et al. Infliximab versus ciclosporin for steroid-resistant acute severe ulcerative colitis (CONSTRUCT): a mixed methods, open-label, pragmatic randomised trial. Lancet Gastroenterol Hepatol 2016;1:15–24.
29. Bartels SA, Gardenbroek TJ, Bos L, et al. Prolonged hospital stay is a risk factor for complications after emergency colectomy for severe colitis. Colorectal Dis 2013;15(11):1392–8.
30. Sheth SG, LaMont JT. Toxic megacolon. Lancet 1998;351(9101):509–13.
31. Heppell J, Farkouh E, Dube S, et al. Toxic megacolon an analysis of 70 cases. Dis Colon Rectum 1986;29(12):789–92.
32. Keighley MRB. Acute fulminating colitis and emergency colectomy. In: Keighley MRB, Williams NS, editors. Surgery of the anus, rectum and colon. London: WB Saunders; 1993. p. 1379–97.
33. Bundred NJ, Dixon JM, Lumsden AB, et al. Free perforation in Crohn's colitis: a ten year review. Dis Colon Rectum 1985;28:35–7.
34. Johnston WF, Stafford C, Francone T, et al. What is the risk of anastomotic leak after repeat intestinal resection in patients with Crohn's disease? Dis Colon Rectum 2017;60(12):1299–306.

35. Yamamoto T, Allan RN, Keighley MR. Risk factors for intra-abdominal sepsis after surgery in Crohn's disease. Dis Colon Rectum 2000;43:1141–5.
36. Crowell KT, Messaris E. Risk factors and implications of anastomotic complications after surgery for Crohn's disease. World J Gastrointest Surg 2015;7:237–42.
37. Bemelman WA, Warusavitarne J, Sampeitro GM, et al. ECCO-ESCP consensus on surgery for Crohn's disease. J Crohns Colitis 2018;12(1):1–16.
38. Muldoon R, Herline AJ. Crohn's disease: surgical management. In: Steele SR, Hull TL, Read TE, et al, editors. The ASCRS textbook of colon and rectal surgery. 3rd edition. New York: Springer International Publishing; 2016. p. 843–68.
39. de Groof EJ, Carbonnel F, Buskens CJ, et al. Abdominal abscess in Crohn's disease: multidisciplinary management. Dig Dis 2014;32(Suppl 1):103–9.
40. Alos R, Hinojosa J. Timing of surgery in Crohn's disease: a key issue in the management. World J Gastroenterol 2008;14(36):5532–9.
41. Gervais DA, Hahn PF, O'Neill MJ, et al. Percutaneous abscess drainage in Crohn disease: technical success and short- and long-term outcomes during 14 years. Radiology 2002;222(3):645–51.
42. Yamazaki Y, Ribeiro MB, Sachar DB, et al. Malignant strictures in Crohn's disease. Am J Gastroenterol 1991;86:882–5.
43. Bessissow T, Reinglas J, Aruljothy A, et al. Endoscopic management of Crohn's strictures. World J Gastroenterol 2018;24(17):1859–67.
44. Michelassi F, Mege D, Rubin M, et al. Long-term results of the side-to-side isoperistaltic strictureplasty in Crohn disease: 25-year follow-up and outcomes. Ann Surg 2019. [Epub ahead of print].
45. Bettenworth D, Gustavsson A, Atreja A, et al. A pooled analysis of efficacy, safety, and long-term outcome of endoscopic balloon dilation therapy for patient with stricturing Crohn's disease. Inflamm Bowel Dis 2017;23:133–42.
46. Morar PS, Faiz O, Warusavitarne J, et al. Systematic review with meta-analysis: endoscopic balloon dilation for Crohn's disease strictures. Aliment Pharmacol Ther 2015;42:1137–48.
47. Lan N, Shen B. Endoscopic stricturotomy versus balloon dilation in the treatment of anastomotic strictures in Crohn's disease. Inflamm Bowel Dis 2018;24(4):897–907.
48. Gumaste V, Sachar DB, Greenstein AJ. Benign and malignant colorectal strictures in ulcerative colitis. Gut 1992;33(7):938–41.
49. Robert JR, Sachar DB, Greenstein AJ. Severe gastrointestinal hemorrhage in Crohn's disease. Ann Surg 1991;213(3):207–11.
50. Pare R, Roger V, Penna C. Management of hemorrhage. In: Michelassi F, Milsom JW, editors. Operative strategies in inflammatory bowel disease. New York: Springer-Verlag; 1999. p. 229–33.
51. Robert JH, Sachar DB, Aufses AH, et al. Management of severe hemorrhage in ulcerative colitis. Am J Surg 1990;159:550–5.
52. Cirocco WC, Reilly JC, Rusin LC. Life-threatening hemorrhage and exsanguination from Crohn's disease. Report of four cases. Dis Colon Rectum 1995;38(1):85–95.
53. Leowardi C, Heuschen G, Kienle P, et al. Surgical treatment of severe inflammatory bowel diseases. Dig Dis 2003;21(1):54–62.
54. Remzi FH, Dietz DW, Unal E, et al. Combined use of preoperative provocative angiography and highly selective methylene blue injection to localize an occult small-bowel bleeding site in a patient with Crohn's disease: report of a case. Dis Colon Rectum 2003;46(2):260–3.

Anorectal Crohn's Disease

Adam Truong, MD, Karen Zaghiyan, MD, Phillip Fleshner, MD*

KEYWORDS

- Anorectal • Anal • Crohn disease • IBD • Fistula

KEY POINTS

- The incidence of perianal Crohn's disease is 74% within 10 years of initial diagnosis.
- Medical treatment of anorectal disease is the mainstay, but surgical management is often necessary for severe or recurrent disease.
- Minimally invasive fistula treatments have become increasingly diverse and show promise as an emerging field, particularly the application of mesenchymal stem cells.
- Severe anorectal disease may require fecal diversion to achieve adequate palliation of symptoms. When determining timing of ostomy reversal, cessation of proctitis is the most important factor to consider.

INTRODUCTION

Inflammatory bowel disease (IBD) affects approximately 1 to 1.3 million people in the United States and is divided into 2 distinct pathologies, ulcerative colitis (UC) and Crohn's disease (CD).[1,2] Although prevalence of UC and CD are similar (201 per 100,000 adults vs 238 per 100,000 adults, respectively), their clinical progression differs dramatically. Patients with UC typically have mild to moderate disease isolated to their lower gastrointestinal (GI) tract at time of diagnosis, and overall treatment is largely medical, including steroids and biological immunomodulators, with only a subset (20%–30%) requiring surgical therapy.[3] In contrast, patients with CD experience progressive disease throughout their entire GI tract, with one meta-analysis quoting 50% of patients with CD ultimately requiring surgical therapy[4] and 18% to 33% requiring surgery within 5 years of diagnosis.[5] Despite the distal to proximal extension of UC, the rate of perianal disease is markedly lower compared with CD. The prevalence of perianal involvement in CD is reportedly 74% within 10 years of initial diagnosis and increases with more distal disease.[6] In 20% to 36% of patients with CD, perianal disease precedes intestinal disease.[6–8] This overview of perianal CD will focus on clinically actionable information for the general and colorectal surgeon.

All authors have no relevant disclosures.
Division of Colorectal Surgery, Cedars-Sinai Medical Center, 8737 Beverly Blvd., Suite 101, Los Angeles, CA 90048, USA
* Corresponding author.
E-mail address: Pfleshner@aol.com

Surg Clin N Am 99 (2019) 1151–1162
https://doi.org/10.1016/j.suc.2019.08.012
surgical.theclinics.com

ANAL DISEASE TYPES
Skin Tags

Skin tags are the most common perianal lesion in CD, present in 40% to 70% of cases, and can vary in appearance and activity.[9,10] Although most often soft, mobile, and asymptomatic, they may become inflamed during a flare. Although skin tags may persist for years, they remain a benign entity and are typically treated only for persistent symptoms.

Hemorrhoids

Symptomatic hemorrhoids are thought to be uncommon in CD with an incidence of approximately 7% compared with the general population (24%).[11] This estimate is likely an understatement owing to symptom crossover with CD itself.[8] Some investigators consider hemorrhoid symptoms independent of Crohn's-related inflammatory pathology, instead caused by chronic diarrhea.[12] Anal skin lesions often resemble and are sometimes mistaken for hemorrhoids. Similarly, treatment is typically recommended for symptom control (mainly bleeding or prolapse) after failure of medical management. Although there is disagreement about the rates and risk of severe complications following hemorrhoidectomy in CD, complications tend to be much higher in those patients whom the diagnosis of IBD had not been established at the time of hemorrhoidectomy, emphasizing the importance of considering IBD in any patient undergoing hemorrhoidectomy.[13]

Fissure

Anal fissures are the second most common reason for outpatient anal evaluation.[14] Whereas noninflammatory fissures may be due to ischemia or sphincter spasm and relieved with lateral sphincterotomy, fissures associated with IBD have no increase in sphincter tone.[15] Although an off-midline fissure is concerning for IBD, anal fissures associated with CD are most commonly posterior with only a small subset off-midline (9%–20%).[16–18] Multiple fissures dramatically increase the likelihood of CD. Fissures are on an ulcer spectrum, considered superficial anal ulceration with the potential to progress to a cavitating ulcer or an abscess. Other causes of anal ulcers include acute immunodeficiency syndrome, infection (eg, Neisseria gonorrhea or chlamydia trachomatis), tuberculosis, carcinoma, or radiation.[19]

Cavitating Ulcer

Cavitating ulcers are large deep irregular defects in the anal canal affecting 5% to 10% of patients with CD.[16] They typically cause severe symptoms with unremitting pain, typically treated with local injection of steroids, which produces durable relief with minimal complications.[20] In the most aggressive cases, ulcers may extend beyond the anal canal to the perineal skin. Location is factored into the Cardiff classification for nonfistulizing perianal CD and is an important consideration in treatment planning.[21] Exclusion of frank sepsis is critical during workup to ensure proper treatment choice.

Abscess/Fistula

Anorectal abscesses and fistulas are penetrating lesions occurring in about 18% of all CD perineal lesions.[22] The cumulative probability of developing perineal fistulas increases with time after CD diagnosis.[23] Perineal fistulas are not specific to CD and other causes include infection, hidradenitis suppurativa, and malignancy. The presence of fistulizing perineal disease is a predictor of poor long-term outcome in patients with CD.[24] The prevalence of fistulas in CD varies according to disease location with fistulas least common in isolated ileal disease (12%) and most common in colonic disease (41%) with a predilection for rectal disease (92%).[25] Among factors that influence fistula healing rates, active proctitis is an independent predictor of both poor healing as well as increased recurrence.[26]

In contrast to the cryptoglandular perianal fistulas that develop following an abscess, the pathophysiology of Crohn's-related fistulas is not well understood although believed to arise secondary to 2 mechanisms: epithelial to mesenchymal transition (EMT) and matrix remodeling enzymes.[27,28] In EMT, differentiated epithelial cells transform into mesenchymal-type cells that gain the ability to penetrate deeper tissues. Matrix metalloproteinases can degrade extracellular matrix components and have been shown to have increased activity in IBD.[29]

The 2 major anatomic classifications of perianal fistulas are the Park's classification[30] and the St. James's University Hospital classification.[31,32] The Park's classification describes anatomic fistula location in relation to sphincter muscles; however, it does not include information of tract complexity or proctitis.[27] In contrast, the St. James's University Hospital classification considers further elements such as fistula complexity, but this index is clinically onerous. The American Gastroenterology Association classification offers a simplified approach by dividing fistulas into 2 categories: simple and complex based on presence of high, multiple, or vaginal openings, abscess presence, or stricture.[33] The authors recommend using the anatomic Park's classification when characterizing fistulas together with other essential information including internal and external opening locations and presence or clinical severity of an associated abscess.

Rectovaginal Fistula

Most rectovaginal fistulas are low and may sometimes be considered anovaginal fistulas. In 85% of cases, the opening is located anteriorly on the rectum or anus.[34] In comparison, high fistulas are less frequent but produce worse symptoms and are most commonly associated with CD. High fistulas involving the sigmoid colon or small bowel are rare and are often a result of CD. Although manual examination will often reveal dimpling indicating a rectovaginal fistula, anoscopic and speculum examination offers size and location of the fistula. If the diagnosis remains elusive, observation of vaginal bubbling during rigid proctoscopy or blue dye passage between organs is a useful adjunct.

Stricture

Anorectal stenosis or stricture occurs when pliable tissues are replaced with scarred fibrotic tissue, occurring in either the anus (34%) or the rectum (50%).[11] Symptoms typically contain functional detriments including defecation difficulty, tenesmus, incontinence, or urgency.[33] In the absence of symptoms, strictures do not require treatment.[35] When strictures are symptomatic, dilation should be done with extreme caution, as these patients are at high risk for subsequent perforation and abscess/fistula.

Carcinoma

Similar to UC, patients with CD are at increased risk of neoplasia. With a 3.7% overall risk of carcinoma for CD, the incidence of carcinoma in isolated perianal CD is 0.7% for both adenocarcinoma as well as squamous carcinoma.[36,37] Human papilloma virus (HPV) vaccination is recommended because vaccination may reduce the incidence of HPV-related lesions.[38] Although a screening program for perianal carcinoma is not recommended given lack of knowledge for optimal frequency or modality, vigilance must be exercised to differentiate clinical symptoms of cancer from fissures or fistulas, which are largely similar. Devon and colleagues[39] reported in their series that all patients with fistula-related cancers had a history of increasing and/or intractable pain.

DISEASE ASSESSMENT

The comprehensive assessment of perianal CD starts with a thorough assessment of the disease history and physical examination; however, consideration of intestinal pathology such as terminal ileitis and infectious etiologies is paramount. The history should include anorectal pain, purulent or bloody discharge, persistent drainage, incontinence or stool changes, urinary symptoms or urinary tract infection, and gynecologic concerns. Although adjunctive imaging may be helpful, the gold standard for evaluation of perianal CD is examination under anesthesia (EUA), allowing both diagnostic and therapeutic opportunities.

Endoanal Ultrasound

Endoanal ultrasound (EUS) is excellent for assessing sphincter structure and integrity. It has also shown increasing utility in fistulizing disease by identifying internal openings and secondary fistula tracts with a concordance between endoanal ultrasound and surgical findings in more than 91% of cases.[40] Injection of hydrogen peroxide enhances detection of internal fistula openings when using ultrasound by improving contrast and conspicuity of the fistula tract.

Pelvic MRI

MRI is considered the gold standard for noninvasive perianal fistula assessment with a sensitivity of 0.87 and specificity of 0.59 for fistula detection.[41,42] In CD specifically, the addition of MRI may alter surgical decision-making in up to 40% of patients with complex fistulizing disease.[43] In their practice, the authors reserve usage of MRI for complex abscess or recurrent fistulas in CD.

Examination Under Anesthesia

In cases of severe disease, clinical examination of the anus may be prohibitive due to pain, necessitating an examination under anesthesia. Complex fistula anatomy may be elucidated through probing with a stylet, often a lacrimal probe, and is aided through adjuncts such as hydrogen peroxide. Hydrogen peroxide will fill a tract and identify internal fistula openings by visible bubbling. Although the gold standard in fistula evaluation, EUA may fail to identify a fistula tract in up to 10% of cases.[44] In these cases, EUS and MRI serve as useful aides where the combination of 2 of these 3 tools are sufficient to achieve higher diagnostic accuracy.[45]

SCORING SYSTEMS

Scoring systems offer objective evaluation of CD activity. The Crohn's Disease Activity Index[46] and the simple Harvey-Bradshaw Activity Index[47] measure intestinal and extraintestinal disease manifestations, but they lack specific criteria for perianal pathology, and so they are not suitable for fistula surveillance activity.[48,49] Perhaps the most widely used assessment tool is the Perianal Disease Activity Index (PDAI), which quantifies 5 fistula-specific categories: discharge, pain, restriction of sexual activity, disease type, and degree of inflammation; each category is graded on a 5-point Likert scale from no symptoms (score of 0) to severe symptoms (score of 4) (**Table 1**).[50] Critics point out that this scale has not been validated in a randomized clinical trial,

Table 1 Perianal Crohn's disease activity index	
Categories Affected by Fistulas	**Score**
Discharge	
No discharge	0
Minimal mucous discharge	1
Moderate mucous or purulent discharge	2
Substantial discharge	3
Gross fecal soiling	4
Pain/restriction of activities	
No activity restriction	0
Mild discomfort, no restriction	1
Moderate discomfort, some limitation activities	2
Marked discomfort, marked limitation	3
Severe pain, severe limitation	4
Restriction of sexual activity	
No restriction in sexual activity	0
Slight restriction in sexual activity	1
Moderate limitation in sexual activity	2
Marked limitation in sexual activity	3
Unable to engage in sexual activity	4
Type of perianal disease	
No perianal disease/skin tags	0
Anal fissure or mucosal tear	1
<3 Perianal fistulae	2
≥3 Perianal fistulae	3
Anal sphincter ulceration or fistulae with significant undermining of skin	4
Degree of induration	
No induration	0
Minimal induration	1
Moderate induration	2
Substantial induration	3
Gross fluctuance/abscess	4

From Irvine EJ. Usual therapy improves perianal Crohn's disease as measured by a new disease activity index. McMaster IBD Study Group. J Clin Gastroenterol. 1995;20(1):27-32; with permission.

and it lacks standardization. The PDAI value is improved by incorporating quality of life parameters using the Inflammatory Bowel Disease Questionnaire.[51]

SURGICAL TECHNIQUES

Despite medical therapy, anorectal disease can recur or remain unhealed.[17,33] Overall, combined medical and surgical management with drainage, seton, and infliximab therapy has been shown to be superior to either medical or surgical treatment alone.[52]

Skin Tags/Fissures/Ulcers/Hemorrhoids

Surgery for skin tags, anal fissures, ulcers, or hemorrhoids is not recommended because of poor healing and other infectious complications. Surgery should be reserved as a last resort. The authors recommend removing skin tags or hemorrhoids by simple ligation amputation. If the lesion is large or grossly inflamed, apply local anesthetic widely around the base and excise it sharply or with cautery if available. Although some have suggested that hemorrhoidopexy is never indicated due to the possibility of sepsis and bleeding,[53] stapled procedures seem to be safe in the authors' experience.[54]

Abscess

Superficial or ischiorectal abscesses are drained externally by cruciate incision and intersphincteric or supralevator abscesses are drained internally (**Fig. 1**).[55] Even in CD the authors do not routinely recommend antibiotic treatment after drainage of an anorectal abscess. They advise waiting for symptomatic relief and resolution of skin erythema before starting or continuing biological therapy.

Modified Hanley Procedure

Deep postanal abscesses comprise less than 15% of all types of anorectal abscesses.[56] For treatment of deep postanal abscesses with unilateral or bilateral horseshoe extension, the authors recommend using the modified-Hanley procedure. The borders of the postanal space are the levator muscles superiorly, the external anal sphincter inferiorly, anal canal medially, and anococcygeal ligament posteriorly. Position the patient in jack-knife position. Incise the skin approximately halfway between the tip of the coccyx and the anal canal large enough to gain adequate and comfortable exposure. Divide the posterior anococcygeal ligament to gain access to the deep posterior space. The abscess cavity should be easily accessed. Fully debride any septations being careful to not create false passages or violate the rectum. Create 2 relaxing incisions approximately 3 to 4 cm lateral to the anus. Penrose or seton drains

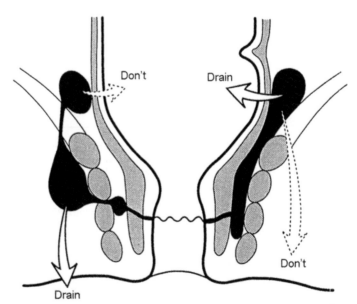

Fig. 1. Drainage of a supralevator abscess. (*From* Beck DE, Roberts PL, Rombeau JL, et al. Benign Anorectal: Abscess and Fistula. In: Wexner S., Stamos M., Rombeau J., Roberts P., Beck D. eds. The ASCRS Manual of Colon and Rectal Surgery. New York, NY. Springer; 2009. p. 273–309.)

may be passed from the posterior incision through the lateral incisions on both affected sides. Additional Malecot drains can be placed within the abscess cavity as well. Most patients will have a posterior midline fistula, which can be defined with gentle probing, but great caution should be excercised to avoid creation of false passages. When present, the fistula can be controlled with a draining seton.

Fistula

Complex fistulas undergo a median of 6 procedures and "simple" fistulas undergo a median of 3 procedures.[57] The initial approach to Crohn's fistulas involves controlling sepsis and placing a seton to prevent recurrent abscess.[58] Although there are no guidelines for timing of removal, noncutting setons may be kept long term (months to years) without negative consequences depending on clinical scenario and patient factors. Cutting setons are generally not recommended due to their risk of damage to the sphincter and deformation of the anus.[59]

Fistulotomy is appropriate for superficial or low transphincteric fistulas without associated proctitis. However, incontinence rates vary from 0% to 50%, so surgeons should remain conservative. Partial fistulotomy with seton placement is an alternative approach.[60]

First described in 2007, many of the earlier studies on Ligation of the Intersphincteric Fistula Tract (LIFT) procedure omitted patients with CD and few observational studies have looked further at this population.[61,62] The authors' group prospectively evaluated 15 patients with CD undergoing LIFT for transphincteric fistulas and found improvements from 14.0 to 3.8 and 10.4 to 1.8 in Wexner Perianal Crohn's Disease Activity Index and McMaster Perianal Crohn's Disease Activity Index quality of life scores, respectively.[63] BioLIFT combines the placement of a prosthetic graft between the ligated and divided tract ends, but this has not been studied in CD.[62,64]

Endorectal advancement flap (ERAF) is a reasonable approach to fistulas in the absence of proctitis or stenosis.[65] A major advantage to this procedure is that it avoids external wounds that are difficult to heal. For CD, ERAF is associated with a cure rate of approximately 65%.[66,67] Healing rates have improved over time, as patients are treated with biological therapy and platelet-rich plasma adjuncts.[68–70] Patients who fail an initial flap procedure are candidates for a repeat procedure, although failure rates expectedly increase with repeat attempts.[71]

Fibrin glue and fistula plugs have both been studied in CD with unfavorable results, and both techniques have largely been abandoned.[57,72–74] An area of emerging research is the injection of stem cells into fistula tracts. The phase-III randomized controlled ADMIRE-CD trial found that injection of mesenchymal stem cells directly into treatment-refractory fistula tracts of 212 patients with CD produced 50% versus 36% remission at 24 weeks compared with saline placebo.[75] More recently, the phase-I STOMP trial studied the application of mesenchymal stem cell–coated fistula plugs into 12 patients with cryptoglandular fistulas and showed promising results.[76]

Diversion/Proctectomy

Patients with refractory perianal disease may require temporary fecal diversion, but such a treatment is not always "temporary." A systematic review of 15 studies with 556 patients found a low rate of restoration of bowel continuity,[77] and this must be discussed with the patient. Proctectomy is a last-resort option for severe perianal CD that has not responded to both aggressive medical and surgical management. In cases with concomitant Crohn's colitis and perineal disease, proctocolectomy is preferred over rectal preservation due to the high incidence of persistent rectal stump disease when left in situ.[78] A dreaded complication following proctectomy or proctocolectomy is poor wound healing or a persistent draining perineal sinus. Risk factors associated with a persistent sinus are a younger patient age, fecal contamination, and extra-sphincteric dissection, needed in cases of severe anorectal disease.[79] Dealing with this complication is difficult, with Yamamoto and colleagues[79] achieving success in only 9 of 24 patients. A variety of methods can be used to combat a persistent sinus, including gracilis muscle flap, abdominal muscle flap, and even omentoplasty.[79,80]

SUMMARY

Medical treatment remains the mainstay of perianal disease management for CD; however, aggressive surgical management should be considered for severe or recurrent disease. In all cases of perianal CD, medical and surgical treatments should be used in tandem by a multidisciplinary team. Significant development has been made in the treatment of Crohn's-related fistulas, particularly minimally invasive options with recent clinical trials showing success with mesenchymal stem cell applications. Inevitably, some patients with severe refractory disease may require fecal diversion or proctectomy. When considering reversal of a diverting or end ileostomy, cessation of proctitis is the most important factor.

REFERENCES

1. Kappelman MD, Rifas-shiman SL, Kleinman K, et al. The prevalence and geographic distribution of Crohn's disease and ulcerative colitis in the United States. Clin Gastroenterol Hepatol 2007;5(12):1424–9.
2. Loftus EV. Clinical epidemiology of inflammatory bowel disease: incidence, prevalence, and environmental influences. Gastroenterology 2004;126(6):1504–17.
3. Langholz E, Munkholm P, Davidsen M, et al. Colorectal cancer risk and mortality in patients with ulcerative colitis. Gastroenterology 1992;103(5):1444–51.
4. Peyrin-biroulet L, Loftus EV, Colombel JF, et al. The natural history of adult Crohn's disease in population-based cohorts. Am J Gastroenterol 2010;105(2):289–97.
5. Bouguen G, Peyrin-biroulet L. Surgery for adult Crohn's disease: what is the actual risk? Gut 2011;60(9):1178–81.
6. Williams DR, Coller JA, Corman ML, et al. Anal complications in Crohn's disease. Dis Colon Rectum 1981;24(1):22–4.
7. Sangwan YP, Schoetz DJ, Murray JJ, et al. Perianal Crohn's disease. Results of local surgical treatment. Dis Colon Rectum 1996;39(5):529–35.
8. D'ugo S, Franceschilli L, Cadeddu F, et al. Medical and surgical treatment of haemorrhoids and anal fissure in Crohn's disease: a critical appraisal. BMC Gastroenterol 2013;13:47.
9. Keighley MR, Allan RN. Current status and influence of operation on perianal Crohn's disease. Int J Colorectal Dis 1986;1(2):104–7.
10. Buchmann P, Keighley MR, Allan RN, et al. Natural history of perianal Crohn's disease. Ten year follow-up: a plea for conservatism. Am J Surg 1980;140(5):642–4.
11. Lewis RT, Maron DJ. Anorectal Crohn's disease. Surg Clin North Am 2010;90(1):83–97.
12. Johanson JF. Association of hemorrhoidal disease with diarrheal disorders: potential pathogenic relationship? Dis Colon Rectum 1997;40(2):215–9.
13. Cracco N, Zinicola R. Is haemorrhoidectomy in inflammatory bowel disease harmful? An old dogma re-examined. Colorectal Dis 2014;16(7):516–9.
14. Higuero T. Update on the management of anal fissure. J Visc Surg 2015; 152(2 Suppl):S37–43.

15. Alexander-williams J, Buchmann P. Perianal Crohn's disease. World J Surg 1980; 4(2):203–8.
16. Bouguen G, Siproudhis L, Bretagne JF, et al. Nonfistulizing perianal Crohn's disease: clinical features, epidemiology, and treatment. Inflamm Bowel Dis 2010; 16(8):1431–42.
17. Fleshner PR, Schoetz DJ, Roberts PL, et al. Anal fissure in Crohn's disease: a plea for aggressive management. Dis Colon Rectum 1995;38(11):1137–43.
18. Sweeney JL, Ritchie JK, Nicholls RJ. Anal fissure in Crohn's disease. Br J Surg 1988;75(1):56–7.
19. Pfenninger JL, Zainea GG. Common anorectal conditions. Obstet Gynecol 2001; 98(6):1130–9.
20. Hughes LE, Donaldson DR, Williams JG, et al. Local depot methylprednisolone injection for painful anal Crohn's disease. Gastroenterology 1988;94(3):709–11.
21. Hughes LE. Clinical classification of perianal Crohn's disease. Dis Colon Rectum 1992;35(10):928–32.
22. Schwartz DA, Loftus EV, Tremaine WJ, et al. The natural history of fistulizing Crohn's disease in Olmsted County, Minnesota. Gastroenterology 2002;122(4): 875–80.
23. Eglinton TW, Barclay ML, Gearry RB, et al. The spectrum of perianal Crohn's disease in a population-based cohort. Dis Colon Rectum 2012;55(7):773–7.
24. Beaugerie L, Seksik P, Nion-larmurier I, et al. Predictors of Crohn's disease. Gastroenterology 2006;130(3):650–6.
25. Hellers G, Bergstrand O, Ewerth S, et al. Occurrence and outcome after primary treatment of anal fistulae in Crohn's disease. Gut 1980;21(6):525–7.
26. Makowiec F, Jehle EC, Starlinger M. Clinical course of perianal fistulas in Crohn's disease. Gut 1995;37(5):696–701.
27. Panés J, Rimola J. Perianal fistulizing Crohn's disease: pathogenesis, diagnosis and therapy. Nat Rev Gastroenterol Hepatol 2017;14(11):652–64.
28. Siegmund B, Feakins RM, Barmias G, et al. Results of the fifth scientific workshop of the ECCO (II): pathophysiology of perianal fistulizing disease. J Crohns Colitis 2016;10(4):377–86.
29. Von lampe B, Barthel B, Coupland SE, et al. Differential expression of matrix metalloproteinases and their tissue inhibitors in colon mucosa of patients with inflammatory bowel disease. Gut 2000;47(1):63–73.
30. Parks AG, Gordon PH, Hardcastle JD. A classification of fistula-in-ano. Br J Surg 1976;63(1):1–12.
31. Spencer JA, Ward J, Beckingham IJ, et al. Dynamic contrast-enhanced MR imaging of perianal fistulas. AJR Am J Roentgenol 1996;167(3):735–41.
32. Morris J, Spencer JA, Ambrose NS. MR imaging classification of perianal fistulas and its implications for patient management. Radiographics 2000;20(3):623–35.
33. Sandborn WJ, Fazio VW, Feagan BG, et al. AGA technical review on perianal Crohn's disease. Gastroenterology 2003;125(5):1508–30.
34. Radcliffe AG, Ritchie JK, Hawley PR, et al. Anovaginal and rectovaginal fistulas in Crohn's disease. Dis Colon Rectum 1988;31(2):94–9.
35. Singh B, George BD, Mortensen NJ. Surgical therapy of perianal Crohn's disease. Dig Liver Dis 2007;39(10):988–92.
36. Singh B, Mcc mortensen NJ, Jewell DP, et al. Perianal Crohn's disease. Br J Surg 2004;91(7):801–14.
37. Chaikhouni A, Regueyra FI, Stevens JR. Adenocarcinoma in perineal fistulas of Crohn's disease. Dis Colon Rectum 1981;24(8):639–43.

38. Wisniewski A, Fléjou JF, Siproudhis L, et al. Anal neoplasia in inflammatory bowel disease: classification proposal, epidemiology, carcinogenesis, and risk management perspectives. J Crohns Colitis 2017;11(8):1011–8.

39. Devon KM, Brown CJ, Burnstein M, et al. Cancer of the anus complicating perianal Crohn's disease. Dis Colon Rectum 2009;52(2):211–6.

40. Ratto C, Grillo E, Parello A, et al. Endoanal ultrasound-guided surgery for anal fistula. Endoscopy 2005;37(8):722–8.

41. Kelley KA, Kaur T, Tsikitis VL. Perianal Crohn's disease: challenges and solutions. Clin Exp Gastroenterol 2017;10:39–46.

42. Siddiqui MR, Ashrafian H, Tozer P, et al. A diagnostic accuracy meta-analysis of endoanal ultrasound and MRI for perianal fistula assessment. Dis Colon Rectum 2012;55(5):576–85.

43. Beets-tan RG, Beets GL, Van der hoop AG, et al. Preoperative MR imaging of anal fistulas: does it really help the surgeon? Radiology 2001;218(1):75–84.

44. Molteni RA, Bonin EA, Baldin júnior A, et al. Usefulness of endoscopic ultrasound for perianal fistula in Crohn's disease. Rev Col Bras Cir 2019;45(6):e1840.

45. Schwartz DA, Wiersema MJ, Dudiak KM, et al. A comparison of endoscopic ultrasound, magnetic resonance imaging, and exam under anesthesia for evaluation of Crohn's perianal fistulas. Gastroenterology 2001;121(5):1064–72.

46. Best WR, Becktel JM, Singleton JW, et al. Development of a Crohn's disease activity index. National Cooperative Crohn's Disease Study. Gastroenterology 1976; 70(3):439–44.

47. Harvey RF, Bradshaw JM. A simple index of Crohn's-disease activity. Lancet 1980;1(8167):514.

48. Sandborn WJ, Feagan BG, Hanauer SB, et al. A review of activity indices and efficacy endpoints for clinical trials of medical therapy in adults with Crohn's disease. Gastroenterology 2002;122(2):512–30.

49. Present DH, Rutgeerts P, Targan S, et al. Infliximab for the treatment of fistulas in patients with Crohn's disease. N Engl J Med 1999;340(18):1398–405.

50. Irvine EJ. Usual therapy improves perianal Crohn's disease as measured by a new disease activity index. McMaster IBD Study Group. J Clin Gastroenterol 1995;20(1):27–32.

51. Irvine EJ, Feagan B, Rochon J, et al. Quality of life: a valid and reliable measure of therapeutic efficacy in the treatment of inflammatory bowel disease. Canadian Crohn's Relapse Prevention Trial Study Group. Gastroenterology 1994;106(2): 287–96.

52. Bouguen G, Siproudhis L, Gizard E, et al. Long-term outcome of perianal fistulizing Crohn's disease treated with infliximab. Clin Gastroenterol Hepatol 2013; 11(8):975–81.e1-4.

53. Mccloud JM, Jameson JS, Scott AN. Life-threatening sepsis following treatment for haemorrhoids: a systematic review. Colorectal Dis 2006;8(9):748–55.

54. Koh S, Barnajian M, Zaghiyan K, et al. Excisional haemorrhoidectomy: safe in patients with Crohn's disease (CD)? Colorectal Dis 2015;17(S2):38–101.

55. Beck DE, Roberts PL, Rombeau JL, et al. Benign anorectal: abscess and fistula. In: Wexner S, Stamos M, Rombeau J, et al, editors. The ASCRS manual of colon and rectal surgery. New York: Springer; 2009. p. 273–309.

56. Hamilton CH. Anorectal problems: the deep postanal space–surgical significance in horseshoe fistula and abscess. Dis Colon Rectum 1975;18(8):642–5.

57. Geltzeiler CB, Wieghard N, Tsikitis VL. Recent developments in the surgical management of perianal fistula for Crohn's disease. Ann Gastroenterol 2014;27(4): 320–30.

58. Zalieckas JM. Treatment of perianal Crohn's disease. Semin Pediatr Surg 2017; 26(6):391–7.

59. Thornton M, Solomon MJ. Long-term indwelling seton for complex anal fistulas in Crohn's disease. Dis Colon Rectum 2005;48(3):459–63.

60. Williams JG, Rothenberger DA, Nemer FD, et al. Fistula-in-ano in Crohn's disease. Results of aggressive surgical treatment. Dis Colon Rectum 1991;34(5):378–84.

61. Rojanasakul A, Pattanaarun J, Sahakitrungruang C, et al. Total anal sphincter saving technique for fistula-in-ano; the ligation of intersphincteric fistula tract. J Med Assoc Thai 2007;90(3):581–6.

62. Mahmoud NN, Halwani Y, Montbrun S, et al. Current management of perianal Crohn's disease. Curr Probl Surg 2017;54(5):262–98.

63. Gingold DS, Murrell ZA, Fleshner PR. A prospective evaluation of the ligation of the intersphincteric tract procedure for complex anal fistula in patients with Crohn's disease. Ann Surg 2014;260(6):1057–61.

64. Ellis CN. Outcomes with the use of bioprosthetic grafts to reinforce the ligation of the intersphincteric fistula tract (BioLIFT procedure) for the management of complex anal fistulas. Dis Colon Rectum 2010;53(10):1361–4.

65. Sordo-mejia R, Gaertner WB. Multidisciplinary and evidence-based management of fistulizing perianal Crohn's disease. World J Gastrointest Pathophysiol 2014; 5(3):239–51.

66. El-gazzaz G, Hull T, Church JM. Biological immunomodulators improve the healing rate in surgically treated perianal Crohn's fistulas. Colorectal Dis 2012;14(10): 1217–23.

67. Rozalén V, Parés D, Sanchez E, et al. Advancement flap technique for anal fistula in patients with Crohn's disease: a systematic review of the literature. Cir Esp 2017;95(10):558–65.

68. Bessi G, Siproudhis L, Merlini l'héritier A, et al. Advancement flap procedure in Crohn and non-Crohn perineal fistulas: a simple surgical approach. Colorectal Dis 2019;21(1):66–72.

69. Schwandner O. Video-assisted anal fistula treatment (VAAFT) combined with advancement flap repair in Crohn's disease. Tech Coloproctol 2013;17(2):221–5.

70. Göttgens KW, Smeets RR, Stassen LP, et al. Treatment of Crohn's disease-related high perianal fistulas combining the mucosa advancement flap with platelet-rich plasma: a pilot study. Tech Coloproctol 2015;19(8):455–9.

71. Nielsen OH, Rogler G, Hahnloser D, et al. Diagnosis and management of fistulizing Crohn's disease. Nat Clin Pract Gastroenterol Hepatol 2009;6(2):92–106.

72. Hjortrup A, Moesgaard F, Kjaergård J. Fibrin adhesive in the treatment of perineal fistulas. Dis Colon Rectum 1991;34(9):752–4.

73. Grimaud JC, Munoz-bongrand N, Siproudhis L, et al. Fibrin glue is effective healing perianal fistulas in patients with Crohn's disease. Gastroenterology 2010; 138(7):2275–81, 2281.e1.

74. Al-maawali AK, Nguyen P, Phang PT. Modern treatments and stem cell therapies for perianal Crohn's fistulas. Can J Gastroenterol Hepatol 2016;2016:1651570.

75. Panés J, García-olmo D, Van assche G, et al. Expanded allogeneic adipose-derived mesenchymal stem cells (Cx601) for complex perianal fistulas in Crohn's disease: a phase 3 randomised, double-blind controlled trial. Lancet 2016; 388(10051):1281–90.

76. Dietz AB, Dozois EJ, Fletcher JG, et al. Autologous mesenchymal stem cells, applied in a bioabsorbable matrix, for treatment of perianal fistulas in patients with Crohn's disease. Gastroenterology 2017;153(1):59–62.e2.

77. Singh S, Ding NS, Mathis KL, et al. Systematic review with meta-analysis: faecal diversion for management of perianal Crohn's disease. Aliment Pharmacol Ther 2015;42(7):783–92.

78. Guillem JG, Roberts PL, Murray JJ, et al. Factors predictive of persistent or recurrent Crohn's disease in excluded rectal segments. Dis Colon Rectum 1992;35(8):768–72.

79. Yamamoto T, Bain IM, Allan RN, et al. Persistent perineal sinus after proctocolectomy for Crohn's disease. Dis Colon Rectum 1999;42(1):96–101.

80. Rius J, Nessim A, Nogueras JJ, et al. Gracilis transposition in complicated perianal fistula and unhealed perineal wounds in Crohn's disease. Eur J Surg 2000;166(3):218–22.

Other Surgeries in Patients with Inflammatory Bowel Disease

Danica N. Giugliano, MD[a], Greta V. Bernier, MD[b],
Eric K. Johnson, MD[c],*

KEYWORDS

- Chronic pain • Hernia • Inflammatory bowel disease • Parastomal hernia

KEY POINTS

- Patients with inflammatory bowel disease (IBD) are at risk for incisional and parastomal hernias due to increased rates of multiple abdominal operations, immunosuppression, and malnutrition.
- Multiple incisional hernia repair options exist including primary repair and mesh repair with a sublay, onlay, or preperitoneal approaches.
- The rate of gallstone formation and cholecystectomy in patients with Crohn disease is higher than the general population, due to several physiologic changes that occur after ileal resection.
- Surgery should be performed in patients with chronic pain only when there are objective indications for surgery, with or without a history of chronic abdominal pain.
- Desmoid disease is rare in Crohn disease, with only a few case reports in the literature, and can be treated by medical management, or by surgery for large, symptomatic lesions.

INTRODUCTION

Patients with inflammatory bowel disease (IBD) will often require abdominal surgical intervention for indications not directly related to their IBD. Because these patients often have a history of multiple previous abdominal operations and/or ostomies, they are at increased risk for incisional and parastomal hernias. Many different techniques for repairing these types of hernias have been proposed and continue to evolve

There are no commercial or financial conflicts for any of the authors, nor was any outside funding provided for the production of this article.
[a] Cooper University Hospital, Department of Surgery, 3 Cooper Plaza, Suite 411, Camden, NJ 08103, USA; [b] UW Medicine- Valley Medical Center, Colorectal Surgery Clinic, 4011 Talbot Road South, #420, Renton, WA 98055, USA; [c] Cleveland Clinic Colorectal Surgery, 6770 Mayfield Road #348, HC31, Mayfield Heights, OH 44124, USA
* Corresponding author.
E-mail address: JOHNSOE7@ccf.org

as recurrence and complication rates improve. Patients with Crohn disease (CD) are also at increased risk for gallstone formation and are more likely to undergo cholecystectomies in their lifetime. Desmoid disease is reported, but is extremely rare in patients with IBD, and may in some cases require surgical intervention. Finally, chronic pain in patients with IBD is not uncommon and can be multifactorial. Although patients who are on chronic pain medication are more likely to require an operation for their IBD, surgery should not be recommended if objective indications for surgery do not exist. A combination of oral pain medications and psychotherapy can improve the abdominal pain in patients with IBD who do not undergo surgery.

INCISIONAL HERNIAS

Approximately 70% of patients with CD and 35% of patients with ulcerative colitis (UC) will undergo abdominal surgery during their lifetime.[1,2] One of the most common complications of abdominal surgery is an incisional hernia, with an incidence of 3% to 17%.[3,4] Risk factors for hernia include body mass index (BMI), history of smoking, male gender, older age, and a history of a postoperative wound infection.[5,6] The rate of incisional hernias in IBD patients is slightly higher than the general population (4%–27%), and these individuals are at a particularly higher risk for developing hernias due to their increased likelihood of having a history of multiple abdominal operations, underlying malnutrition, and use of immunosuppressive medications such as corticosteroids.[6–11] The highest risk factor is a greater number of previous abdominal operations.[7]

A history of open bowel surgery for IBD has also been shown to be a higher risk factor than a history of laparoscopic bowel surgery.[6] This could be because the incisions created during laparoscopic surgery are often smaller than those created during open abdominal surgery. However, the location and length of the bowel extraction site in laparoscopic bowel resections influences hernia rates.[5,8,9,12–15] A vertical midline extraction site of 4 cm or greater increases the risk of hernia compared with a smaller, transverse incision (either a Pfannenstiel incision or an incision near the periumbilical trocar site).[5,14]

There are several different approaches to repairing incisional hernias, which include primary repair and various types of repairs using mesh. Primary repair has been shown to be inferior to a mesh repair with respect to hernia recurrence rates and is therefore not used often.[7] There are various approaches to mesh placement, as well as many different types of mesh that can be used. Mesh can be placed as an onlay, sublay, or in the retrorectus plane. Mesh can essentially be placed on or between any tissue plane that can be developed, and caution should be taken when interpreting mesh placement from documentation, as debate among definitions exists. There are many different types of mesh with different weaves, porosities, strengths, thicknesses, size of interstices, and adhesiogenicity. There are coated meshes made of almost every conceivable material created in an effort to prevent adhesions to the construct. These meshes handle differently and can be made of synthetic, synthetic absorbable, biological, or hybrid materials. Biological mesh has a collagen framework and can potentially integrate into tissue more effectively than synthetic mesh.[11] However, biological mesh has been shown to have a higher rate of hernia recurrence than synthetic mesh.[16] Biological mesh was also originally believed to be superior to synthetic mesh when used in a contaminated field due to decreased wound infection rates,[16,17] but more recent studies have shown low rates of mesh removal and wound infection rates when using synthetic mesh.[18,19] Currently there is lack of any real convincing data that biological meshes truly integrate into host tissue or handle contamination better than macroporous synthetics. Despite this, there are still situations where a biologic can be useful.

The retrorectus repair is a common approach to incisional hernias.[11] Incising the posterior rectus sheath close to the midline exposes the retrorectus space. This plane is then developed laterally toward the linea semilunaris. If there is concern for difficulty closing the midline incision, an anterior component separation can be performed by incising the external oblique muscle. A transversus abdominis release (TAR) can also be used and avoids the creation of subcutaneous flaps that are needed for anterior component separation. After the component separation is complete, the mesh is secured into the retrorectus plane, excluding the bowel. Drains can be left anterior to the mesh, and the midline incision is reapproximated using the anterior rectus sheath. Performance of a TAR allows for a much larger piece of mesh to be placed extraperitoneally.

Either synthetic or biological mesh can be used within the retrorectus space. With the placement of the mesh in the retrorectus space, the mesh is not exposed to bowel and can reduce the incidence of postoperative bowel adhesions or mesh erosions. This type of repair can also be used for patients who have both incisional and parastomal hernias. One factor that should be considered before undertaking a component separation is the fact that once a true separation of parts of the abdominal wall has been performed, the proverbial "bridge" may have been burned. Although some expert complex hernia surgeons will perform redo component separations or a TAR after an anterior component separation technique or vice versa, this is controversial and can be associated with dramatic failure if performed incorrectly or inappropriately.

Complications

Complications after a hernia repair can include surgical site infections (SSIs) and surgical site occurrences such as seroma or wound separation, bowel obstructions, enterocutaneous fistulas, and hernia recurrence. In patients with IBD, the incidence of SSIs after hernia surgery has been reported to be 15% to 18%.[11,20] Most often the SSIs that occur after a retrorectus repair can be treated with antibiotics plus or minus drainage.[11] Even with exposed mesh (**Fig. 1**A–D), prudent debridement and wound care and occasional use of negative pressure wound therapy may salvage the situation.

Enterocutaneous fistulas have been reported after using a sublay mesh for incisional hernias in both patients with and without IBD (**Fig. 2**). Heimann and colleagues[7] reported a late-onset (3–7 years) of enterocutaneous fistulas in 10% of patients with IBD who underwent mesh repair using synthetic underlay. In patients who have enterocutaneous fistulas, abdominal wall reconstruction at the time of fistula takedowns can result in recurrence of fistulas in 12% to 41% of patients treated with biological mesh, 10% to 24% of patients treated with synthetic mesh, and 1.6% of patients treated with primary repair.[21,22] It is for this reason that many surgeons addressing the combination of incisional hernia and enterocutaneous fistula will stage the repairs using fistula closure first with primary closure, followed by definitive hernia repair several months later.

Hernia recurrence can be as high as 27% for patients with IBD who undergo incisional hernia repairs,[7] which is similar to that seen in those without IBD.[23,24] Compared with UC, patients with CD undergoing mesh repair have an increased risk of recurrence.[7] Open and laparoscopic repairs have similar rates of recurrence.[25,26]

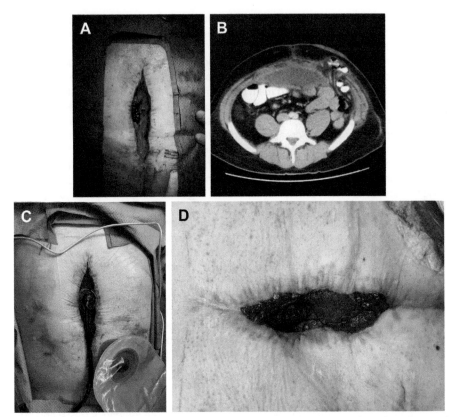

Fig. 1. (*A–D*) A male patient with CD who underwent a complex repair of combined ventral midline and parastomal hernias using a combination of the TAR and Sugarbaker techniques (Pauli repair). (*A*) An open wound with fascial defect and exposed mesh. (*B*) The computed tomographic (CT) scan reveals the appearance of the repair before drainage of an infected seroma (abscess). (*C*) A negative pressure wound system in place. (*D*) A nearly healed wound. This was managed with drainage and negative pressure with intravenous antibiotics, and never required mesh explantation.

Need for Disease to be Quiescent

Elective hernia repair is best attempted when patients with IBD have clinically quiescent disease. For patients with recurrent or persistent disease, repair of an incisional hernia should be undertaken with caution. Consider use of techniques that place mesh in an extraperitoneal location, consider use of absorbable material, and avoid techniques requiring component separation. Hernia recurrence is more common in this group, and the likelihood for reintervention secondary to IBD is high.

Impact of Biologics

There is concern that biological therapy increases the risk of surgical complications with hernia re2pair, but there is very little data on the subject. The data that are available suggest that immunosuppression does not negatively affect short-term outcomes,[27,28] but it is likely best to time surgery for more than one half-life after administration.

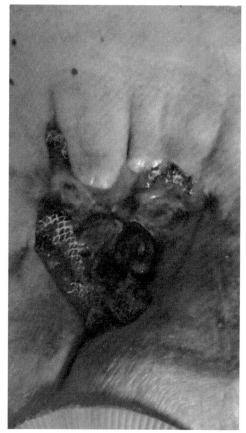

Fig. 2. A patient who has developed exposed synthetic mesh and an enteroatmospheric fistula after a complicated hernia repair.

PARASTOMAL HERNIAS

For all patients with ostomies, the incidence of parastomal hernias is up to 50%.[29,30] Risk factors include BMI, waist circumference, cigarette smoking, steroid use, chemotherapy, malnutrition, postoperative sepsis, age, and gender.[31,32] Increased duration of time after stoma placement is also a known risk factor.[32] Although it was once believed that colostomies have a higher risk of hernia formation than ileostomies (4%–48% vs 1.8%–28%[31]), several studies have challenged this belief.[30,33] In addition, loop ostomies have lower rates of hernia formation compared with end ostomies, which may be explained by the likelihood of loop ostomies to be less permanent than end ostomies, and therefore may not be in place long enough for a hernia to occur.

Although most of the parastomal hernias are managed nonoperatively, up to 30% require surgical repair. Those patients who require repair have symptoms such as bleeding, obstruction, pain, leakage, or poor fitting appliances.

Prophylactic Mesh

Prophylactic mesh placement during ostomy creation for prevention of hernia has been well described.[32,34,35] Use of synthetic mesh has been shown to have some benefit in reducing hernia rates,[36–38] whereas the effectiveness of biological mesh is not as clear.[39,40] Several complications from the use of prophylactic mesh have been reported, including mesh erosion, peristomal abscess, stoma necrosis, and wound infection.[40–45] Several systematic reviews and meta-analyses have shown that these complication rates are low, and therefore, prophylactic mesh placement may be effective in reducing hernia occurrence.[46,47] Virtually all studies of prophylactic mesh placement have used a cut keyhole technique or retrorectus placement of an uncut keyhole of mesh through which the stoma is pulled.

Stoma Relocation

Rubin and colleagues[29] compared stoma relocation with direct fascial repair and found that relocation was superior to repair for patients who had their first parastomal hernia. However, for patients with recurrent parastomal hernias, the use of mesh was superior to stoma relocation. Similarly, Riansuwan and colleagues[48] compared direct repair and stoma relocation for patients with recurrent parastomal hernias and found that relocation to the opposite side of the abdomen had good short-term results, but long-term results were unknown. The logic of relocating the stoma in hopes of a better outcome is somewhat flawed. One would have to assume that they are creating a technically superior stoma or that some other modifiable risk factor for hernia recurrence had been eliminated, which is not typically the case. It is for this reason that the authors would recommend stoma relocation as a primary option only in those requiring a shorter procedure or in those with a parastomal hernia that is so large that it prevents repair in situ (**Fig. 3**).

Types of Repair

Primary repair

Primary repair of a parastomal hernia can be used for patients who are unable to tolerate a laparotomy incision or for patients who would benefit from a shorter operative time. However, similar to incisional hernia repairs, hernia recurrence rates are high after primary repair of parastomal hernias.[29] Although primary repair is sometimes used in a contaminated field, recent studies have shown that wound infection rates are low when using a mesh as a sublay or as an onlay in a contaminated field.[49]

Mesh

The first described use of mesh to repair a parastomal hernia was by Rosin and Bonardi in 1977.[50] They described using a polyethylene mesh as an onlay. Since then, different techniques of mesh placement for parastomal hernia repairs have been described in the literature, such as placement of the mesh circumferentially as an onlay,[34] intraperitoneal mesh placement lateral to the hernia site,[51] mesh placement at the midline,[52] or mesh placement as an incomplete ring of mesh.[53] A funnel-shaped prosthetic mesh placement using either an open technique or a laparoscopic technique has also been described.[42]

Sublay The first reported use of intraperitoneal mesh placement for parastomal hernia repair was by Sugarbaker in 1985.[54] The technique uses a laparotomy incision, and a circular piece of mesh is placed around the fascial defect. It is secured around the margins of the defect except laterally, where the stoma exits the abdominal wall. Other studies have described methods of intraperitoneal mesh placement, including creating a slit or keyhole within the mesh or using modification of the Sugarbaker technique.[55–57]

Keyhole repair has been associated with high rates of recurrence, and so the modified Sugarbaker technique is preferred.[57–60] The modified Sugarbaker technique uses

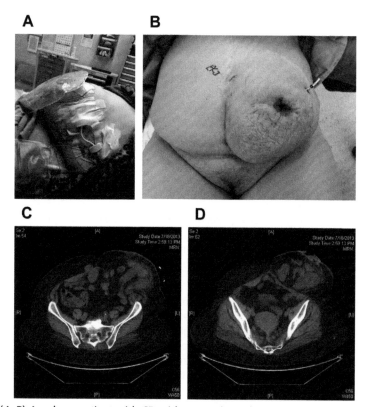

Fig. 3. (*A–D*) An obese patient with CD with a complicated parastomal hernia as well as a ventral midline hernia. (*A*) A lateral view of the large hernia with a drain in place that is draining a chronic abscess (mesh had been previously placed). (*B*) An anterior view just before surgery demonstrating a very large parastomal hernia with redundant overlying skin. (*C* and *D*) CT scan images of this same patient demonstrating the size of the defect as well as the midline component.

primary closure of the parastomal defect to an appropriate size and then intraperitoneal onlay placement of a piece of mesh with adequate overlap around the stoma. The ostomy itself is lateralized such that it travels through a "tunnel" of mesh before entering and exiting the abdominal wall. This lateralization is in theory what reduces recurrence. One must take care to effectively lateralize the bowel so that an acute angulation against the mesh is avoided. This acute angulation may lead to erosion or bowel obstruction.

Fascial onlay Many types of fascial onlay techniques have been described.[51,54,61,62] When placing the mesh, a local incision around the ostomy at the mucocutaneous junction can be used, or an incision further from the ostomy can be used to access the hernia sac. A major concern using a mesh onlay is the risk for infection due to placement of mesh in a field that is contaminated and has been reported in the literature.[53] Placing the incision further from the ostomy site can, in theory, lessen the risk of surgical site infection, but this has not been shown in the literature.

Preperitoneal mesh Preperitoneal mesh placement for parastomal hernia repair has been described and may be best for patients who have both parastomal and incisional hernias.[11] A retrorectus mesh repair with relocation of the stoma can be carried out using retrorectus dissection similar to the dissection for an incisional hernia. After placement of the mesh into this space, a cruciate incision is created in both the posterior rectus sheath and the mesh at the stoma relocation site to allow for the passage of the ostomy. The stoma is then passed through the layers of both the abdominal wall and mesh in a way that allows for no kinking or scissoring of the bowel.

A modification combining aspects of both a TAR repair and a modified Sugarbaker repair in the preperitoneal space has been described and is in use, but we lack robust long-term data. This is a useful repair in the setting of combined ventral incisional and parastomal hernias but should be used with caution unless a surgeon has extensive experience with TAR.[63]

Laparoscopic repair Several studies have described laparoscopic repair techniques using an intraperitoneal mesh, including keyhole and Sugarbaker techniques.[32,64–67] Although these studies are small, they have shown low complication rates and recurrence rates, as compared with open techniques. Among the types of laparoscopic repairs, studies have reported a higher recurrence when using laparoscopic keyhole technique (37%) compared with the laparoscopic Sugarbaker technique (6.6%).[57–59]

Recurrent parastomal hernias Up to 60% of initial parastomal hernia repairs will have a hernia recurrence.[29] Repair options for hernias that recur are the same for initial hernias. Primary repair without the use of mesh is rarely used, as repair failure has been reported to be as high as 100%.[29] Laparoscopic techniques for recurrent hernias have also shown to have promising results, with recurrence rates as low as 4% to 12%.[68,69] One must consider all factors mentioned in the incisional hernia section when repairing parastomal hernias in the IBD population.

GALLBLADDER DISEASE

The prevalence of asymptomatic gallstones in patients with CD is 13% to 34%,[70] which is greater than that in the general population (7%–20%).[71,72] Up to 22% of patients with CD eventually require a cholecystectomy.[71] Risk factors for patients with CD include ileocolonic disease, disease for more than 15 years, more than 3 clinical recurrences of CD, history of greater than 30 cm of ileum resected, use of total parenteral nutrition, and prolonged or recurrent hospitalizations.[70–72]

Ileal disease and/or ileal resection can result in decreased bile salt absorption, increasing bilirubin secretion into bile and subsequent gallstone formation. Another cause of cholelithiasis is reduced emptying of the gallbladder leading to supersaturation of cholesterol in the bile.[70,73–77] Reresection of ileum and resection of at least 10 cm of ileum has also been shown to increase the risk of cholecystectomy.[70,78,79]

There is a lack of literature to support prophylactic cholecystectomy in the IBD population, but one must be aware of the possibility of gallbladder disease in this population, as symptoms may be confused with IBD exacerbation delaying the diagnosis and treatment, which may lead to an increased complication rate.

CHRONIC PAIN

The symptomatology for patients with IBD is diverse and can be nonspecific. They can experience fever, weakness, weight loss, abdominal pain, and diarrhea. When patients have exacerbations of their disease, nearly 70% will have abdominal pain.[80] The degree of pain that these patients experience, however, does not always correlate with objective findings of the disease process that is seen on endoscopy or radiological imaging. Furthermore, nearly 20% to 50% of patients continue to experience pain even when they are in remission from exacerbations.[81] Therefore, the pathogenesis of pain in patients with IBD is likely multifactorial. Exploratory surgery is rarely beneficial and can result in several adverse outcomes and worsen quality of life.

Studies have shown that in patients with chronic IBD, recurrent inflammation can release mucosal signaling molecules and increase ion channel expression and can cause visceral hypersensitivity and chronic visceral pain.[80] Disturbance in the brain-gut axis can also cause hyperalgesia and chronic pain. Lastly, emotional and cognitive processes in the prefrontal cortex of the brain can modulate inhibitory signals and can play a role in chronic pain.

Certain medications for pain control, such as COX-2 inhibitors, tricyclic antidepressants, and antispasmodics, if used long term, can have negative effects on IBD symptoms, exacerbate symptoms, and affect motility.[82] Nonsteroidal antiinflammatory drugs (NSAIDs) that are nonselective can reduce prostaglandin production and can damage mucosal integrity of the bowel.[80] Therefore, traditionally NSAIDs have not been used in patients with IBD. More recent studies suggest that only select patients with IBD may experience flares from chronic NSAID use,[83] but the data are limited and lack long-term efficacy in patients with IBD who use NSAIDs regularly. Therefore, a limited use of NSAIDs in patients with IBD is recommended.

The rates of chronic opioid use in patients with IBD can be higher in those who experience exacerbations of their IBD symptoms more often. Furthermore, patients who are taking opiates chronically have been shown to be twice as likely to require surgery for their disease.[84,85] In the acute setting, however, half of the patients with IBD who use opiates for an acute flare will be able to discontinue opiate use when their exacerbations go into remission.[84] Therefore, chronic opiate use may indicate disease severity, and these patients may be more likely to undergo surgery for their IBD.

Psychotherapy has been shown to be effective in patients with IBD who have chronic pain, especially in patients who have chronic opioid use.[80] Psychotherapy techniques include stress management techniques and coping mechanisms, as well as techniques to target pain catastrophizing and fear avoidance.[86] When psychotherapy is used in combination with the use of multimodal pain control, patients with IBD will have improvement in abdominal pain. Therefore, surgery should be reserved for those patients who experience pain due to intestinal inflammation, obstruction, or fistulizing disease that would require operative intervention.

SUMMARY

Patients with IBD, especially those who have undergone prior surgery, may often present with disease processes that may be directly or indirectly related to IBD. Many of these individuals will require surgery or at least a surgical evaluation to treat this disease process. It is critical to examine these patients with caution, always taking into account the fact that they have IBD and consider how this may affect the treatment plan.

REFERENCES

1. Maggiori L, Panis Y. Surgical management of IBD -from an open to a laparoscopic approach. Nat Rev GastroenterolHepatol 2013. https://doi.org/10.1038/nrgastro.2013.30.

2. Solina G, Mandalà S, La Barbera C, et al. Current management of intestinal bowel disease: the role of surgery. Updates Surg 2016. https://doi.org/10.1007/s13304-016-0361-4.

3. Fischer JP, Basta MN, Mirzabeigi MN, et al. A risk model and cost analysis of incisional hernia after elective abdominal surgery based on 12,373 cases. the case for targeted prophylactic intervention. Ann Surg 2016. https://doi.org/10.1097/SLA.0000000000001394.

4. Llaguna OH, Avgerinos DV, Lugo JZ, et al. Incidence and risk factors for the development of incisional hernia following elective laparoscopic versus open colon resections. Am J Surg 2010. https://doi.org/10.1016/j.amjsurg.2009.08.044.

5. Heimann TM, Swaminathan S, Greenstein AJ, et al. Can laparoscopic surgery prevent incisional hernia in patients with Crohn's disease: a comparison study of 750 patients undergoing open and laparoscopic bowel resection. SurgEndosc 2017;31(12):5201–8.

6. Heimann TM, Swaminathan S, Greenstein AJ, et al. Incidence and factors correlating with incisional hernia following open bowel resection in patients with inflammatory bowel disease. Ann Surg 2018;267(3):532–6.

7. Heimann TM, Swaminathan S, Greenstein AJ, et al. Outcome of incisional hernia repair in patients with inflammatory bowel disease. Am J Surg 2017;214(3):468–73.

8. Stocchi L, Milsom JW, Fazio VW. Long-term outcomes of laparoscopic versus open ileocolic resection for Crohn's disease: follow-up of a prospective randomized trial. Surgery 2008. https://doi.org/10.1016/j.surg.2008.06.016.

9. Benlice C, Stocchi L, Costedio M, et al. Laparoscopic IPAA is not associated with decreased rates of incisional hernia and small-bowel obstruction when compared with open technique: long-term follow-up of a case-matched study. Dis Colon-Rectum 2015. https://doi.org/10.1097/DCR.0000000000000287.

10. Bartels SAL, Vlug MS, Henneman D, et al. Less adhesiolysis and hernia repair during completion proctocolectomy after laparoscopic emergency colectomy for ulcerative colitis. SurgEndosc 2012. https://doi.org/10.1007/s00464-011-1880-1.

11. Wang J, Majumder A, Fayezizadeh M, et al. Outcomes of retromuscular approach for abdominal wall reconstruction in patients with inflammatory bowel disease. Am Surg 2016.

12. Lee L, Mappin-Kasirer B, Liberman AS, et al. High incidence of symptomatic incisional hernia after midline extraction in laparoscopic colon resection. SurgEndosc 2012. https://doi.org/10.1007/s00464-012-2311-7.

13. Singh R, Omiccioli A, Hegge S, et al. Does the extraction-site location in laparoscopic colorectal surgery have an impact on incisional hernia rates? SurgEndoscOtherInterv Tech 2008. https://doi.org/10.1007/s00464-008-9845-8.

14. DeSouza A, Domajnko B, Park J, et al. Incisional hernia, midline versus low transverse incision: what is the ideal incision for specimen extraction and hand-assisted laparoscopy? SurgEndosc 2011. https://doi.org/10.1007/s00464-010-1309-2.

15. Benlice C, Stocchi L, Costedio MM, et al. Impact of the specific extraction-site location on the risk of incisional hernia after laparoscopic colorectal resection. Dis ColonRectum 2016. https://doi.org/10.1097/DCR.0000000000000632.

16. Rosen MJ, Krpata DM, Ermlich B, et al. A 5-year clinical experience with single-staged repairs of infected and contaminated abdominal wall defects utilizing biologic mesh. Ann Surg 2013. https://doi.org/10.1097/SLA.0b013e3182849871.

17. Bachman S, Ramshaw B. Prosthetic material in ventral hernia repair: how do I choose? SurgClin North Am 2008. https://doi.org/10.1016/j.suc.2007.11.001.

18. Carbonell AM, Criss CN, Cobb WS, et al. Outcomes of synthetic mesh in contaminated ventral hernia repairs. J Am Coll Surg 2013. https://doi.org/10.1016/j.jamcollsurg.2013.07.382.
19. Cobb WS, Criss C, Matthews BD, et al. A multicenter prospective observational cohort study of permanent synthetic mesh versus biologic mesh reinforcement for open ventral hernia repair in clean-contaminated and contaminated surgical sites. J Am Coll Surg 2013. https://doi.org/10.1016/j.jamcollsurg.2013.07.041.
20. Taner T, Cima RR, Larson DW, et al. The use of human acellular dermal matrix for parastomal hernia repair in patients with inflammatory bowel disease. Dis Colon-Rectum 2009;52(2):349–54.
21. Hodgkinson JD, Maeda Y, Leo CA, et al. Complex abdominal wall reconstruction in the setting of active infection and contamination: a systematic review of hernia and fistula recurrence rates. Colorectal Dis 2017. https://doi.org/10.1111/codi.13609.
22. Connolly PT, Teubner A, Lees NP, et al. Outcome of reconstructive surgery for intestinal fistula in the open abdomen. Ann Surg 2008. https://doi.org/10.1097/SLA.0b013e3181612c99.
23. Hawn MT, Snyder CW, Graham LA, et al. Long-term follow-up of technical outcomes for incisional hernia repair. J Am Coll Surg 2010. https://doi.org/10.1016/j.jamcollsurg.2009.12.038.
24. Majumder A, Winder JS, Wen Y, et al. Comparative analysis of biologic versus synthetic mesh outcomes in contaminated hernia repairs. Surgery 2016. https://doi.org/10.1016/j.surg.2016.04.041.
25. Asti E, Sironi A, Lovece A, et al. Open versus laparoscopic management of incisional abdominal hernia: cohort study comparing quality of life outcomes. J LaparoendoscAdvSurg Tech A 2016. https://doi.org/10.1089/lap.2016.0060.
26. Al Chalabi H, Larkin J, Mehigan B, et al. A systematic review of laparoscopic versus open abdominal incisional hernia repair, with meta-analysis of randomized controlled trials. Int J Surg 2015. https://doi.org/10.1016/j.ijsu.2015.05.050.
27. Haskins IN, Krpata DM, Prabhu AS, et al. Immunosuppression is not a risk factor for 30-day wound events or additional 30-day morbidity or mortality after open ventral hernia repair: an analysis of the Americas Hernia Society Quality Collaborative. Surgery 2018. https://doi.org/10.1016/j.surg.2018.05.023.
28. Tastaldi L, Blatnik JA, Krpata DM, et al. Posterior component separation with transversusabdominis release (TAR) for repair of complex incisional hernias after orthotopic liver transplantation. Hernia 2019. https://doi.org/10.1007/s10029-019-01918-8.
29. Rubin MS, Schoetz DJ, Matthews JB. Parastomalhernia: is stoma relocation superior to fascial repair? Arch Surg 1994. https://doi.org/10.1001/archsurg.1994.01420280091011.
30. Williams JG, Etherington R, Hayward MWJ, et al. Paraileostomy hernia: a clinical and radiological study. Br J Surg 1990. https://doi.org/10.1002/bjs.1800771212.
31. Carne PWG, Robertson GM, Frizelle FA. Parastomal hernia. Br J Surg 2003;90(7):784–93.
32. O'Neill CH, Borrazzo EC, Hyman NH. Parastomalhernia repair. J Gastrointest Surg 2015. https://doi.org/10.1007/s11605-014-2717-8.
33. Makela JT, Turku PH, Laitinen ST. Analysis of late stomal complications following ostomy surgery. Ann ChirGynaecol 1997.
34. Franks ME, Hrebinko RL. Technique of parastomal hernia repair using synthetic mesh. Urology 2001. https://doi.org/10.1016/S0090-4295(00)01014-1.

35. Hotouras A, Murphy J, Thaha M, et al. The persistent challenge of parastomal herniation: a review of the literature and future developments. Colorectal Dis 2013. https://doi.org/10.1111/codi.12156.

36. López-Cano M, Lozoya-Trujillo R, Quiroga S, et al. Use of a prosthetic mesh to prevent parastomal hernia during laparoscopic abdominoperineal resection: A randomized controlled trial. Hernia 2012. https://doi.org/10.1007/s10029-012-0952-z.

37. Serra-Aracil X, Bombardo-Junca J, Moreno-Matias J, et al. Randomized, controlled, prospective trial of the use of a mesh to prevent parastomal hernia. Ann Surg 2009. https://doi.org/10.1097/SLA.0b013e31819ec809.

38. Jänes A, Cengiz Y, Israelsson LA. Preventing parastomal hernia with a prosthetic mesh: a 5-year follow-up of a randomized study. World J Surg 2009;33(1):118–21 [discussion: 122–3].

39. Fleshman JW, Beck DE, Hyman N, et al. A prospective, multicenter, randomized, controlled study of non-cross-linked porcine acellular dermal matrix fascialsublay for parastomal reinforcement in patients undergoing surgery for permanent abdominal wall ostomies. Dis ColonRectum 2014. https://doi.org/10.1097/DCR.0000000000000106.

40. Hammond TM, Huang A, Prosser K, et al. Parastomal hernia prevention using a novel collagen implant: A randomised controlled phase 1 study. Hernia 2008. https://doi.org/10.1007/s10029-008-0383-z.

41. Gögenur I, Mortensen J, Harvald T, et al. Prevention of parastomal hernia by placement of a polypropylene mesh at the primary operation. Dis ColonRectum 2006. https://doi.org/10.1007/s10350-006-0615-1.

42. Berger D. Prevention of parastomal hernias by prophylactic use of a specially designed intraperitonealonlay mesh (DynameshIPST®). Hernia 2008. https://doi.org/10.1007/s10029-007-0318-0.

43. Janson AR, Jänes A, Israelsson LA. Laparoscopic stoma formation with a prophylactic prosthetic mesh. Hernia 2010. https://doi.org/10.1007/s10029-010-0673-0.

44. Marimuthu K, Vijayasekar C, Ghosh D, et al. Prevention of parastomal hernia using preperitoneal mesh: a prospective observational study. Colorectal Dis 2006. https://doi.org/10.1111/j.1463-1318.2006.00996.x.

45. Vijayasekar C, Marimuthu K, Jadhav V, et al. Parastomal hernia: is prevention better than cure? Use of preperitoneal polypropylene mesh at the time of stoma formation. Tech Coloproctol 2008. https://doi.org/10.1007/s10151-008-0441-7.

46. Shabbir J, Chaudhary BN, Dawson R. A systematic review on the use of prophylactic mesh during primary stoma formation to prevent parastomal hernia formation. Colorectal Dis 2012. https://doi.org/10.1111/j.1463-1318.2011.02835.x.

47. Sajid MS, Kalra L, Hutson K, et al. Parastomal hernia as a consequence of colorectal cancer resections can prophylactically be controlled by mesh insertion at the time of primary surgery: a literature based systematic review of published trials. Minerva Chir 2012;67(4):289–96.

48. Riansuwan W, Hull TL, Millan MM, et al. Surgery of recurrent parastomal hernia: direct repair or relocation? Colorectal Dis 2010. https://doi.org/10.1111/j.1463-1318.2009.01868.x.

49. Steele SR, Lee P, Martin MJ, et al. Is parastomal hernia repair with polypropylene mesh safe? Am J Surg 2003;185(5):436–40. Available at: http://www.ncbi.nlm.nih.gov/pubmed/12727563. Accessed January 26, 2019.

50. Rosin JD, Bonardi RA. Paracolostomy hernia repair with Marlex mesh: a new technique. Dis ColonRectum 1977. https://doi.org/10.1007/BF02586428.

51. Byers JM, Steinberg JB, Postier RG. Repair of parastomal hernias using polypropylene mesh. Arch Surg 1992. https://doi.org/10.1001/archsurg.1992.01420100112019.

52. Kasperk R, Klinge U, Schumpelick V. The repair of large parastomal hernias using a midline approach and a prosthetic mesh in the sublay position. Am J Surg 2000. https://doi.org/10.1016/S0002-9610(00)00309-3.

53. Tekkis PP, Kocher HM, Payne JG. Parastomal hernia repair: modified Thorlakson technique, reinforced by polypropylene mesh. Dis ColonRectum 1999. https://doi.org/10.1007/BF02235057.

54. Sugarbaker PH. Peritoneal approach to prosthetic mesh repair of paraostomy hernias. Ann Surg 1985. https://doi.org/10.1097/00000658-198503000-00015.

55. Muysoms FE, Hauters PJ, Van Nieuwenhove Y, et al. Laparoscopic repair of parastomal hernias: a multi-centre retrospective review and shift in technique. ActaChir Belg 2008. https://doi.org/10.1080/00015458.2008.11680249.

56. Yang F. A modified sublay-keyhole technique for in situ parastomal hernia repair. SurgToday 2012. https://doi.org/10.1007/s00595-011-0095-3.

57. Hansson BME, Morales-Conde S, Mussack T, et al. The laparoscopic modified Sugarbaker technique is safe and has a low recurrence rate: a multicenter cohort study. SurgEndosc 2013. https://doi.org/10.1007/s00464-012-2464-4.

58. Hansson BME, Slater NJ, van der Velden AS, et al. Surgical techniques for parastomal hernia repair. Ann Surg 2012. https://doi.org/10.1097/SLA.0b013e31824b44b1.

59. Hansson BME, Bleichrodt RP, De Hingh IH. Laparoscopic parastomal hernia repair using a keyhole technique results in a high recurrence rate. SurgEndosc 2009. https://doi.org/10.1007/s00464-008-0253-x.

60. Hansson BME, De Hingh IHJT, Bleichrodt RP. Laparoscopic parastomal hernia repair is feasible and safe: early results of a prospective clinical study including 55 consecutive patients. SurgEndoscOtherInterv Tech 2007. https://doi.org/10.1007/s00464-007-9244-6.

61. Morris-Stiff G, Hughes LE. The continuing challenge of parastomal hernia: failure of a novel polypropylene mesh repair. Ann R CollSurg Engl 1998;80(3):184–7.

62. Hofstetter WL, Vukasin P, Ortega AE, et al. New technique for mesh repair of paracolostomy hernias. Dis ColonRectum 1998. https://doi.org/10.1007/BF02237400.

63. Pauli EM, Juza RM, Winder JS. How I do it: novel parastomalherniorrhaphy utilizing transversusabdominis release. Hernia 2016. https://doi.org/10.1007/s10029-016-1489-3.

64. Kozlowski PM, Wang PC, Winfield HN. Laparoscopic repair of incisional and parastomal hernias after major genitourinary or abdominal surgery. J Endourol 2001. https://doi.org/10.1089/089277901750134520.

65. Bickel A, Shinkarevsky E, Eitan A, et al. Laparoscopic repair of paracolostomy hernia. J LaparoendoscAdvSurg Tech A 1999. https://doi.org/10.1089/lap.1999.9.353.

66. Porcheron J, Payan B, Balique JG. Mesh repair of paracolostomal hernia by laparoscopy. SurgEndosc 1998. https://doi.org/10.1007/s004649900838.

67. Voitk A. Simple technique for laparoscopic paracolostomy hernia repair. Dis ColonRectum 2000. https://doi.org/10.1007/BF02236646.

68. Mancini GJ, McClusky DA, Khaitan L, et al. Laparoscopic parastomal hernia repair using a nonslit mesh technique. SurgEndoscOtherInterv Tech 2007. https://doi.org/10.1007/s00464-007-9419-1.

69. Berger D, Bientzle M. Laparoscopic repair of parastomal hernias: A single sur-geon's experience in 66 patients. Dis ColonRectum 2007. https://doi.org/10.1007/s10350-007-9028-z.

70. Fraquelli M, Losco A, Visentin S, et al. Gallstone disease and related risk factors in patients with Crohn disease: analysis of 330 consecutive cases. Arch Intern Med 2001. https://doi.org/10.1001/archinte.161.18.2201.

71. Parente F, Pastore L, Bargiggia S, et al. Incidence and risk factors for gallstones in patients with inflammatory bowel disease: a large case-control study. Hepatol-ogy 2007. https://doi.org/10.1002/hep.21537.

72. Chew SSB, Ngo TQ, Douglas PR, et al. Cholecystectomy in patients with Crohn's ileitis. Dis ColonRectum 2003;46(11):1484-8.

73. Lapidus A, Åkerlund JE, Einarsson C. Gallbladder bile composition in patients with Crohn's disease. World J Gastroenterol 2006. https://doi.org/10.3748/wjg.v12.i1.70.

74. Brink MA, Slors JFM, Keulemans YCA, et al. Enterohepatic cycling of bilirubin: a putative mechanism for pigment gallstone formation in ilealCrohn's disease. Gastroenterology 1999. https://doi.org/10.1016/S0016-5085(99)70507-X.

75. Pereira SP, Bain IM, Kumar D, et al. Bile composition in inflammatory bowel dis-ease: Ileal disease and colectomy, but not colitis, induce lithogenic bile. Aliment PharmacolTher 2003. https://doi.org/10.1046/j.1365-2036.2003.01529.x.

76. Hutchinson R, Tyrrell PNM, Kumar D, et al. Pathogenesis of gall stones in Crohn's dis-ease: an alternative explanation. Gut 1994. https://doi.org/10.1136/gut.35.1.94.

77. Vu MK, Gielkens HA, van Hogezand RA, et al. Gallbladder motility in Crohn dis-ease: influence of disease localization and bowel resection. Scand J Gastroen-terol 2000;35(11):1157-62.

78. Goet JC, Beelen EMJ, Biermann KE, et al. Cholecystectomy risk in Crohn's-disease patients after ileal resection: a long-term nationwide cohort study. J GastrointestSurg 2018. https://doi.org/10.1007/s11605-018-4028-y.

79. Hill GL, Mair WSJ, Goligher JC. Gallstones after ileostomy and ileal resection. Gut 1975. https://doi.org/10.1136/gut.16.12.932.

80. Zielińska A, Sałaga M, Włodarczyk M, et al. Focus on current and future manage-ment possibilities in inflammatory bowel disease-related chronic pain. Int J Colo-rectal Dis 2019;34(2):217-27. https://doi.org/10.1007/s00384-018-3218-0.

81. Schirbel A, Reichert A, Roll S, et al. Impact of pain on health-related quality of life in patients with inflammatory bowel disease. World J Gastroenterol 2010. https://doi.org/10.3748/WJG.V16.I25.3168.

82. Makharia GK. Understanding and treating abdominal pain and spasms in organic gastrointestinal diseases: Inflammatory bowel disease and biliary dis-eases. J ClinGastroenterol 2011;45Suppl:S89-93.

83. Kaufmann HJ, Taubin HL. Nonsteroidal anti-inflammatory drugs activate quies-cent inflammatory bowel disease. Ann Intern Med 1987. https://doi.org/10.7326/0003-4819-107-4-513.

84. Hanson KA, Loftus EV, Hármsen WS, et al. Clinical features and outcome of patients with inflammatory bowel disease who use narcotics: a case-control study. InflammBowel Dis 2009. https://doi.org/10.1002/ibd.20847.

85. Grunkemeier DMS, Cassara JE, Dalton CB, et al. {A figure is presented}Thenar-cotic bowel syndrome: clinical features, pathophysiology, and management. ClinGastroenterolHepatol 2007. https://doi.org/10.1016/j.cgh.2007.06.013.

86. Regueiro M, Greer JB, Szigethy E. Etiology and treatment of pain and psychoso-cial issues in patients with inflammatory bowel diseases. Gastroenterology 2017. https://doi.org/10.1053/j.gastro.2016.10.036.

Pediatric Inflammatory Bowel Disease
Special Considerations

Megan K. Fuller, MD[a,b],*

KEYWORDS

- Pediatric inflammatory bowel disease • Very early onset IBD (VEOIBD)
- Pediatric Crohn's disease • Pediatric ulcerative colitis • Pediatric IBD–unclassified

KEY POINTS

- Very early onset inflammatory bowel disease (IBD) (diagnosis less than age 6 years) and infantile IBD (diagnosis less than age 2 years) more commonly than adult-onset IBD have a colitis phenotype. Underlying monogenic disorders or immunologic disorders are more likely in this subset of pediatric IBD and should be excluded.
- Computed tomography scans should be used judiciously and only with as low as reasonably achievable protocols in children and young adults (up to age 35 years) due to cumulative radiation exposure and risk of malignancy.
- Nonadherence to medical regimens should be excluded during flares.
- Careful attention should be given to growth and developmental parameters, including missed days of school, in developing treatment plans.
- Transition to adult care for long-term follow-up should be planned carefully.

INTRODUCTION

For patients with inflammatory bowel disease (IBD), approximately 20% to 30% are diagnosed in childhood or adolescence.[1] Studies suggest that the incidence is increasing over time. Incidence in Germany has increased from 13.6/100,000 in 2009 to 17.4/100,000 in 2012.[2] This incidence is the highest reported in literature, but it parallels trends seen in other countries[2,3] Incidence seems to increase for both Crohn's disease (CD) and ulcerative colitis (UC) at approximately age 7 years. The incidence of CD is higher than that of UC, and in pediatrics there is a male-to-female predominance up to a ratio of 1.8:1.[3]

Disclosure Statement: There are no commercial or financial conflicts of interest to report for any listed authors.
[a] Department of Surgery, University of Nebraska Medical Center, Children's Hospital and Medical Center, Omaha, NE, USA; [b] Boys Town National Research Hospital, Boystown, NE, USA
* Pediatric Surgery, 14080 Boystown Hospital Road, Boystown, NE 68010.
E-mail address: megan.fuller@boystown.org

surgical.theclinics.com

PRESENTATION

Childhood IBD often presents with more extensive disease and a more aggressive course than adult-onset disease.[4] One study reported a 90% incidence of pancolitis in children diagnosed with UC in contrast to 37% of those diagnosed in adulthood.[5] Of pediatric IBD patients, there is a 34% risk of need for surgery within 5 years of diagnosis.[3] The most common presenting symptoms include abdominal pain, diarrhea, hematochezia, and anemia; however, they also include more systemic symptoms of weight loss, anorexia, growth delay, delayed puberty, joint pains, skin changes, depression, and anxiety.[6] Family history remains a strong risk factor for IBD. Of children with very early onset IBD (VEOIBD), defined by diagnosis less than age 6 years, this history is even stronger.[7]

DIAGNOSIS

In children with suspected IBD, it is recommended to exclude enteric infections and send serum studies, including complete blood cell count, inflammatory markers, fecal calprotectin, albumin, transaminases, and γ-glutamyl transferase.[8] Subsequent evaluation should include ileocolonoscopy and esophagogastroduodenoscopy with multiple biopsies and careful documentation of mucosal appearance. The small bowel also should be evaluated by magnetic resonance enterography for most patients. Wireless capsule endoscopy also may be used for small bowel evaluation.[8] Ultrasound is becoming the standard for diagnosis of pediatric appendicitis and also visualizes the terminal ileum. Ultrasound may be a reasonable screening test for suspected CD of the terminal ileum, demonstrating changes, including thickened mesentery, enlarged lymph nodes, mural thickening, hyperemia, and loss of stratification. Computed tomography (CT) should be used with caution, balancing the benefits against the risk of radiation exposure. CT should be as low as reasonably achievable protocoled to minimize radiation exposure. Patients with IBD, in particular those diagnosed early in life, are at risk from repeated radiation exposures over a lifetime. Exposures greater than 50 mSv are associated with an increased risk of malignancy; radiation from CT ranging from 4 mSv to 45 mSv. The cancer risk associated with radiation decreases with age, but it does not flatten out until age 35.[9]

In contrast to adult-onset IBD, a polygenic disorder, children with VEOIBD (diagnosis age <6 years) and infantile IBD (diagnosis age <2 years) have an increased risk of monogenic disorders. They also are more likely to present with colonic disease, with 20% to 35% of these being classified as IBD–unclassified.[7,10] Infantile IBD represents approximately 1% and VEOIBD 15% of pediatric IBD patients. VEOIBD has an incidence of approximately 4/100,000.[7] Defects in genes that control the epithelial barrier, phagocytes, interleukin 10, T cells and B cells, immunoregulation, and inflammation represent most of the pathways implicated in monogenic disorders.[7] A pneumonic has been proposed by Uhlig and colleagues[7] to remember factors that should raise suspicion and exclusion of these monogenic disorders in the diagnosis of pediatric IBD: YOUNG AGE MATTERS MOST (young age, multiple family members or consanguinity, autoimmunity, thriving failure, treatment with conventional medication failure, endocrine concerns, recurrent infections or unexplained fever, severe perianal disease, macrophage activation syndrome and hemophagocytic lymphohistiocytosis, obstruction and atresia of intestine, skin lesions and dental or hair abnormalities, and tumors). Strong suspicion, especially in infantile-onset disease, is key to diagnosis and appropriate treatment of these mimickers of IBD.

CLASSIFICATION OF DISEASE

Pediatric IBD is classified by the revised Porto criteria (2014) into 1 of 5 categories: typical UC, atypical UC, clear CD including colonic CD, normal, or IBD–unclassified.[8] For exact classification schemes, refer to the article by Birimberg-Schwartz and colleagues,[11] but, in short, to help differentiate between groups, they defined 23 features of typical CD grouped into 3 classes: incompatible with UC, present rarely in UC (<5%), and present uncommonly in UC (5%–10%). Features of disease are then weighted by class to aid in classification.

Pediatric IBD is categorized further using the Paris pediatric modification of the Montreal classification of phenotypic characteristics of IBD.[12] Features for classification CD include

- Age at diagnosis in years: A1a, 0 to less than 10 years; A1b, 10 years to less than 17 years; A2, 17 years to 40 years; and A3, greater than 40 years
- Location of disease: L1, distal one-third ileal with or without limited cecal disease; L2, colonic; L3, ileocolonic; L4a, upper disease proximal to the ligament of Treitz; L4b, upper disease distal to the ligament of Treitz and proximal to the distal one-third ileum; *L4a and L4b disease may coexist
- Behavior of disease: B1, nonstricturing nonpenetrating; B2, stricturing; B3, penetrating; * if structuring and penetrating disease are present at the same or different times, use designation B2B3; * if perianal disease, add modifier p
- Growth: G0, no evidence of growth delay, and G1, growth delay defined by impaired linear growth

Features for classification of UC include

- Age at diagnosis (A1a–A3)
- Extent of disease: E1, ulcerative proctitis; E2, left sided (distal to the splenic flexure); E3, extensive (distal to hepatic flexure); and E4, pancolitis (proximal to the hepatic flexure); severity: S0, never severe, and S1, severe at any time during disease course
- Severity: defined by the pediatric ulcerative colitis activity index (PUCAI) greater than or equal to 65

The A1a group has been subdivided further into VEOIBD (age <6) and infantile IBD (age <2).[7]

TREATMENT AND MONITORING
Ulcerative Colitis (Typical, Atypical, and Inflammatory Bowel Disease–Unclassified)

Severity of disease should be graded using the PUCAI score, which provides points based on abdominal pain, rectal bleeding, consistency of the majority of stools, the number of stools per 24 hours, presence of nocturnal stools, and activity level. The maximum score is 85, with remission defined as score less than 10, mild disease 10 to 35, moderate disease 40 to 60, and severe disease 65 to 85.[13] Severe disease in the first 3 months after diagnosis places a child at increased risk of refractory disease and should prompt tight monitoring.

Choice of agent to induce remission is guided by severity of presentation and is similar to that in adults. Severe disease also is treated with steroids; however, steroid dependency is to be avoided. When transitioning to maintenance therapy, factors that may impede compliance should be considered, including the number of doses daily and ability to swallow pills. If unable to wean steroids on 5-aminosalicylic acid therapy, escalation to biologics or thiopurines should be considered.[13] Low doses of steroids can suppress growth, and children with UC have increased complications in comparison to their adult counterparts, even after adjusting dose for weight; complications include osteopenia, acne, glaucoma, and cataracts.[13] In addition to its adverse reactions, including pancreatitis, thiopurine use also has been implicated in the development of hepatosplenic T-cell lymphoma. Combination therapy of thiopurines with anti-tumor necrosis factor (TNF) agents increases the risk of lymphoma more than either treatment alone.[14] Vedolizumab has limited pediatric data and is still off-label in pediatrics but also has shown promise in children with failure of other therapy.[15]

Despite significant earlier use of anti–TNF-α agents in recent years, there have been no significant decreases in the rate of surgery[16]; 10% to 30% of patients still require surgery within 5 years of diagnosis.[16,17] Indications for surgery are similar to adults, including toxic megacolon, perforation, and hemorrhage. In children, the indications for ulcerative colitis also may include failure to wean off steroids, development of dysplasia, and growth failure.[13] Surgery is not without its own risks, and studies in children have quoted complication rates of 15% to 40%.[5,17] Children typically have very low rate of venous thromboembolism; however, up to 4% developed symptomatic abdominal venous thromboembolism in 1 study. Strong consideration should be made for prophylactic anticoagulation.[18] Techniques may need to be adapted depending on the size of the child and require hand-sewn anastomosis. There is no evidence on whether postponing restorative pouch surgery influences long-term outcomes. Overall rates of pouch abandonment are similar to those in adult series.[12]

Screening for dysplasia with colonoscopy should begin 5 years to 10 years after diagnosis. Children with primary sclerosing cholangitis are at increased risk of malignancy and screening should follow guidelines of increased frequency.[12] Childhood-onset IBD is associated with a low absolute risk of cancer but a hazard ratio of 18 (colorectal, small intestinal, liver, lymphoma, and skin cancer).[19]

Crohn's Disease

CD is monitored via the Pediatric Crohn's Disease Activity Index, which accounts for abdominal pain (patient reported and on physical examination), stools per day, activity level, laboratory values (hematocrit, erythrocyte sedimentation rate, and albumin), weight, height, height velocity, perirectal disease, and extraintestinal manifestations. Score ranges from in remission (<10) to mild (<30) to moderate (≥30–40) to severe (≥40). A change in score of greater than or equal to 12.5 points reflects clinically significant response to therapy.[20]

Exclusive enteral nutrition is recommended as first-line induction therapy, and recent studies suggest it may be more effective in achieving early remission than steroids.[21] Linear growth improvement also seems superior to other therapies.[21] Other therapies remain similar to adults with usage of biologics, immunomodulators, and steroids.[16,22,23] Despite the introduction of biologics and data that they slow progression of disease, the risk of surgery within 5 years of diagnosis has not changed.[21] Surgery rates remain between 14% and 34% within 5 years of diagnosis.[24] Investigators believe that this is secondary to significant disease progression before diagnosis, and they advocate early effective treatment. Surgical indications for CD include failure of medical management, inability to wean steroids, perforation, refractory stricture, diversion, and treatment of perianal disease.[17]

SPECIAL CONSIDERATIONS

IBD diagnosis in children and adolescents has an impact on their growth and development. Bone density peak in adolescence determines lifelong skeletal health, so avoidance of nutritional deficiency and promoting weight-bearing exercise are important for lifelong health.[13] IBD diagnosis is associated with decreased quality of life, missed days of school, reduced participation in extracurricular activities and subjective school underperformance.[25,26] School accommodations should be considered early. Children qualify for 504 plans or individualized education plans. Medical professionals should actively advocate for their patients and encourage early social work involvement. Finding reasons for missed school can help individualize plans and promote school attendance. Children with illnesses leading to potential incontinence miss school more frequently than expected.[27] Missed school can affect both school performance and social functioning.[28] Screening for depression and anxiety should be part of routine care.[26] Early-onset IBD often delays vaccination in a patient group at increased risk for infection. Inactive vaccines have demonstrated safety. Although there is decreased response while on immunosuppressive medications in comparison to healthy controls, a majority of patients do achieve protective immunity.[29]

ImproveCareNow (ICN) is a collaborative network to help improve the quality of life and care of children with IBD. They have numerous resources available for families, including example accommodation plans. Providers should consider timing of nonemergent surgeries to minimize school absenteeism and account for things that children consider important like a potential sports season or trip to camp. Body image also may be of concern and finding support groups can aid adolescents, in particular those who may have stomas. A toolkit is also available via ICN to help address common questions about stomas, such as how to build an emergency kit or play sports with a stoma.[30]

When assessing flares, it is important to examine adherence to treatment plans because up to 50% to 66% of children demonstrate nonadherence for a variety of reasons.[13] As children age, an individualized plan for transition to adult care is also important. Most sources recommend starting assessment for readiness at approximately age 12 and to finish transition in a period of disease stability. Successful transition promotes self-reliance and adherence to therapy.[31] Tools exist to facilitate transition because pediatric patients often lack knowledge about their medical history and medication regimens. Teaming up adult and pediatric providers can aid in the transition. Skills for independence also may need to be taught, including how to schedule appointments, check in at appointments, and how to reach providers during a flare.

SUMMARY

Pediatric IBD may present differently than adult-onset disease. It is important to consider a broader differential diagnosis in very early onset disease. Of pediatric patients with A1a disease, those with VEOIBD and infantile IBD have the greatest risk of monogenic cause of disease. Allergic colitis and infectious colitis should be excluded. Treatment plans should promote growth, development, and adherence to therapy. Diagnostic and treatment decisions must consider the long-term risks and benefits over a lifetime. Collaborative care networks like ICN promote best practice and have been effective in increasing rates of steroid-free remission. Surgical triggers in children may include impaired growth and inability to wean from steroids in addition to standard adult indications. Transition to adult care encompasses much more than transferring a medical record. Good transition of care promotes patient adherence to therapy and is crucial to developing lifelong care patterns.

REFERENCES

1. Benchimol EI, Fortinsky KJ, Gozdyra P, et al. Epidemiology of pediatric inflammatory bowel disease: a systematic review of international trends. Inflamm Bowel Dis 2011;17:423–9.
2. Wittig R, Albers L, Koletzko S, et al. Pediatric inflammatory bowel disease in a German statutory health INSURANCE-Incidence rates from 2009-2012. J Pediatr Gastroenterol Nutr 2019;68:244–50.
3. Moon JS. Clinical aspects and treatments for pediatric inflammatory bowel diseases. Pediatr Gastroenterol Hepatol Nutr 2019;22(1):50–6.
4. Duricova D, Burisch J, Jess T, et al. Age-related differences in presentation and course of pediatric inflammatory bowel disease; an update on the population-based literature. J Crohns Colitis 2014;8(11):1351–61.
5. Ponsky T, Hindle A, Sandler A. Inflammatory bowel disease in the pediatric patient. Surg Clin North Am 2007;87:643–58.
6. Keethy D, Mrakotsky C, Szigethy E. Pediatric inflammatory bowel disease and depression: treatment implications. Curr Opin Pediatr 2014;26:561–7.
7. Uhlig HH, Schwerd T, Koletzko S, et al. The diagnostic approach to monogenic very early onset inflammatory bowel disease. Gastroenterology 2014;147:990–1007.
8. Levine A, Koletzko S, Turner D, et al. ESPGHAN revised porto criteria for the diagnosis of inflammatory bowel disease in children and adolescents. J Pediatr Gastroenterol Nutr 2014;58(6):795–806.
9. Govani SM, Higgins PDR, Rubenstein JH, et al. CT utilization abruptly increases at age 18 among patients with inflammatory bowel diseases in the hospital. PLoS One 2018;13(3):e0195022.
10. Snapper SB. Very-early onset inflammatory bowel disease. Gastroenterol Hepatol 2015;11(8):554–6.
11. Birimberg-Schwartz L, Zucker DM, Akriv A, et al. Development and validation of diagnostic criteria for IBD subtypes with an emphasis on IBD-Unclassified in children: a multicenter study from the pediatric IBD Porto group of ESPGHAN. J Crohns Colitis 2017;11:1078–84.
12. Levine A, Griffiths A, Markowitz J, et al. Pediatric modification of the Montreal classification for inflammatory bowel disease: the Paris classification. Inflamm Bowel Dis 2011;17(6):1314–21.
13. Turner D, Ruemmele FM, Orlanski-Meyer E, et al. Management of paediatric ulcerative colitis, part 1: ambulatory care-an evidence based guideline from European crohn's and colitis organization and European society of paediatric gastroenterology, hepatology and nutrition. J Pediatr Gastroenterol Nutr 2018;67(2):257–91.
14. Lemaitre M, Kirchgesner J, Rudnichi A, et al. Association between use of thiopurines or tumor necrosis factor antagonists alone or in combination and risk of lymphoma in patients with inflammatory bowel disease. JAMA 2017;318(17):1679–86.
15. Schneider A-M, Weghuber D, Hezer B, et al. Vedolizumab use after failure of TNF-α antagonists in children and adolescents with inflammatory bowel disease. BMC Gastroenterol 2018;18:140.
16. Guilcher K, Fournier N, Schoepfer A, et al. Change of treatment modalities over the last 10 years in pediatric patients with inflammatory bowel disease in Switzerland. Eur J Gastroenterol Hepatol 2018;30(10):1159–67.

17. Fehmel E, Teague WJ, Simpson D, et al. The burden of surgery and postoperative complications in children with inflammatory bowel disease. J Pediatr Surg 2018; 53:2440–3.
18. Antiel RM, Hashim Y, Moir CR, et al. Intrabdominal venous thrombosis after colectomy in pediatric patients with chronic ulcerative colitis: incidence, treatment, and outcomes. J Pediatr Surg 2014;49(4):614–7.
19. Olen O, Askling J, Sachs MC, et al. Childhood onset inflammatory bowel disease and risk of cancer. A Swedish nationwide cohort study 1964-2014. BMJ 2017; 358:j3951.
20. Hyams J, Markowitz J, Otley A, et al. Evaluation of the pediatric Crohn disease activity index: a prospective multicenter experience. J Pediatr Gastroenterol Nutr 2005;41(4):416–21.
21. Connors J, Basseri S, Grant A, et al. Exclusive enteral nutrition therapy in paediatric Crohn's disease results in long-term avoidance of corticosteroids: results of a propensity-score matched cohort analysis. J Crohns Colitis 2017;11(9): 1063–70.
22. Alvisi P, Arrigo S, Cucchiara S, et al. Efficacy of adalimumab as second-line therapy in a pediatric cohort of Crohn's disease patients who failed infliximab therapy: the Italian Society of Pediatric Gastroenterology, Hepatology, and Nutrition experience. Biologics 2019;13:13–21.
23. Walters TD, Kim M-O, Denson LA, et al. Increased effectiveness of early therapy with anti-tumor necrosis factor-α vs an immunomodulatory in children with Crohn's disease. Gastroenterology 2014;146:383–91.
24. Kerur B, Machan JT, Shapiro JM, et al. Biologics delay progression of Crohn's disease, but not early surgery, in children. Clin Gastroenterol Hepatol 2018;16: 1467–73.
25. Egberg MD, Kappelman MD, Gulati AS. Improving care in pediatric inflammatory bowel disease. Gastroenterol Clin North Am 2018;47:909–19.
26. Mackner LM, Greenley RN, Szigethy E, et al. Psychosocial issues in pediatric inflammatory bowel disease: a clinical report of North American Society for Pediatric Gastroenterology, Hepatology, and Nutrition. J Pediatr Gastroenterol Nutr 2013;56(4):449–58.
27. Filce HG, LaVergne L. Abseentism, educational plans, and anxiety among children with incontinence and their parents. J Sch Health 2015;85(4):241–50.
28. Emerson ND, Distelberg B, Morrell HER, et al. Quality of life and school absenteeism in children with chronic illness. J Sch Nurs 2016;32(4):258–66.
29. Nguyen H-T, Minar P, Jackson K, et al. Vaccinations in immunosuppressive-dependent pediatric inflammatory bowel disease. World J Gastroenterol 2017; 23(42):7644–52.
30. David JG, Jofriet A, Seid M, et al. 'A guide to gutsy living": patient-driven development of a pediatric ostomy toolkit. Pediatrics 2018;141(5):e20172789.
31. Kim J, Ye BD. Successful transition from pediatric to adult care in inflammatory bowel disease: what is the key? Pediatr Gastroenterol Hepatol Nutr 2019;22(1): 28–40.

Ileal Pouch Complications

Jennifer A. Leinicke, MD, MPHS

KEYWORDS

- Ileal pouch • Complications • Postoperative • IPAA • IBD
- Inflammatory bowel disease • Ulcerative colitis • Continent ileostomy

KEY POINTS

- Complications after ileal pouch surgery can be categorized based on timing and etiology.
- Postoperative pelvic sepsis increases the risk of poor pouch function and pouch failure.
- Prompt treatment of septic complications increases the likelihood of pouch salvage.
- Development of Crohn's disease after ileal pouch anal anastomosis has significant symptom overlap with postoperative septic complications and pouchitis.
- Patients with an ileal pouch anal anastomosis have a small but significant risk of developing dysplasia and carcinoma of the pouch, rectal cuff, or anal transitional zone and require routine postoperative endoscopic surveillance.

The creation of an ileal pouch reservoir with ileal pouch anal anastomosis (IPAA) is a well-accepted method of restoration of intestinal continuity after total proctocolectomy. In patients who are not candidates for IPAA, a Koch pouch or continent ileostomy (CI) may be performed. The most common indications for IPAA are ulcerative colitis (UC) and familial adenomatous polyposis syndrome, whereas Crohn's disease remains controversial and a relative contraindication. In experienced hands, IPAA has a high primary success rate with acceptable functional results, high patient satisfaction, and improved quality of life. A subset of patients will develop complications unique to this procedure that can significantly affect functional outcomes and result in pouch failure.

The etiology of pouch complications can be broadly classified as infectious, inflammatory, or mechanical. Infectious complications include pelvic sepsis and anastomotic leak with resulting abscess, fistulae, or sinus tracts. Inflammatory complications include pouchitis, cuffitis, and Crohn's disease. Mechanical causes of failure result in obstruction and/or pouch disfunction. These causes include pouch stricture or fibrosis, pouch prolapse, and technical errors in construction, such as a small volume pouch, pouch volvulus, pouch septae, or a long efferent limb. The timing of pouch complications can be categorized as intraoperative—technical concerns during

Disclosures: The author has nothing to disclose.
Department of Surgery, University of Nebraska Medical Center, 983280 Nebraska Medical Center, Omaha, NE 68198-3280, USA
E-mail address: jennifer.leinicke@unmc.edu

pouch creation—versus postoperative. Early postoperative complications occur within 3 months of IPAA creation or stoma reversal, whereas late complications occur more than 3 months postoperatively. This article focuses on early and late postoperative complications of IPAA and CI.

COMPLICATIONS OF CONTINENT ILEOSTOMY

Originally described by Koch, a CI may be performed for patients who wish to avoid permanent conventional end ileostomy after proctocolectomy. The intussuscepted valve in the ileal pouch creates a functional obstruction allowing for continence, and therefore creation of a stoma that does not require the application of an appliance to collect stool. Patients intubate the stoma several times per day to empty the pouch contents. CI are most commonly used for patients with UC with a failed IPAA or in situations where primary IPAA is not possible. CIs are associated with a high reoperation rate of 30% to 58%, mostly owing to valve slippage.[1–3] Valve slippage results in progressive difficulty with pouch intubation because it creates an increasingly sharp angulation through which the tube must pass. Ultimately, valve slippage results in bowel obstruction or valve leakage (loss of continence).

The diagnosis of a slipped valve as the cause of bowel obstruction can be made clinically based on patient history and confirmed with either computed tomography scan with intravenous or oral contrast or small bowel follow through using water-soluble contrast demonstrating a diffusely dilated small bowel and ileal pouch without evidence of upstream mechanical obstruction. Initial treatment includes nasogastric tube decompression and fluid resuscitation followed by urgent endoscopic decompression with flexible pouchoscopy.[4] A 24F Medina catheter or equivalent sized silastic chest tube is placed over the pediatric esophagogastroduodenoscopy scope and the valve traversed. The catheter can then be slid over the scope into the pouch in a Seldinger technique and secured to the skin. Definitive management of the slipped valve requires pouch revision or excision.

EARLY POSTOPERATIVE COMPLICATIONS OF THE ILEAL POUCH ANAL ANASTOMOSIS
Pelvic Sepsis and Anastomotic Leak

Pelvic sepsis refers to abdominal, pelvic, or perianal infections occurring within 3 months of IPAA creation or stoma reversal. These infections can represent deep organ space surgical site infections, but usually are related to a leak in the IPAA or pouch. Pelvic sepsis occurs in up to 6% to 37% of patients,[5–8] with more recent case series reporting lower rates of 6% to 8%.[9] It is the most common cause of pouch failure. The timely diagnosis and treatment of pelvic sepsis gives the patient the best chance for a good functional outcome. Delay in diagnosis and treatment results in a scarred, noncompliant pouch with a high likelihood of pouch excision.

Ileal J pouch leaks are most frequently located at the IPAA or at the tip of the j pouch, although a leak along the body of the pouch is much less common.[10] A small leak may not become symptomatic until after stomal reversal. Most patients with pelvic sepsis and abdominopelvic abscess present with signs of infection: fever, new or increasing abdominal pain, leukocytosis, ileus, or systemic signs of sepsis, namely, tachycardia, hypotension, oliguria, or anuria. The diagnosis is confirmed by computed tomography scan of the abdomen and pelvis with oral and intravenous contrast demonstrating an abscess with an associated leak. The integrity of the pouch and anastomosis can be evaluated by either administration of transanal water-soluble contrast during the computed tomography scan or with a water-soluble contrast enema.

The treatment of an IPAA leak with pelvic sepsis depends on patient condition and includes source control and broad spectrum intravenous antibiotics (**Fig. 1**). Patients who are hemodynamically unstable with diffuse peritonitis may require return to the operating room for laparotomy and washout. If the pouch is not already defunctionalized, fecal diversion will be necessary. Stable patients may be treated with broad spectrum intravenous antibiotics and percutaneous (image guided) and/or transanal abscess drainage. Image-guided drainage is preferable if the anastomosis is intact; however, abscesses associated with an anastomotic leak are better drained transanally. One caveat of image-guided drain placement is the possibility of creating an extrasphincteric fistula.[11] Transgluteal, transperineal, and transvaginal drainage approaches are may create chronic fistulae and should be avoided.

Transanal and transanstomotic drain placement can be done during an examination under anesthesia. Typically a small mushroom or Malecot catheter is guided through the anastomotic defect and secured with suture to the anal verge. Many IPAA leaks will heal over time. Leaks that do not heal will require a redo IPAA to attempt to salvage the pouch. Ultimately, pouch salvage options depend on the patient's condition, the degree of the defect, and the presence of associated abscess.

The tip of the J leak is a less common cause of pelvic sepsis and represents a leak from the transanal or gastrointestinal anastomosis staple line on the distal ileum[10] (**Fig. 2**). These are often small and may be unrecognized until after stoma reversal. Initial management is similar to IPAA leak and includes broad spectrum antibiotics, percutaneous or endoscopic drainage, and pouch decompression. If the pouch is undiverted, fecal diversion may be required.

For leaks that do not heal with time and diversion, there are several options for salvage. The size and location of the leak dictates the salvage options. If there is sufficient length, the tip of the J can be restapled. Otherwise, the leak can be repaired primarily and imbricated. If the leak is large, not amenable to local revision, or local revision fails, the pouch will either need to be excised or redone.

Pouch sinuses are relatively uncommon and occur in 2% to 8% of patients.[12–14] The sinus represents a contained anastomotic leak. Many are asymptomatic and found incidentally on imaging or endoscopy before ileostomy closure, although they may cause symptoms of pain and pouch dysfunction (**Fig. 3**). Most pouch sinuses identified before stoma reversal close spontaneously with time and continued fecal

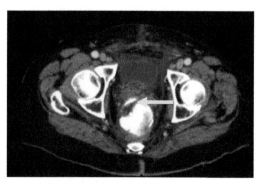

Fig. 1. Pouch–anal anastomotic leak. In the selected computed tomography cuts, the yellow arrow demonstrates the leak site, with the majority of contrast filling the pouch but leaking through an anterior defect in the pouch anal anastomosis.

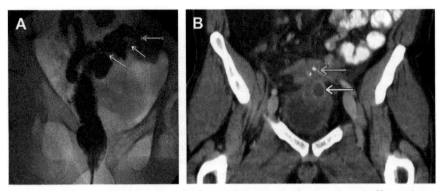

Fig. 2. Tip of the J leak. (*A*) Water-soluble contrast enema. The pouch and afferent bowel are distended with contrast. The yellow arrows are demonstrating the contrast leaking from the tip of the J. (*B*) Computed tomography scan. The green arrow indicates the pouch and the yellow arrow indicates the leak from the tip of the J.

diversion. Symptomatic sinus tracts are associated with poorer rates of healing. Treatment for sinuses that fail to close spontaneously depend on size, symptoms, location, and whether the patient is proximally diverted. Fibrin glue can be injected with very modest success rates. Other times, the sinus tract can be unroofed or incorporated into the lumen. If maneuvers these are unsuccessful, and the patient is symptomatic, the pouch may require excision and revision.

LATE POSTOPERATIVE COMPLICATIONS
Pouchitis and Cuffitis

Pouchitis is an inflammation of the ileal pouch in the absence of local complications such as a stricture or abscess. It is the most common complication after IPAA and occurs in 23% to 46% of patients.[10,15,16] Pouchitis has a wide range of disease severity. Approximately 40% of patients have a have single episode lasting less than 4 weeks without recurrence (acute pouchitis), whereas 60% of patients will have a relapsing course. Of the patients with relapsing pouchitis, 10% to 30% will develop unremitting or refractory pouchitis (chronic pouchitis). Cuffitis occurs in 2% to 6% of patients and

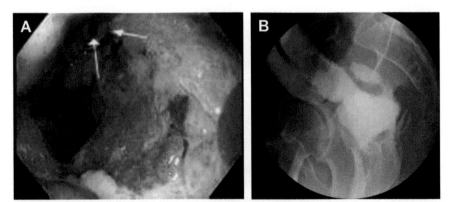

Fig. 3. Pouch sinus. (*A*). Pouchoscopy. The yellow arrows indicate the pouch sinus. (*B*) Contrast enema. The yellow arrow indicates contrast filling the sinus tract.

refers to inflammation of the retained rectal columnar mucosa above the anal transition zone. It is thought to represent recurrent or residual UC in the rectal cuff.[15]

Pouchitis results from an abnormal immune response to altered small bowel mucosal and/or luminal bacteria in a genetically susceptible individual. Genetic factors, adaptive changes in the gut mucosal structure, and alterations in the gut microbiome are also associated with pouchitis. Genetic factors clearly play a role in development of pouchitis because it occurs almost exclusively in patients with underlying UC and very rarely in those with familial adenomatous polyposis syndrome.[17,18] The reservoir function of an ileal pouch creates in fecal stasis on the small bowel mucosa resulting in metaplastic changes of villus blunting and chronic inflammation.[19] The microbiome of the pouch transitions with an increase in colonization by bacterial species more typical of colonic flora.[20] It is the combination of these factors, and likely others yet to be elucidated, that result in the syndrome of pouchitis.

For patients with UC, the risk of pouchitis is higher for those with more severe disease (pancolitis, backwash ileitis).[21,22] Extraintestinal manifestations of UC, especially primary sclerosing cholangitis, also increase risk of pouchitis.[23,24] Postoperative use of nonsteroidal anti-inflammatory drugs is associated with the development of pouchitis, and withdrawal has been demonstrated to improve symptoms.[25] Presence of perinuclear antineutrophil cytoplasmic antibodies is associated with an increased risk of chronic pouchitis.[26] Other potential risk factors include male sex, smoking, and pouch configuration.[27]

Patients with pouchitis present with nonspecific symptoms of increased stool frequency, new urgency or fecal incontinence, bloody stools, tenesmus, abdominal cramping or pelvic pain, and malaise. Pouchitis is a diagnosis of exclusion; patients with suspected pouchitis require a detailed evaluation to rule out alternative diagnoses, including a history and physical examination, stool studies, and endoscopic evaluation with biopsy.[15] A history of significant bleeding with bowel movements is more typical of cuffitis than pouchitis. New symptoms of obstructed defecation may indicate anastomotic stricture, pouch prolapse, or pelvic floor dysfunction. Pouchitis infrequently causes systemic symptoms such as fever or weight loss, which are more suggestive of infection (eg, cytomegalovirus, *Clostridium difficile*) or Crohn's disease. New or increasing mucopurulent drainage with or without fever may indicate a postoperative complication (anastomotic leak, pouch sinus, or fistula) or perianal Crohn's disease. Stool testing should be performed to rule out infection by common intestinal pathogens such as *Salmonella*, *Shigella*, *Yersinia*, *Campylobacter*, *Escherichia coli* O157:H7, and *C difficile*.

Pouchoscopy with biopsy is a crucial part of the diagnostic evaluation. On endoscopy, the pouch should be inspected for the location and severity of inflammation as well as pouch anatomy (configuration, presence of fistula, sinus, or strictures), the prepouch ileum inspected for evidence of Crohn's disease, and the anal transitional zone and rectal cuff inspected for cuffitis or neoplasia (**Figs. 4** and **5**). Multiple biopsies should be obtained to rule out Crohn's disease, ischemia, or cytomegalovirus infection. Endoscopic findings typical for pouchitis reflect the diffuse inflammatory nature of the condition and are located throughout the entire pouch, including erythema, friability with contact bleeding, erosions, ulcerations, granularity, and/or exudates. Nodularity and pseudopolyps may be seen with chronic pouchitis. Inflammatory findings occurring only in the distal pouch or that demarcate along suture lines should raise suspicion for ischemia. Cuffitis occurs as an inflammation of the rectal cuff and IPAA, and can be associated with concurrent pouchitis.

Oral antibiotics are the mainstay of treatment for pouchitis.[15,28] First-line therapy is generally either ciprofloxacin (250 mg twice daily) or metronidazole (500 mg 3 times

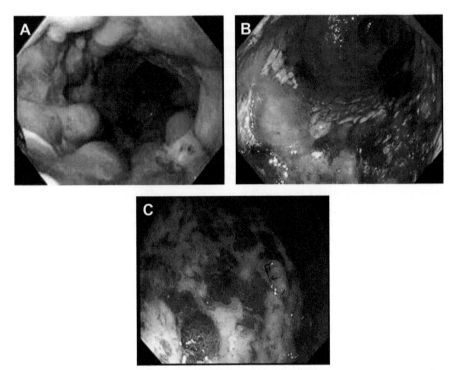

Fig. 4. Pouchitis. (*A*) Erythema, nodularity, and ulcerations. (*B*) Erythema, edema, and friability with bleeding, erosions, and ulcerations. (*C*) Erythema, edema, granularity, and exudate.

daily) for 14 days, with most patients experiencing improvement in symptoms within 3 to 4 days of initiation of therapy. Patients with refractory symptoms after first line antibiotic treatment are generally treated with either an extended course of ciprofloxacin and metronidazole for 4 weeks, or an alternative antibiotic such as rifaximin or

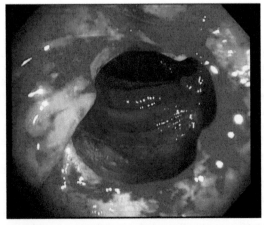

Fig. 5. Cuffitis. Pouchoscopy demonstrating inflammatory changes of the rectal remnant.

tinidazole. Patients with chronic pouchitis symptoms refractory to an extended course of antibiotics should have fecal coliform culture and sensitivity testing to guide future antibiotic therapy.[29] Additionally, alternative causes should be evaluated and treated, such as nonsteroidal anti-inflammatory drugs, Crohn's disease, primary sclerosing cholangitis, *C difficile* or cytomegalovirus infection, or concurrent mechanical complications (eg, anastomotic stricture, sinus, chronic leak, or outlet obstruction). Subsequent medical treatment for chronic pouchitis includes oral or topical 5-amino-salicylic acid, steroids (budesonide, beclomethasone), immunomodulators (azathioprine, mercaptopurine), or anti-tumor necrosis factor agents (infliximab, adalimumab).

There is conflicting evidence regarding the efficacy of probiotics for prevention and treatment of pouchitis. The most studied bacterial formulation is VSL#3 (*Lactobacillus* spp, *Bifidobacterium* spp, *Streptococcus salivarius* spp, and *Thermophilus* spp).[30–34] However, these studies are limited by small sample size, a high risk of bias, and inadequate power. A Cochrane systematic review and metaanalysis by Singh and colleagues[35] in 2015 concluded that VSL#3 may be more effective than placebo for prevention and treatment of pouchitis, but that the quality of available data is low.

Ultimately, inflammation from chronic pouchitis can cause fibrosis and scarring of the pouch, resulting in poor pouch function and pouch failure. Patients who have failed medical management and remain symptomatic may require diverting ileostomy, pouch excision, or possible redo pouch surgery.

Cuffitis is generally treated medically with topical steroids or 5-aminosalicylic acid in form of suppositories or enemas. Refractory cuffitis may require transanal mucosectomy with pouch advancement or redo IPAA.[15]

Fistula

Pouch vaginal fistulas are relatively common, occurring in 3% to 15% of women who undergo pouch surgery.[36,37] The causes of pouch vaginal fistula include separation of the IPAA owing to hematoma or abscess, pelvic sepsis, technical error (vagina inadvertently stapled into the anastomosis), staple line erosion, and development of Crohn's disease. Fistulae which occur early (within the first year after surgery) are more likely to be due to a septic complication of the IPAA, whereas fistulas that occur beyond 1 year from surgery are highly suspicious for Crohn's disease.[38] Patients with pouch vaginal fistulas present with vaginal or anal pain or discomfort, recurrent vaginal or urinary tract infections, and leakage of stool or gas through the vagina.

A diagnosis of a pouch vaginal fistula is primarily made by patient history and findings on anovaginal examination. Pelvic MRI is very sensitive in detecting fistulae and will also provide detailed information about surrounding anatomy, such as the presence of a sphincter defect. Water-soluble contrast enema with or without a vaginogram may also reveal the location of an occult fistula.

The treatment of pouch vaginal fistula depends on the timing, severity of symptoms, underlying etiology, and individual patient anatomy.[39–41] Active inflammation and induration with associated abscess is best treated initially with drainage and seton placement. Antibiotics may be necessary. If the patient has Crohn's disease, she should be treated medically with a goal of remission before attempted repair.

Before definitive repair, fecal diversion should be considered. There are several approaches for the treatment of pouch vaginal fistula. Short, low fistulae without inflammation and healthy surrounding tissue may be managed by a transanal or transvaginal advancement flap. Perineal pouch advancement with can also be considered, but is often limited by surrounding tissue fibrosis hindering mobility. A combined abdominoperineal approach with redo IPAA may be required. In experienced hands, surgical repair is successful in only 56% of cases.[41]

Pouch perineal fistula has a similar pathophysiology to pouch vaginal fistula. The diagnostic evaluation, management, and surgical options are also the similar.

Crohn's Disease

Approximately 10% to 15% of patients with presumed UC or indeterminate colitis develop Crohn's disease after IPAA.[42–44] Patients with Crohn's disease have a high risk of pouch complications resulting in pouch failure. A diagnosis of Crohn's disease after IPAA can be challenging given the similarities and overlap in symptoms between Crohn's disease and postoperative septic complications or pouchitis. Technical errors made at the time of the primary surgery are the most common cause of IPAA failure but are often mislabeled as Crohn's disease.[45]

Crohn's disease after IPAA may manifest as new perianal or vaginal fistulas unrelated to the pouch anal anastomosis, ulcerations and atypical fissures of the anal canal, inflammation of the ileal pouch with symptoms of pouchitis, or inflammation of the afferent limb or proximal small bowel. Endoscopic biopsies demonstrating nonnecrotizing granulomas or inflammatory changes in the proximal small bowel in the absence of nonsteroidal anti-inflammatory drugs use would be pathognomonic on histopathology.[44]

Treatment for Crohn's disease in the patient with an IPAA depends on the severity of the patient's symptoms, the nature of disease (fistulizing, fibrostenotic, inflammatory), and the disease location.[43] A combination of medical therapy, typically with anti-tumor necrosis factor agents, endoscopic interventions, and surgical treatments are often necessary.

Outlet Obstruction

Obstructed defecation symptoms manifest as difficulty with pouch evacuation or incomplete evacuation. This is usually due to mechanical or anatomic cause, such as anastomotic stricture, pouch prolapse, or kinking of the pouch inflow or outflow. Anastomotic strictures occur in 10% to 17% of patients.[46–48] In addition to difficulty with emptying, patients with anastomotic stricture may have nocturnal seepage. Nonfibrotic web-type strictures are often identified at stoma closure and are easily dilated. Fibrotic strictures are usually related to intraoperative or postoperative complications, such as ischemia and anastomotic leak, abscess or fistula. Chronic inflammation, from cuffitis or Crohn's disease, may also result in stricturing. Diagnosis is based on physical examination and pouchoscopy (**Fig. 6**). Symptomatic IPAA strictures may be treated with periodic endoscopic dilation, or patients may be taught to perform daily self-dilation with Hegar dilators. Refractory IPAA strictures may require advancement flap, stricturoplasty, or pouch excision.

Pouch prolapse is a rare complication of IPAA and can either be a full-thickness or mucosa-only prolapse.[49,50] Examination of the patient during Valsalva or while on the commode will confirm the diagnosis. Partial thickness prolapse is treated with mucosal resection, whereas full-thickness prolapse may be treated with transabdominal tacking of the pouch to the sacral promontory.

Inflow obstruction, or afferent limb syndrome, is caused by scar tissue creating an acute angulation or prolapse of the afferent limb at the pouch inlet. This can occur with any pouch configuration (J or S), and is diagnosed by abdominal imaging and pouchoscopy. An S pouch configuration will have an efferent limb or spout connecting the pouch to the anus. As pouches empty owing to gravity, a long efferent limb will preserve the anorectal angle and make spontaneous emptying difficult.[51] The J pouch

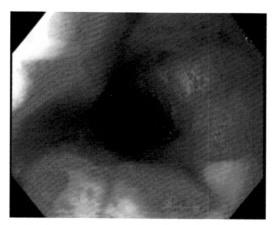

Fig. 6. IPAA stricture. Pouchoscopy demonstrating short, fibrotic stricture of a J pouch IPAA.

configuration overcomes this problem by attaching just above the dentate line, removing the anorectal angulation to facilitate emptying. However, a long rectal stump associated with a J pouch can create the same difficulty with angulation and emptying as the efferent limb of the S pouch.[51] Twisting of the pouch at the time of creation can also create outlet obstruction. Keeping stools a liquid consistency, spending increased time on the commode to empty as completely as possible, use of enemas, or self-intubation may improve symptoms. Pouch revision or excision may be required in severely symptomatic patients.

Neoplasia

Dysplasia and cancers can develop in the ileal pouch, the anal transition zone, or retained rectal mucosa after IPAA.[52] The overall risk of neoplasia is small, but increases with time, ranging from 1.3% to 2.1% at 10 years, and 3.3% to 4.2% at 20 years.[53,54] A personal or family history of colorectal cancer, UC-associated dysplasia, primary sclerosing cholangitis, familial adenomatous polyposis syndrome, and chronic pouchitis or cuffitis are risk factors for the development of pouch neoplasia. Mucosectomy at time of IPAA does not prevent development of dysplasia and cancers.[55] Even with a complete mucosectomy, small islands of rectal mucosa are left in situ. There is a lack of consensus guidelines regarding frequency of endoscopic surveillance for neoplasia after IPAA for UC. Some experts suggest that, given the relatively poor prognosis for cancers occurring after IPAA, routine surveillance with pouchoscopy and biopsy is indicated every 1 to 3 years.[52] If dysplasia is identified, ablation or excision is indicated, followed by shorter surveillance intervals of 3 to 6 months. Patients who develop carcinoma require pouch excision versus exenteration to achieve local control.

SUMMARY

Complications after ileal pouch surgery can result in poor pouch function and can have a significant negative impact on a patient's quality of life. Timely diagnosis and appropriate management of complications allows for the best chance of pouch salvage. Many complications require a multimodal approach. As with any reoperative surgery, the success of surgical revision or redo of an ileal pouch is highly dependent on the skill, judgment, and experience of the surgeon and requires an extremely motivated patient.

REFERENCES

1. Castillo E, Thomassie LM, Whitlow CB, et al. Continent ileostomy: current experience. Dis Colon Rectum 2005;48:1263–8.
2. Wasmuth HH, Myrvold HE. Durability of ileal pouch–anal anastomosis and continent ileostomy. Dis Colon Rectum 2009;52:1285–9.
3. Lan L, Fazio VW, Remzi FH, et al. Outcomes for patients undergoing continent ileostomy after a failed ileal pouch-anal anastomosis. Dis Colon Rectum 2009; 52:1409–16.
4. Church JM, Fazio VW, Lavery IC. The role of fiberoptic endoscopy in the management of the continent ileostomy. Gastrointest Endosc 1987;33(3):203–9.
5. Reissman P, Teoh TA, Weiss EG, et al. Functional outcome of the double stapled ileoanal reservoir in patients more than 60 years of age. Am Surg 1996;62: 178–83.
6. Mikkola K, Luukkonen P, Jarvinen HJ. Long-term results of restorative proctocolectomy for ulcerative colitis. Int J Colorectal Dis 1995;10:10–4.
7. Tan HT, Connolly AB, Morton D, et al. Results of restorative proctocolectomy in the elderly. Int J Colorectal Dis 1997;12:319–22.
8. Lim M, Sagar P, Abdulgader A, et al. The impact of preoperative immunomodulation on pouch-related septic complications after ileal pouch-anal anastomosis. Dis Colon Rectum 2007;50:943–51.
9. Kiely JM, Fazio VW, Remzi FH, et al. Pelvic sepsis after IPAA adversely affects function of the pouch and quality of life. Dis Colon Rectum 2012;55:387–92.
10. Emmanouil PP, Kiran RP. The failed j pouch. Clin Colon Rectal Surg 2016;29: 123–9.
11. Kirat HT, Remzi FH, Shen B, et al. Pelvic abscess associated with anastomotic leak in patients with ileal pouch-anal anastomosis (IPAA): transanastomotic or CT-guided drainage? Int J Colorectal Dis 2011;26:1469.
12. Akbari RP, Madoff RD, Parker SC, et al. Anastomotic sinuses after ileoanal pouch construction: incidence, management, and outcome. Dis Colon Rectum 2009;52: 452–5.
13. Nyam DC, Wolff BG, Dozois RR, et al. Does the presence of a pre-ileostomy closure asymptomatic pouch-anastomotic sinus tract affect success of ileal pouch anal anastomosis? J Gastrointest Surg 1997;1:274–7.
14. Swain BT, Ellis CN. Fibrin glue treatment of low rectal and pouch-anal anastomotic sinuses. Dis Colon Rectum 2004;47:253–5.
15. Shen B. Diagnosis and management of postoperative ileal pouch disorders. Clin Colon Rectal Surg 2010;23(4):259–68.
16. Coffey JC, McCarthy E, Kavanagh E, et al. Pouchitis: an evolving clinical enigma-a review. Dis Colon Rectum 2009;52(1):140–53.
17. Tjandra JJ, Fazio VW, Church JM, et al. Similar functional results after restorative proctocolectomy in patients with familial adenomatous polyposis and mucosal ulcerative colitis. Am J Surg 1993;165:322–5.
18. Penna C, Tiret E, Kartheuser A, et al. Function of ileal J pouch-anal anastomosis in patients with familial adenomatous polyposis. Br J Surg 1993;80:765–7.
19. Stallmach A, Moser C, Hero-Gross R, et al. Pattern of mucosal adaptation in acute and chronic pouchitis. Dis Colon Rectum 1999;42:1311–7.
20. Kohyama A, Ogawa H, Funayama Y, et al. Bacterial population moves toward a colon-like community in the pouch after total proctocolectomy. Surgery 2009; 145(4):435–47.

21. Achkar JP, Al-Haddad M, Lashner B, et al. Differentiating risk factors for acute and chronic pouchitis. Clin Gastroenterol Hepatol 2005;3(1):60.
22. Hashavia E, Dotan I, Rabau M, et al. Risk factors for chronic pouchitis after ileal pouch anal anastomosis: a prospective cohort study. Colorectal Dis 2012;14(11):1365–71.
23. Seril DN, Yao Q, Lashner BA, et al. Autoimmune features are associated with chronic antibiotic-refractory pouchitis. Inflamm Bowel Dis 2015;21(1):110–20.
24. Penna C, Dozois R, Tremaine W, et al. Pouchitis after ileal pouch anal anastomosis for ulcerative colitis occurs with increasing frequency in patients with associated primary sclerosing cholangitis. Gut 1996;38(2):234.
25. Shen B, Fazio VW, Remzi FH, et al. Effect of withdrawal of non-steroidal anti-inflammatory drug use on ileal pouch disorders. Dig Dis Sci 2007;52(12):3321–8.
26. Singh S, Sharma PK, Loftus EV Jr, et al. Meta-analysis: serological markers and the risk of acute and chronic pouchitis. Aliment Pharmacol Ther 2013;37(9):867.
27. Mukewar S, Wu X, Lopez R, et al. Comparison of long-term outcomes of S and J pouches and continent ileostomies in ulcerative colitis patients with restorative proctocolectomy-experience in subspecialty pouch center. J Crohns Colitis 2014;8(10):1227–36.
28. Pardi DS, D'Haens G, Shen B, et al. Clinical guidelines for management of pouchitis. Inflamm Bowel Dis 2009;15:1424.
29. McLaughlin SD, Clark SK, Shafi S, et al. Fecal coliform testing to identify effective antibiotic therapies for patients with antibiotic-resistant pouchitis. Clin Gastroenterol Hepatol 2009;7:545.
30. Gionchetti P, Rizello F, Helwig U, et al. Prophylaxis of pouchitis onset with probiotic therapy: a double-blind, placebo controlled trial. Gastroenterology 2003;124:1202.
31. Pronio A, Montesani C, Butteroni C, et al. Probiotic administration in patients with ileal pouch anal anastomosis for ulcerative colitis is associated with expansion of mucosal regulatory cells. Inflamm Bowel Dis 2008;14:662.
32. Shen B, Brzezinski A, Fazio VW, et al. Maintenance therapy with a probiotic in antibiotic-dependent pouchitis: experience in clinical practice. Aliment Pharmacol Ther 2005;22:721.
33. Mimura T, Rizello F, Helwig U, et al. Once daily high dose probiotic therapy (VSL3#) for maintaining remission in recurrent or refractory pouchitis. Gut 2004;53:108.
34. McLaughlin SD, Johnson MW, Clark SK, et al. VSL#3 for chronic pouchitis: experience in UK clinical practice. Gastroenterology 2008;134(Suppl 1):A711.
35. Singh S, Stroud AM, Holubar SD, et al. Treatment and prevention of pouchitis after ileal pouch-anal anastomosis for chronic ulcerative colitis. Cochrane Database Syst Rev 2015;(11):CD001176.
36. Lolohea S, Lynch AC, Robertson GB, et al. Ileal pouch anal anastomosis-vaginal fistula: a review. Dis Colon Rectum 2005;48:1802–10.
37. Johnson PM, O'Connor BI, Cohen Z, et al. Pouch-vaginal fistula after ileal pouch-anal anastomosis: treatment and outcomes. Dis Colon Rectum 2005;48:1249–53.
38. Nisar PJ, Kiran RP, Shen B, et al. Factors associated with ileoanal pouch failure in patients developing early or late pouch related fistula. Dis Colon Rectum 2011;54:446–53.
39. Mallick IH, Hull TL, Remzi FH, et al. Management and outcome of pouch vaginal fistulas after IPAA surgery. Dis Colon Rectum 2014;57:490–6.
40. Heriot AG, Tekkis PP, Smith JJ, et al. Management and outcome of pouch vaginal fistulas following restorative proctocolectomy. Dis Colon Rectum 2005;48:451–8.

41. Sapci I, Akeel N, DeLeon M, et al. What is the best surgical treatment of pouch-vaginal fistulas? Dis Colon Rectum 2019;62:595–9.
42. Shen B, Remzi FH, Brzezinski A, et al. Risk factors for pouch failure in patients with different phenotypes of Crohn's disease of the pouch. Inflamm Bowel Dis 2008;14:942–8.
43. Shen B, Remzi FH, Lavery IC, et al. A proposed classification of ileal pouch disorders and associated complications after restorative proctocolectomy. Clin Gastroenterol Hepatol 2008;6:145–58.
44. Goldstein NS, Sanford WW, Bodzin JH. Crohn's-like complications in patients with ulcerative colitis after total proctocolectomy and ileal pouch-anal anastomosis. Am J Surg Pathol 1997;21:1343–53.
45. Garrett KA, Remzi FH, Kirat HT, et al. Outcome of salvage surgery for ileal pouches referred with a diagnosis of Crohn's disease. Dis Colon Rectum 2009; 52(12):1967–74.
46. Lewis WG, Kuzu A, Sagar PM, et al. Stricture at the pouch-anal anastomosis after restorative proctocolectomy. Dis Colon Rectum 1994;37(2):120–5.
47. Prudhomme M, Dozois RR, Godlewski G, et al. Anal canal strictures after ileal pouch-anal anastomosis. Dis Colon Rectum 2003;46(1):20–3.
48. Kirat HT, Kiran RP, Lian L, et al. Influence of stapler size used at ileal pouch-anal anastomosis on anastomotic leak, stricture, long-term functional outcomes, and quality of life. Am J Surg 2010;200(1):68–72.
49. Joyce MR, Fazio VW, Hull TT, et al. Ileal pouch prolapse: prevalence, management, and outcomes. J Gastrointest surg 2010;14(6):993–7.
50. Ehsan M, Isler JT, Kimmins MH, et al. Prevalence and management of prolapse of the ileoanal pouch. Dis Colon Rectum 2004;47(6):885–8.
51. Church J. Implications of pouch physiology. Dis Colon Rectum 2019;62(4):510–2.
52. Khan F, Shen B. Inflammation and neoplasia of the pouch in inflammatory bowel disease. Curr Gastroenterol Rep 2019;21:10.
53. Kariv R, Remzi FH, Lian L, et al. Preoperative colorectal neoplasia increases risk for pouch neoplasia in patients with restorative proctocolectomy. Gastroenterologia 2010;139:806–12.
54. Derikx LA, Kievit W, Drenth JP, et al. Prior colorectal neoplasia is associated with increased risk of ileoanal pouch neoplasia in patients with inflammatory bowel disease. Gastroenterologia 2014;146:119–28.
55. Selvaggi F, Pellino G, Canonico S, et al. Systematic review of cuff and pouch cancer in patients with ileal pelvic pouch for ulcerative colitis. Inflamm Bowel Dis 2014;20:1296–308.

Genetic and Environmental Considerations for Inflammatory Bowel Disease

Angela Kuhnen, MD

KEYWORDS

- Inflammatory bowel disease • Crohn's disease • Ulcerative colitis • Gut microbiome
- Heritability • Fecal microbial transplantation • Pouchitis
- Ileal pouch–anal anastomosis

KEY POINTS

- Inflammatory bowel disease is an inflammatory disorder of the gastrointestinal tract driven by an exaggerated immune response to the luminal microbiota and environmental influences in a genetically susceptible individual.
- Several single-nucleotide polymorphisms have been identified that increase risk for but incompletely account for occurrence Crohn's disease, ulcerative colitis, and pouchitis.
- Several specific bacteria have been identified to increase or decrease risk of both inflammatory bowel disease and pouchitis. Decreased diversity of the intestinal microbiota correlates with intestinal inflammation, both preoperatively in ulcerative colitis and postoperatively in pouchitis.

INTRODUCTION

Inflammatory bowel disease (IBD), composed of ulcerative colitis (UC), and Crohn's disease (CD), is a chronic inflammatory disorder of the gastrointestinal tract driven by an exaggerated immune response to the luminal microbiota in a susceptible individual. It presents with a heterogenous pattern of disease severity, location, and behavior. Understanding the interaction between the host genome, the gut microbiome, and further environmental exposures in the development of IBD is in the early stages, and the factors that trigger the onset of disease in a susceptible individual remain unknown. With up to 12% of IBD patients having a family history of IBD,[1] there is a clear heritable component to IBD that is incompletely explained by genetics,[2] and the extent to which family clustering of IBD is due to pure genetic inheritance versus shared environmental and dietary factors is unclear.[3] Expanding knowledge of the gut microbiome, including changes in the microbiome that result

No disclosures.
Lahey Hospital and Medical Center, 41 Mall Road, Burlington, MA 01805, USA
E-mail address: angela.h.kuhnen@lahey.org

after surgery for IBD, lends hope for a better understanding of this complex disease process.

GENETIC AND HERITABILITY CONSIDERATIONS IN INFLAMMATORY BOWEL DISEASE

There exists a clear familial inheritance of IBD in some but not all patients, with up to 12% of IBD patients having a family history of IBD,[1] but unraveling the contribution of pure genetics versus environmental factors is challenging. The concordance rate of CD in monozygotic twins is 30% to 35%, significantly higher than the 10% to 15% observed in UC.[4] Furthermore, patients with CD at higher risk of having a first degree relative with IBD than patients with UC,[1] with the incidence rate ratio in CD 7.77 (95% CI, 7.05–8.56) and in UC 4.08 (95% CI, 3.81–4.38). A 25-year population-based cohort study of familial risk of IBD by Moller and colleagues[1] found that 20% of families with 2 or more affected members were pure CD families, 43% were pure UC families, and 36% were mixed UC and CD families.

On a population level, genome-wide association studies have compared defined ethnic populations with variable IBD risk. More than 230 single-nucleotide polymorphisms (SNPs) have been associated with IBD,[2,5] with varying risk ascribed to these polymorphisms (**Table 1**). A large common core of SNPs associated with IBD risk exists across ethnic populations,[2] with only small differences noted in the specific SNPs associated with IBD in different ethnicities. Noting that many individuals carry IBD risk alleles but never develop disease, it is clear that genetics play only a partial role in heritability of IBD.

The first risk allele variant identified for IBD was located in the nucleotide oligomerization domain containing protein 2 gene (*NOD2*). *NOD2* is cell surface receptor on gut epithelial cells, monocytes, macrophages, and lamina propria lymphocytes that binds to muramyl dipeptide, a peptidoglycan in bacterial cell walls. This results in activation of nuclear factor κB and mitogen-activated protein kinase and downstream transcription of proinflammatory cytokines.[6] The common IBD-associated *NOD2* mutations occur in the leucine-rich domain that binds muramyl dipeptides, suggesting that the loss of bacterial sensing is involved in development of IBD.[7,8] Mutations in the *NOD2* allele impart a 3.1-fold increased risk of developing CD disease.[2]

Several other risk-associated alleles have been associated with features of gut immunity, including autophagy and gut mucosal barrier function, highlighting the

Table 1 Sample of short nucleotide polymorphisms associated with inflammatory bowel disease	
	Odds Ratio for Inflammatory Bowel Disease
NOD2 (nucleotide oligomerization domain containing protein 2 gene)	3.1 for CD
IL23R (interleukin 23 receptor)	2.0
rsl748195 on *DOCK7* gene	1.07
FUT2	1.1 for CD

Data from Liu JZ, van Sommeren S, Huang H, Ng SC, Alberts R, Takahashi A, et al. Association analyses identify 38 susceptibility loci for inflammatory bowel disease and highlight shared genetic risk across populations. Nat Genet. 2015;47(9):979-86; and Jostins L, Ripke S, Weersma RK, Duerr RH, McGovern DP, Hui KY, et al. Host-microbe interactions have shaped the genetic architecture of inflammatory bowel disease. Nature. 2012;491(7422):119-24.

complex interaction between the host immune system and the gut microbiome in the pathogenesis of IBD.[3,5]

THE GUT MICROBIOME IN INFLAMMATORY BOWEL DISEASE

It has long been presumed that the gut microbiome plays a role in IBD disease activity, given the clinical improvement in IBD seen with diversion of the fecal stream and treatment with broad-spectrum antibiotics. In addition, several animal models that normally develop spontaneous colitis remain colitis-free under germ-free conditions.[9] To date, the vast majority of research on the impact of the gut microbiome on development of IBD has focused on the composition and function of bacterial populations in the gut, with the understanding that other members of the microbiome, such has fungi and viruses, likely also play a role.[3,10]

The gut microbiome is first introduced in the newborn at childbirth, after which both the gut microbiome and immune system develop in parallel over the first few years of life.[11,12]

From there, the composition of the microbiome is influenced by environmental factors, including medications, especially antimicrobials, diet, smoking, and pollution.[13,14] The Human Microbiota Project, working to define the composition and function of the gut microbiome in healthy subjects, offers an early glimpse into the interplay between the microbiome and the human host.[15]

In comparing alterations in the gut microbiome between IBD cases and healthy controls, determination of causality is limited, because active inflammation itself can alter the microbiome. Differences in microbiome profiles, however, hopefully will provide insight into the etiology and possible treatments of IBD.[10] In case-control studies, IBD patients have higher counts of bacteria belonging to the phyla Proteobacteria and Actinobacteria and fewer bacteria belonging to the phyla Bacteroidetes and Firmicutes[16] (**Table 2**). In addition, alterations in the microbiota of patients with colonic CD are different from the changes seen in ileal CD.[17]

The specific impact of host IBD risk-associated allele variants on the microbiome has been investigated on a variety of levels with mixed results. Imhann and

Table 2
Changes in abundance of gut bacteria in inflammatory bowel disease compared with healthy controls

Increased in Inflammatory Bowel Disease	Decreased in Inflammatory Bowel Disease
Proteobacteria	**Bacteroidetes**
• *Enterococcus*	• *Bacteroides*
• *Escherichia coli*	• *Prevotella*
Actinobacteria	**Firmicutes**
	• *Faecalibacterium*
	• *Roseburia*
	• *Blautia*
	• *Ruminococcus*
	• *Coprococcus*
	Actinobacteria
	• *Bifidobacterium*

Phyla in bold. Genus in italics.
Data from Frank DN, St Amand AL, Feldman RA, Boedeker EC, Harpaz N, Pace NR. Molecular-phylogenetic characterization of microbial community imbalances in human inflammatory bowel diseases. Proc Natl Acad Sci U S A. 2007;104(34):13780-5

colleagues[17] compared genotypes and gut microbiomes of IBD patients to the healthy individuals and calculated an IBD genetic risk score based on 11 allele variants known to be associated with IBD. They found that healthy individuals with a high genetic risk for IBD had alterations in their microbiome similar to changes seen in patients with active IBD, with a relative decrease in the acetate-to-butyrate converter *Roseburia*.[17] Other IBD risk-associated alleles, such as *NOD2* and the alpha^{1,2}-fucosyltransferase 2 gene (*FUT2*), have not been definitively shown to be associated with changes in the gut microbiome.[17,18] The study of the interaction between the host genome and the microbiome is still in its infancy, and this complex question is further confounded when observing this interplay in the setting of active inflammation, which in itself influences the composition of the microbiome.[3]

ENVIRONMENTAL CONSIDERATIONS FOR INFLAMMATORY BOWEL DISEASE

In addition to the heritable component of the gut microbiome, several other environmental factors have an impact on risk for IBD, many of which may confound apparent heritable effects. With migration from and industrialization of regions with traditionally low IBD prevalence, including Asia, South America, and the Middle East, IBD has arisen as a global disease with a sharp rise in prevalence,[19,20] which may be explained by changes in diet, air pollution and smoking, altitude, and urban versus rural life.[13] Piovani and colleagues[21] recently performed an umbrella review of meta-analyses evaluating 71 environmental factors that might have an impact on IBD risk. They identified 9 factors with high to moderate strength associations of increased risk of IBD and 7 protective factors (**Table 3**), among dozens of other potential risk factors.

Smoking

Smoking has long been recognized as a risk factor for IBD, primarily CD,[21] but no association has been found between childhood or prenatal second-hand smoke and IBD.[22] It is unclear to what extent smoking influences IBD risk through changes in the microbiome, direct toxin effects, or relative ischemia.

Living Conditions

The impact of hygiene and living conditions on risk of IBD is likely related to childhood antigen stimuli, which promote microbiome diversity and support development of a dominant helper T cell type 1–mediated response rather than a helper T cell type 2–mediated proinflammatory immune milieu.[23] Various other childhood exposures have protective associations against IBD to a lesser extent than childhood bed sharing, including living near farm animals, home sharing, having pets, and having 2 or more siblings.[21]

Appendectomy

Risk of developing CD in the 5 years after appendectomy was elevated compared with the general population, although this association diminished significantly 5 years after surgery, raising the question of whether early CD symptoms were interpreted as appendicitis.[21,24] On the contrary, a history of appendectomy has a strong protective association against UC.[21,25]

Dietary and Nutritional Factors

The hazard of interpreting association as causation in observational studies is important to highlight, especially in interpreting dietary and nutritional risk

Table 3
Environmental exposures and inflammatory bowel disease risk

	Increased Risk			Decreased Risk		
	Crohn's Disease	Ulcerative Colitis	Inflammatory Bowel Disease	Crohn's Disease	Ulcerative Colitis	Inflammatory Bowel Disease
Smoking	OR 1.76 (1.40–2.22)	—	—	—	OR 0.58 (0.45–0.75)	—
Physical activity	—	—	—	OR 0.63 (0.50–0.79)	—	—
Urban living	IRR 1.42 (1.26–1.60)	IRR 1.17 (1.03–1.32)	OR 1.35 (1.15–1.58)	—	—	—
Bed sharing in childhood	—	—	—	OR 0.54 (0.43–0.65)	OR 0.53 (0.24–0.82)	—
Breastfeeding	—	—	—	OR 0.71 (0.59–0.85)	OR 0.78 (0.67–0.91)	OR 0.74 (0.66–0.83)
Appendectomy	RR 1.61 (1.28–2.02)	—	—	—	OR 0.39 (0.29–0.52)	—
Tonsillectomy	OR 1.37 (1.16–1.62)	—	—	—	—	—
Antibiotic exposure	OR 1.74 (1.35–2.23) Pediatrics OR, 2.75 (1.72–4.38)	—	OR 1.57 (1.27–1.94)	—	—	—
Oral contraceptive use	OR 1.25 (1.05–1.48)	OR 1.28 (1.08–1.52)	OR 1.31 (1.15–1.50)	—	—	—
Tea consumption	—	—	—	—	RR 0.69 (0.58–0.83)	—
Consumption of soft drinks	—	RR 1.69 (1.24–2.30)	—	—	—	—
High levels of folate	—	—	—	—	OR 0.40 (0.27–0.60)	OR 0.43 (0.31–0.61)
High levels of vitamin D	—	—	—	OR 0.62 (0.46–0.84)	OR 0.40 (0.21–0.76)	—
Vitamin D deficiency	OR 1.63 (1.24–2.13)	2.28 (1.18–4.41)	1.64 (1.30–2.08)	—	—	—
Gastric *H pylori* infection	—	—	—	OR 0.38 (0.31–0.47)	OR 0.53 (0.44–0.65)	OR 0.43 (0.36–0.50)
Non-*H pylori*-like enterohepatic *Helicobacter* species	RR 1.72 (1.20–2.47)	—	—	—	—	—

Measure of association expressed as odds ratio (OR), relative risk (RR), or incidence rate ratio (IRR), all expressed with 95% CI in parentheses
Data from Piovani D, Danese S, Peyrin-Biroulet L, Nikolopoulos G, Lytras T, Bonovas S. Environmental Risk Factors for Inflammatory Bowel Diseases: An Umbrella Review of Meta-analyses. Gastroenterology. 2019(pii: S0016-5085(19)36709-5).

associations for IBD. High levels of vitamin D and folate have a protective association for both CD and UC,[21] which is more likely related to disease state than causation. Similarly, questionnaire-based studies have shown specific dietary factors associated with IBD onset. For instance, milk consumption was associated with decreased risk of CD,[26] which may be a reflection of dietary tolerance rather than causation.

Nonsteroidal Anti-inflammatory Drugs

Nonsteroidal anti-inflammatory drugs (NSAIDs) are one of the most frequently consumed medications and have been linked to the development of IBD.[27] NSAIDs function via inhibition of cyclooxygenase, which reduces synthesis of anti-inflammatory prostaglandins. A higher risk of both CD and UC has been seen in cohorts with chronic frequent NSAID use,[27] and patients with CD who frequently used NSAIDs had a 1.65-fold greater risk of showing active disease at follow-up.[28]

Antibiotic Exposure and Specific Bacteria

Previous antibiotic exposure is associated with CD in a dose-dependent fashion,[21] with greatest effect seen in pediatric CD.[29] The association of tonsillectomy with CD is thought to be a confounder, reflecting previous exposure to antibiotics.[21]

The impact of the microbiome and the immune environment has already been highlighted, but it seems that not only the specific bacteria but also the specific location of bacteria have an impact on risk of IBD. The presence of gastric *Helicobacter pylori* has protective association against CD, UC, and IBD, whereas presence of intestinal *H pylori* and enterohepatic *Helicobacter* species was associated with increased risk of CD.[21]

FECAL MICROBIOTA TRANSPLANTATION AND INFLAMMATORY BOWEL DISEASE

Using fecal microbiota transplantation (FMT) to manipulate the dysbiosis associated with IBD is an enticing approach. A recent metanalysis of 277 participants with UC suggested that FMT increases remission in UC 2-fold compared with controls, with 37% versus 18% (risk ratio [RR] 2.03; 95% CI, 1.07–3.86) achieving remission 8 weeks after FMT.[30]

A recent randomized, double-blinded clinical trial of FMT for treatment of mild to moderately active UC showed steroid-free remission of UC at 8 weeks after treatment in 32% of study patients (who received pooled donor FMT) versus 9% of controls (who received autologous FMT).[31]

Two recent small studies have provided limited insight into the utility of FMT for CD. In 1 recent study that was halted early due to presumed CD flares in 2 patients shortly after FMT, 3 of 10 patients did show clinical improvement 8 weeks after treatment.[32] Another study treated 27 CD patients with FMT and found 67% clinical remission at 8 weeks. In addition, they showed that at baseline CD patients had lower fecal microbiota diversity compared with fecal donors, and 2 weeks after FMT the fecal microbiota diversity was significantly increased in CD patients.[33]

For both UC and CD, data on complication rates and long-term efficacy with FMT are limited, and utility in treatment of pediatric patients has not been reported.

INTESTINAL INFLAMMATION AFTER ILEAL POUCH–ANAL ANASTOMOSIS
Pouchitis

Between 10% and 35% of patients with UC ultimately undergo proctocolectomy with ileal pouch–anal anastomosis (IPAA) reconstruction.[34] Approximately half of these patients suffer at least 1 episode of pouchitis, or inflammation of the ileal pouch, which manifests as increased stool frequency, hematochezia, abdominal cramping, fecal urgency and tenesmus, incontinence, and fever.[35] Over time after IPAA surgery, enterocytes change morphology and become more colon-like. Villi flatten, mucin expression changes, and the microbiome comes to resemble that of the colon.[36] It remains unclear if pouchitis represents recurrence of UC in the neocolonic environment or a unique disease state in an altered small intestinal environment. Understanding of how the microbiome and host genetics interact in IBD is nascent, and pouchitis provides a unique model in which to study these interactions.[37]

Pouchitis Risk and Surgical Indication

Patients who undergo IPAA for UC have an approximately 20% to 32% risk of developing chronic pouchitis.[38,39] In patients with familial adenomatous polyposis who undergo IPAA, however, pouchitis is extremely rare.[40] In contrast, patients with primary sclerosing cholangitis (PSC) and UC who undergo IPAA have rates of pouchitis (63%–75%[41]) compared with UC patients without PSC.[39,41] It has been suggested that pouchitis may be more common in PSC patients due to their higher risk of postoperative complications, such as pelvic sepsis, which increases risk of chronic inflammation.[42]

Impact of Genetics on Pouchitis

The selective development of pouchitis based on indication for IPAA suggests that stasis of intestinal contents in the small intestine does not fully explain the inflammatory changes that occur. Complex host genetics likely play a critical role in pouchitis development and course. Specific alleles of *TNF* and *IL-1* receptor antagonist are associated with lower rates of pouchitis, and certain alleles of *NOD2*, *TLR9*, and *CD14* are associated with increased risk of severe and recurrent pouchitis.[35]

Impact of the Microbiome on Pouchitis

The impact of variations in the microbiome of pouch patients on development of pouchitis is a complex question to address. Research has addressed both the microbiome before surgery and after surgery as well as the of impact of specific bacteria versus global diversity of bacterial populations.

Preoperatively, patients who developed pouchitis in their first year after IPAA had a consistent dysbiosis signature: higher stool levels of *Ruminococcus gnavus*, *Bacteriodes vulgatus*, and *Clostridium perfringens* and a reduction of *Blautia* and *Roseburia* compared with patients who did not develop pouchitis.[43] Notably, *Blautia* and *Roseburia* species produce butyrate, the primary energy source for colonocytes and an important factor in mucosal barrier function.[43] Additionally, patients with a history of preoperative *C difficile* colitis are at higher risk of pouch failure after reconstruction.[44] Many bacterial species have been identified by different studies to have both positive and negative associations with pouchitis.[45]

Decreased microbial diversity both preoperatively and after pouch surgery seems to correlate with inflammation. Li and colleagues[46] studied fecal samples from UC patients with and without IPAA as well as controls without UC and found higher microbial biodiversity in control groups than both UC groups and IPAA groups. In addition, pouchitis patients had less diverse microbiomes than UC patients with severe disease activity. Maharshak and colleagues[47] compared microbial diversity of stool from pouch patients who developed pouchitis within the following year and showed that patients who developed pouchitis had decreased microbial diversity compared with pouch patients who did not develop pouchitis. They also found that in normal pouch patients, microbial diversity was low in the first year after ileostomy closure and steadily increased over the following 3 years.

Morgan and colleagues[37] attempted to gain insight into host-microbe interactions by analyzing paired host transcriptome and microbial metagenome data in pouch patients. The host gene expression between the prepouch ileum and the pouch itself showed large variation within the same individual. They found, however, that despite the transcriptional differences, the microbiome in individuals remained similar between the prepouch ileum and pouch, arguing that the composition of an individual's microbiome may not be shaped by local transcriptional activity. Conversely, variation in the microbiome between individuals did not associate with significant differences in gene expression but rather with history of antibiotic treatment.

Insight from Treatments of Pouchitis

Antibiotics have been widely used for primary treatment of IBD, although supporting data are limited. Broad-spectrum antibiotics are at times used to treat CD flares, both for ileocolonic and perianal disease, with mixed results.[48] A recent retrospective cohort study evaluated a 3-month course of low-dose metronidazole after ileal resection with primary anastomosis for CD and showed a protective effect of metronidazole 1 year after surgery, with 20% of treated patients showing endoscopic recurrence versus 54% of control patients.[49] Use of antibiotics in the treatment of UC has been shown to be ineffective at achieving remission in severe UC.[48] Treatment options for acute pouchitis include both ciprofloxacin and metronidazole, with some evidence that ciprofloxacin may be more effective than metronidazole[50] but generally with more anecdotal than scientific evidence.

Use of probiotics in IPAA has been suggested for both treatment and prevention of pouchitis.[35] One prospective randomized double-blind, placebo-controlled trial of VSL#3 (Alfasigma USA, inc, Covington, LA) versus placebo for 1 year starting immediately after ileostomy closure found pouchitis rates were 10% in VSL#3 treated patients versus 40% in placebo patients during the treatment year.[51] A recent metanalysis of treatment strategies for chronic pouchitis suggested that VSL#3 may effective at maintaining remission,[50] with 85% of treated patients versus 3% of controls maintaining remission at 9 to 12 months. Evidence is weaker for use of VSL#3 for chronic prevention of pouchitis.[50]

A recent small pilot study of FMT for pouchitis showed improvement in bowel movement frequency but no change in pouchitis disease activity index, endoscopy scores, histology findings, or bacterial microbiota profiles 4 weeks after FMT.[52]

SUMMARY

The interaction of the environment, gut microbiome, and host genetics in IBD and pouchitis is multifaceted and challenging to tease apart, but it is clear that the microbiota plays a central role in mediating both healthy and diseased states. Manipulation of the interface between intestinal microbiota and the host immune system will likely allow for further understanding of disease phenotypes and novel therapies for IBD.

REFERENCES

1. Moller FT, Andersen V, Wohlfahrt J, et al. Familial risk of inflammatory bowel disease: a population-based cohort study 1977-2011. Am J Gastroenterol 2015; 110(4):564–71.

2. Liu JZ, van Sommeren S, Huang H, et al. Association analyses identify 38 susceptibility loci for inflammatory bowel disease and highlight shared genetic risk across populations. Nat Genet 2015;47(9):979–86.
3. Turpin W, Goethel A, Bedrani L, et al. Determinants of IBD heritability: genes, bugs, and more. Inflamm Bowel Dis 2018;24(6):1133–48.
4. Brant SR. Update on the heritability of inflammatory bowel disease: the importance of twin studies. Inflamm Bowel Dis 2011;17(1):1–5.
5. Jostins L, Ripke S, Weersma RK, et al. Host-microbe interactions have shaped the genetic architecture of inflammatory bowel disease. Nature 2012; 491(7422):119–24.
6. Barnich N, Aguirre JE, Reinecker HC, et al. Membrane recruitment of NOD2 in intestinal epithelial cells is essential for nuclear factor-{kappa}B activation in muramyl dipeptide recognition. J Cell Biol 2005;170(1):21–6.
7. Eckmann L, Karin M. NOD2 and Crohn's disease: loss or gain of function? Immunity 2005;22(6):661–7.
8. Maeda S, Hsu LC, Liu H, et al. Nod2 mutation in Crohn's disease potentiates NF-kappaB activity and IL-1beta processing. Science 2005;307(5710):734–8.
9. Hudcovic T, Stěpánková R, Cebra J, et al. The role of microflora in the development of intestinal inflammation: acute and chronic colitis induced by dextran sulfate in germ-free and conventionally reared immunocompetent and immunodeficient mice. Folia Microbiol (Praha) 2001;46(6):565–72.
10. Sartor RB, Wu GD. Roles for intestinal bacteria, viruses, and fungi in pathogenesis of inflammatory bowel diseases and therapeutic approaches. Gastroenterology 2017;152(2):327–39.e4.
11. Bokulich NA, Chung J, Battaglia T, et al. Antibiotics, birth mode, and diet shape microbiome maturation during early life. Sci Transl Med 2016;8(343):343ra82.
12. Dominguez-Bello MG, De Jesus-Laboy KM, Shen N, et al. Partial restoration of the microbiota of cesarean-born infants via vaginal microbial transfer. Nat Med 2016;22(3):250–3.
13. Ananthakrishnan AN, Bernstein CN, Iliopoulos D, et al. Environmental triggers in IBD: a review of progress and evidence. Nat Rev Gastroenterol Hepatol 2018; 15(1):39–49.
14. Turpin W, Espin-Garcia O, Xu W, et al. Association of host genome with intestinal microbial composition in a large healthy cohort. Nat Genet 2016;48(11):1413–7.
15. Lloyd-Price J, Mahurkar A, Rahnavard G, et al. Strains, functions and dynamics in the expanded human microbiome project. Nature 2017;550(7674):61–6.
16. Frank DN, St Amand AL, Feldman RA, et al. Molecular-phylogenetic characterization of microbial community imbalances in human inflammatory bowel diseases. Proc Natl Acad Sci U S A 2007;104(34):13780–5.
17. Imhann F, Vich Vila A, Bonder MJ, et al. Interplay of host genetics and gut microbiota underlying the onset and clinical presentation of inflammatory bowel disease. Gut 2018;67(1):108–19.
18. Bonder MJ, Kurilshikov A, Tigchelaar EF, et al. The effect of host genetics on the gut microbiome. Nat Genet 2016;48(11):1407–12.
19. Kaplan GG. The global burden of IBD: from 2015 to 2025. Nat Rev Gastroenterol Hepatol 2015;12(12):720–7.
20. Ananthakrishnan AN. Epidemiology and risk factors for IBD. Nat Rev Gastroenterol Hepatol 2015;12(4):205–17.
21. Piovani D, Danese S, Peyrin-Biroulet L, et al. Environmental risk factors for inflammatory bowel diseases: an umbrella review of meta-analyses. Gastroenterology 2019;157(3):647–59.e4.

22. Jones DT, Osterman MT, Bewtra M, et al. Passive smoking and inflammatory bowel disease: a meta-analysis. Am J Gastroenterol 2008;103(9):2382–93.
23. Kostic AD, Xavier RJ, Gevers D. The microbiome in inflammatory bowel disease: current status and the future ahead. Gastroenterology 2014;146(6):1489–99.
24. Kaplan GG, Jackson T, Sands BE, et al. The risk of developing Crohn's disease after an appendectomy: a meta-analysis. Am J Gastroenterol 2008;103(11): 2925–31.
25. Sahami S, Kooij IA, Meijer SL, et al. The link between the appendix and ulcerative colitis: clinical relevance and potential immunological mechanisms. Am J Gastroenterol 2016;111(2):163–9.
26. Opstelten JL, Leenders M, Dik VK, et al. Dairy products, dietary calcium, and risk of inflammatory bowel disease: results from a european prospective cohort investigation. Inflamm Bowel Dis 2016;22(6):1403–11.
27. Ananthakrishnan AN, Higuchi LM, Huang ES, et al. Aspirin, nonsteroidal anti-inflammatory drug use, and risk for Crohn disease and ulcerative colitis: a cohort study. Ann Intern Med 2012;156(5):350–9.
28. Long MD, Kappelman MD, Martin CF, et al. Role of nonsteroidal anti-inflammatory drugs in exacerbations of inflammatory bowel disease. J Clin Gastroenterol 2016; 50(2):152–6.
29. Ungaro R, Bernstein CN, Gearry R, et al. Antibiotics associated with increased risk of new-onset Crohn's disease but not ulcerative colitis: a meta-analysis. Am J Gastroenterol 2014;109(11):1728–38.
30. Imdad A, Nicholson MR, Tanner-Smith EE, et al. Fecal transplantation for treatment of inflammatory bowel disease. Cochrane Database Syst Rev 2018;(11):CD012774.
31. Costello SP, Hughes PA, Waters O, et al. Effect of fecal microbiota transplantation on 8-week remission in patients with ulcerative colitis: a randomized clinical trial. JAMA 2019;321(2):156–64.
32. Gutin L, Piceno Y, Fadrosh D, et al. Fecal microbiota transplant for Crohn disease: a study evaluating safety, efficacy, and microbiome profile. United European Gastroenterol J 2019;7(6):807–14.
33. Yang Z, Bu C, Yuan W, et al. Fecal microbiota transplant via endoscopic delivering through small intestine and colon: no difference for crohn's disease. Dig Dis Sci 2019. [Epub ahead of print].
34. Landy J, Al-Hassi HO, McLaughlin SD, et al. Etiology of pouchitis. Inflamm Bowel Dis 2012;18(6):1146–55.
35. Lichtenstein L, Avni-Biron I, Ben-Bassat O. The current place of probiotics and prebiotics in the treatment of pouchitis. Best Pract Res Clin Gastroenterol 2016; 30(1):73–80.
36. Young VB, Raffals LH, Huse SM, et al. Multiphasic analysis of the temporal development of the distal gut microbiota in patients following ileal pouch anal anastomosis. Microbiome 2013;1(1):9.
37. Morgan XC, Kabakchiev B, Waldron L, et al. Associations between host gene expression, the mucosal microbiome, and clinical outcome in the pelvic pouch of patients with inflammatory bowel disease. Genome Biol 2015;16:67.
38. Tyler AD, Milgrom R, Stempak JM, et al. The NOD2insC polymorphism is associated with worse outcome following ileal pouch-anal anastomosis for ulcerative colitis. Gut 2013;62(10):1433–9.
39. Penna C, Dozois R, Tremaine W, et al. Pouchitis after ileal pouch-anal anastomosis for ulcerative colitis occurs with increased frequency in patients with associated primary sclerosing cholangitis. Gut 1996;38(2):234–9.

40. McLaughlin SD, Clark SK, Tekkis PP, et al. The bacterial pathogenesis and treatment of pouchitis. Therap Adv Gastroenterol 2010;3(6):335–48.

41. Sinakos E, Samuel S, Enders F, et al. Inflammatory bowel disease in primary sclerosing cholangitis: a robust yet changing relationship. Inflamm Bowel Dis 2013; 19(5):1004–9.

42. Gorgun E, Remzi FH, Manilich E, et al. Surgical outcome in patients with primary sclerosing cholangitis undergoing ileal pouch-anal anastomosis: a case-control study. Surgery 2005;138(4):631–7 [discussion: 7–9].

43. Machiels K, Sabino J, Vandermosten L, et al. Specific members of the predominant gut microbiota predict pouchitis following colectomy and IPAA in UC. Gut 2017;66(1):79–88.

44. Skowron KB, Lapin B, Rubin M, et al. Clostridium difficile infection in ulcerative colitis: can alteration of the gut-associated microbiome contribute to pouch failure? Inflamm Bowel Dis 2016;22(4):902–11.

45. Segal JP, Ding NS, Worley G, et al. Systematic review with meta-analysis: the management of chronic refractory pouchitis with an evidence-based treatment algorithm. Aliment Pharmacol Ther 2017;45(5):581–92.

46. Li KY, Wang JL, Wei JP, et al. Fecal microbiota in pouchitis and ulcerative colitis. World J Gastroenterol 2016;22(40):8929–39.

47. Maharshak N, Cohen NA, Reshef L, et al. Alterations of enteric microbiota in patients with a normal ileal pouch are predictive of pouchitis. J Crohn's Colitis 2017; 11(3):314–20.

48. Gionchetti P, Rizzello F, Lammers KM, et al. Antibiotics and probiotics in treatment of inflammatory bowel disease. World J Gastroenterol 2006;12(21):3306–13.

49. Glick LR, Sossenheimer PH, Ollech JE, et al. Low-dose metronidazole is associated with a decreased rate of endoscopic recurrence of Crohn's disease after ileal resection: a retrospective cohort study. J Crohns Colitis 2019;13(9):1158–62.

50. Singh S, Stroud AM, Holubar SD, et al. Treatment and prevention of pouchitis after ileal pouch-anal anastomosis for chronic ulcerative colitis. Cochrane Database Syst Rev 2015;(11):CD001176.

51. Gionchetti P, Rizzello F, Helwig U, et al. Prophylaxis of pouchitis onset with probiotic therapy: a double-blind, placebo-controlled trial. Gastroenterology 2003; 124(5):1202–9.

52. Selvig D, Piceno Y, Terdiman J, et al. Fecal microbiota transplantation in pouchitis: clinical, endoscopic, histologic, and microbiota results from a pilot study. Dig Dis Sci 2019. [Epub ahead of print].

Inflammatory Bowel Disease and Short Bowel Syndrome

Matthew A. Fuglestad, MD, Jon S. Thompson, MD*

KEYWORDS

- Intestinal failure • Short bowel syndrome • Inflammatory bowel disease
- Crohn's disease • Ulcerative colitis

KEY POINTS

- Inflammatory bowel disease, in particular Crohn's disease, predisposes patients to development of short bowel syndrome/intestinal failure.
- When operative management is required for inflammatory bowel disease, attempts should be made to preserve enough intestinal length for enteral autonomy.
- Both medical and surgical therapies for the treatment of intestinal failure/short bowel syndrome, including intestinal transplantation, have been demonstrated to be safe and feasible in the setting of inflammatory bowel disease.
- Chronic intestinal failure and short bowel syndrome in the setting of inflammatory bowel disease is a rare and complex disease process that mandates a multidisciplinary approach.

INTRODUCTION

Intestinal failure (IF) is an uncommon and highly morbid condition with few definitive treatment options once developed.[1,2] IF is defined by a reduction in gut function below the minimum necessary for absorption of macronutrients and/or water and electrolytes, such that intravenous supplementation (IVS) is required to maintain health and/or growth.[3] This is contrasted with intestinal insufficiency where absorptive function is compromised, resulting in malabsorption, but does not require IVS.[1] Despite its rarity, the societal and personal costs of IF are substantial.[2] Five pathologic mechanisms are commonly responsible for producing IF: short bowel syndrome (SBS), intestinal fistulae, dysmotility disorders (chronic intestinal pseudo-obstruction), mechanical obstruction, and extensive small bowel mucosal disease.[3] Although these pathologies may interact to produce IF, SBS is the primary cause of greater than 60% of

Disclosure Statement: The authors have nothing to disclose.
Department of Surgery, Division of General Surgery, University of Nebraska Medical Center, 983280 Nebraska Medical Center, Omaha, NE 68198-3280, USA
* Corresponding author.
E-mail address: jthompso@unmc.edu

Surg Clin N Am 99 (2019) 1209–1221
https://doi.org/10.1016/j.suc.2019.08.010
0039-6109/19/© 2019 Elsevier Inc. All rights reserved.

documented cases of IF due to benign etiologies and is the most common indication for intestinal transplantation (IT) globally.[4–6]

SBS is diagnosed clinically when patients are unable to maintain protein-energy, fluid, electrolyte, or micronutrient balance, generally in the setting of a total small intestinal length of less than 150 cm to 200 cm.[3] Remnant anatomy is classified by the presence of an enterostomy and the remaining colon in continuity (**Fig. 1**). Nutritional prognosis is closely linked to remnant anatomy, patient demographics, and treatment-related factors (**Fig. 2**). Long-term parenteral nutrition (PN) often is required when the small bowel remnant is less than 120 cm in the presence of an enterostomy. Patients with full colonic continuity, however, may be weaned from PN with less than 60 cm of small bowel. No matter the anatomic configuration, all patients are predisposed to altered intestinal transit and malabsorption.[6,7]

The remnant length, function, and ability for remnant adaptation influence whether SBS results in intestinal insufficiency or failure. Intestinal adaptation plateaus within 1 years to 2 years after the diagnosis of SBS and few patients who require PN beyond 2 years regain enteral autonomy without additional medical or surgical therapy.[8] In these patients, special consideration must be given to optimize the function of supporting digestive organs to promote enteral autonomy.

RISK FACTORS AND RELATION TO INFLAMMATORY BOWEL DISEASE

SBS develops from repeated or massive intestinal resection commonly as a result of malignancy, Crohn's disease (CD), mesenteric ischemia, or surgical complications.[5,8,9] Although risk factors associated with SBS are well known, there is limited information

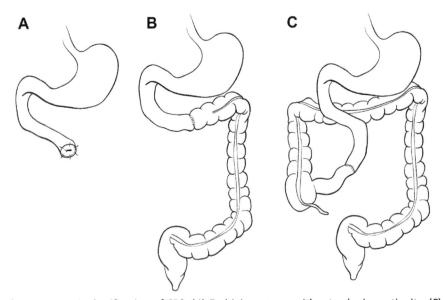

Fig. 1. Anatomic classification of SBS. (*A*) End jejunostomy without colonic continuity. (*B*) Jejunocolic anastomosis without the presence of the ileocecal valve and partial colonic continuity. (*C*) Jejunoileal anastomosis with presence of ileocecal valve and intact colon in continuity. (*From* Thompson JS, Rochling FA, Weseman RA, et al. Current management of short bowel syndrome. *Curr Probl Surg.* 2012 Feb;49(2):52-115. https://doi.org/10.1067/j.cpsurg.2011.10.002; with permission.)

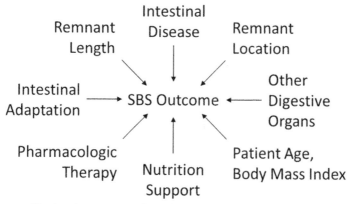

Fig. 2. Factors affecting the outcome of SBS. (*From* Thompson JS, Rochling FA, Weseman RA, et al. Current management of short bowel syndrome. *Curr Probl Surg.* 2012 Feb;49(2):52-115. https://doi.org/10.1067/j.cpsurg.2011.10.002.)

regarding its incidence, in part due to its rarity and evolving definition.[5,10] A review of the United States national home PN registry in 1992 demonstrated SBS was associated with 35% of patients receiving PN.[10,11] More recently, a European study of 65 home PN centers demonstrated that 64% of patients without malignancy required TPN due to SBS.[5] The global incidence and prevalence of SBS/IF, however, remain unknown.[5,10]

SBS may develop as a consequence of both of ulcerative colitis (UC) and CD.[5,12,13] Incorrect or delayed diagnosis of inflammatory bowel disease (IBD), need for excision of continuity-preserving reservoirs, and the propensity for mesenteric venous thrombosis in IBD are risk factors for SBS shared by both UC and CD.[8,14,15] UC, compared with CD, more commonly develops SBS acutely after operative complications or intra-abdominal emergencies as opposed to by direct involvement of the small bowel. Additionally, the increased utilization of continuity-preserving procedures in UC places patients at risk for small bowel loss due to pouch-related complications, such as pelvic adhesive disease, and pouch volvulus. Furthermore, elective colectomy represents the most common initial operation prior to development of postoperative SBS compared with those undergoing other intra-abdominal operations.[8] Lastly, for the UC patient after proctocoloectomy, the loss of colonic continuity significantly alters fluid and sodium balance and eliminates the possibility of recruiting the large intestine to treat SBS.[6]

The nature of CD uniquely predisposes patients to development of SBS as patients at baseline have shortened remnants and often have had colectomy or ileal resections. In addition, the small bowel is frequently involved and patients may develop fistulas, mechanical obstruction(s), and mucosal damage of the remaining intestine. Penetrating and stricturing variants of CD may be at the highest risk for SBS/IF, although initial site of disease is not independently predictive of long-term need for parenteral support.[12,16] This is of particular importance because the incidence of IBD is increasing, with notable increases in the pediatric population.[17–19]

Development of IF due to CD remains rare.[5] A recent review suggests the incidence of SBS is 0.8% at 5 years, 3.6% at 10 years, and 8.5% at 20 years after a patient's index operation for CD.[20] Up to 60% of patients with CD require a resection at some point in their disease course, with up to a third of patients requiring multiple small bowel resections.[21] With this knowledge, the medical community has aimed to reduce the need for operative intervention with the development of novel therapies and changes in treatment paradigms, including top-down management of IBD.

INITIAL MANAGEMENT OF INFLAMMATORY BOWEL DISEASE–RELATED SHORT BOWEL SYNDROME

IBD-related SBS frequently occurs as a result of sequential bowel resection.[12] Reviewing the authors' experience, SBS often develops in middle-aged individuals 18 years after their initial diagnosis of CD.[12] At that time, patients have on average undergone 4 previous resections and likely have been exposed to either immunomodulators or biologicals.[12] Anatomically, patients with SBS commonly possess less than 120 cm of small bowel, and approximately half have a colonic remnant or an ostomy.[12] In addition to strict medical control of their underlying IBD, these patients should electively undergo a full nutritional work-up and assessment of parenteral fluid and nutrition needs and be evaluated by an intestinal rehabilitation program to maximize the chance of regaining enteral autonomy.

IBD-related SBS also may develop as a result of catastrophic intraabdominal processes (perforation, fistula, and perioperative complications) leaving patients critically ill. Early goals in management are centered on controlling sepsis, restoring hemodynamics, and preventing further small bowel loss. No matter the initial insult, only grossly nonviable bowel should be removed in an attempt to preserve intestinal length. Tenuous bowel should be evaluated over time and with appropriate resuscitation. At the time of definitive abdominal closure, the location of all resected bowel, total remaining intestinal length, and presence of an enterostomy should be documented carefully.

After the diagnosis of SBS, a multidisciplinary team familiar with the management of SBS should be involved. Comprehensive care represents an interplay between medical rehabilitation, surgical rehabilitation, and transplantation (**Fig. 3**). Important components of an intestinal rehabilitation program include gastrointestinal/transplant surgeons, gastroenterologists, pharmacists, nutritionists, nurse coordinators, social workers, and psychologists. Enteral nutrition should be implemented early to promote intestinal adaption and prevent mucosal atrophy whenever feasible. The decision to place a permanent feeding tube versus temporary methods of delivery is made primarily based on the perceived duration of time a patient requires supplemental nutrition.

The benefits of enteral nutrition must be weighed against the propensity of SBS patients for malabsorption. PN is needed in approximately 60% of those with SBS in the acute setting to maintain fluid, nutrient, and energy balance.[12] Of these patients, approximately 40% require PN for greater than 1 year.[12] Enteral feeding should be titrated to minimize malabsorptive losses and increased, as able, to support nutritional requirements. Oral feeding should be encouraged avoiding foods with high-fat and simple sugar content. Fluid losses can be improved with use of dietary fiber, agents

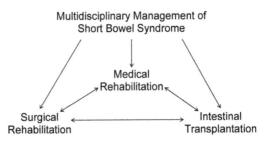

Fig. 3. Multidisciplinary management of SBS. (*From* Thompson JS, Rochling FA, Weseman RA, et al. Current management of short bowel syndrome. *Curr Probl Surg.* 2012 Feb;49(2):52-115. https://doi.org/10.1067/j.cpsurg.2011.10.002.)

to slow intestinal transit (diphenoxylate, loperamide, codeine sulfate, and tincture of opium), and antisecretory medications (proton pump inhibitors, H_2-antagonists, octreotide). Malabsorption and fluid losses often improve over the first 1 year to 2 years as the intestinal remnant adapts and may allow for gradual withdrawal of PN.

The optimal composition of enteral formula in IBD-related SBS has yet to be defined and, therefore, the specific considerations for its use are similar to other situations where enteral supplementation is required.[1] Polymeric isotonic compositions are recommended; however, semielemental and elemental formulas all can be used safely in SBS. Formerly, glutamine-rich formulas and glutamine in combination with the use of growth hormone were thought to promote intestinal adaption. These therapies are not generally recommended, however, because there are reservations regarding the long-term benefits of use.[1,6] Similarly, probiotics and omega-3 fatty acids do not have a clear role in the management of IBD-related SBS.[1,6] Overall, when choosing an enteral formula, the ability of the patient to tolerate feedings that meet nutritional goals and the associated cost should be the major drivers of the decision.

MEDICAL THERAPY FOR INFLAMMATORY BOWEL DISEASE-RELATED SHORT BOWEL SYNDROME
Glucagon-Like Peptide-2 Analogs

Teduglutide is a recombinant, 33-amino acid analog of glucagon-like peptide-2 (GLP-2), which is Food and Drug Administration approved for the treatment of SBS.[22] Administration of GLP-2 has been demonstrated to reduce secretory losses, decrease gastric motility, and stimulate villous hyperplasia, thus making it an attractive target for the treatment of SBS/IF.[23-26] A phase III trial of SBS/IF patients receiving teduglutide achieved higher rates of meaningful reduction in parenteral support (defined as a >20% reduction in optimized baseline parenteral support volume) compared with placebo at 24 weeks of treatment (63% vs 30%, respectively).[27] Further studies have demonstrated similar efficacy in reducing or eliminating PN support, with durable improvements seen out to 3 years.[28-31]

Long-term use of teduglutide seems well tolerated with an acceptable safety profile.[28-31] Common adverse reactions generally are minor and include abdominal pain/distension, nausea, and vomiting.[22,28-31] Obstructive symptoms have been reported, and stoma-related complications, including stomal hypertrophy, were significantly more common in patients receiving teduglutide compared with placebo.[22] Furthermore, teduglutide may increase the propensity for gastrointestinal polyps/neoplasia.[22] Although SBS patients with in situ colon at baseline are not at an elevated risk for colorectal cancer, close endoscopic surveillance is recommended for any patient receiving GLP-2 based therapy with a remaining colonic remnant.[22,32]

There are few data specifically addressing the use of teduglutide in IBD-related SBS/IF. Overall, the results seem favorable and mirror those of SBS patients without IBD. Kochar and colleagues[33] have reported a series of patients with CD-related SBS/IF treated with teduglutide. All 13 patients were able to reduce IVS (median reduction 3.1 L per week) and in 6 patients (46%) IVS no longer was required. Importantly, these results occurred in the setting of high risk CD (stricturing or penetrating disease) and in patients on immunosuppressive medications.[33] Furthermore, George and colleagues[34] have reported 3 cases of teduglutide use in patient with CD who do not meet strict criteria for diagnosis of IF. All reported patient improved their nutritional status and the use of teduglutide was associated with the resolution of an enterocutaneous fistula in both patients with fistulas. The investigators suggested teduglutide may have a role in treatment of CD by enhancing epithelial recovery. These are promising results, especially because teduglutide may represent a potential therapeutic target for CD.[35] Larger and longer duration studies, however, are needed to routinely recommend teduglutide in CD-related SBS.

Immunomodulators and biologics

There has been a trend toward earlier and increased utilization of immunomodulators and biologic agents in patients with CD.[36,37] Although these therapies are effective in achieving disease control, it is unknown if they have led to a decrease in the incidence of SBS/IF or a reduction in SBS/IF-related complications. Comparing the IBDSL cohort during the prebiologic era to 2 postbiologic time periods demonstrates a significant decrease in 5-year need for surgery. CD patients with SBS continue, however, to have a steady rate of resection in the postbiologic era.[37,38]

The success of combination therapy in CD should be weighed against the potential for complications. McKenna and colleagues[39] recently reported preoperative triple immunosuppression (defined as the combination of a biological agent, immunomodulator, and corticosteroid) was independently associated with postoperative intra-abdominal sepsis after ileocecectomy.

SURGICAL MANAGEMENT OF INFLAMMATORY BOWEL DISEASE-RELATED SHORT BOWEL SYNDROME

Primary prevention of functional small bowel loss is the overarching principle for prevention of SBS/IF in IBD patients. Close communication between medical and surgical teams is essential to optimize management. When surgery is necessary, bowel resections should be carried out to visibly and palpably normal tissue. It is not necessary to resect to microscopically negative margins in an attempt to prevent recurrence. Similarly, in patients with Crohn's colitis, segmental colectomy with restoration of intestinal continuity is ideal unless otherwise contraindicated.

Strictureplasty is an effective way to preserve bowel length in CD, but it is used in less than 10% of SBS patients.[12] Strong consideration should be given to strictureplasty in the presence of previously diagnosed SBS. In the absence of active Crohn's colitis or severe perianal disease, recruitment of the remaining in situ colon should be considered in refractory cases of SBS/IF. Recruitment can be accomplished with full restoration of colonic continuity or by creation of a distal colostomy. This promotes additional fluid absorption and increases nutrient absorption by allowing for short chain fatty acid production by intestinal flora, addressing 2 of the major challenges of SBS/IF.[6]

Surgical rehabilitation involves nontransplant procedures to relieve obstructions, increase/recruit additional intestinal length, slow intestinal transit, and optimize intestinal diameter to promote function. Additionally, surgery therapy for SBS aims at prevention of SBS-related complications. The specific procedures available to the SBS/IF patient are influenced by the remaining intestinal anatomy, the presence of bacterial overgrowth, and the clinical status of the patient (**Table 1**). When medical and surgical rehabilitation is insufficient to promote health/growth or complications of PN arise, IT may be considered.

Intestinal Lengthening Procedures

Longitudinal intestinal lengthening and tailoring (LILT [Bianchi procedure]) and serial transverse enteroplasty (STEP) are the standard operations for increasing intestinal surface area, promoting intestinal function, and treating bacterial overgrowth in patients with SBS (**Figs. 4** and **5**).[40–42] LILT was first described in 1980 and STEP later

Table 1		
Surgical therapy for short bowel syndrome		
Intestinal Anatomy	**Clinical Status**	**Surgical Therapy**
Adequate intestinal length (remnant >120 cm)		
Normal diameter bowel	Enteral nutrition only	Optimize intestinal function
Dilated bowel	Bacterial overgrowth	Treat obstruction/intestinal tapering
Marginal length (remnant 60–120 cm)		
Normal diameter bowel	PN/rapid transit	Recruit additional length/ procedure to slow transit
Dilated bowel	PN/bacterial overgrowth	Intestinal lengthening
Short length (remnant <60 cm)		
Normal diameter bowel	PN	Optimize intestinal function
Dilated bowel	PN/bacterial overgrowth	Intestinal lengthening
Short length (remnant <60 cm)	Complications from PN	IT

Adapted from Thompson JS, Rochling FA, Weseman RA, et al. Current management of short bowel syndrome. Curr Probl Surg. 2012 Feb;49(2):52-115. https://doi.org/10.1067/j.cpsurg.2011.10.002.

in 2003.[43,44] The success and lower complexity of STEP, however, have made it the predominant operation for intestinal lengthening today and more attractive for use in CD.[41] In a retrospective comparison of LILT and STEP, both procedures produced similar improvements in weaning PN (STEP, 60%, vs LILT, 55%), with a trend toward earlier resolution of PN requirements in STEP.[41] Although more frequently used in the pediatric population, both procedures are effective at improving intestinal function and length in adults in small bowel that has dilated to 3 cm to 4 cm.[42] In the authors' experience, greater than 50% of adults who are candidates for these procedures regain enteral autonomy while avoiding the need for IT.[45] The most common complication after these operations are adhesive small bowel obstructions or stenosis of the divided bowel.[45]

There are few data regarding the safety of these operations in CD. The authors have performed the STEP procedure in 2 patients with CD-related SBS.[12] Both patients had uneventful recoveries without early staple line leak, fistula formation, or CD recurrence.[12] Long-term outcomes of these procedures are not known in CD and, therefore, should be considered only in patients who are not candidates for IT who are highly motivated to wean from PN.

Segmental Reversal of the Small Bowel

In the setting of rapid intestinal transit and malabsorption, consideration of a reversed intestinal segment is a viable treatment strategy for those with SBS. In the largest series of patients undergoing segmental reversal of the small bowel (SRSB), 45% of patients were able to be weaned from PN support at 5-year follow-up.[46] Patients unable to fully discontinue PN also derived benefit from the operation, with a median decrease from 7 to 4 PN-dependent days per week. Early utilization of SRSB and a reversal segment greater than 10 cm were predictive of successful and more rapid weaning.[46] Complications generally were minor and none of the patients alive at 5 years required takedown of their reversed segment. These results mirror the authors' experience, with 56% of patients weaned from TPN at a mean follow-up of 65 months.[9]

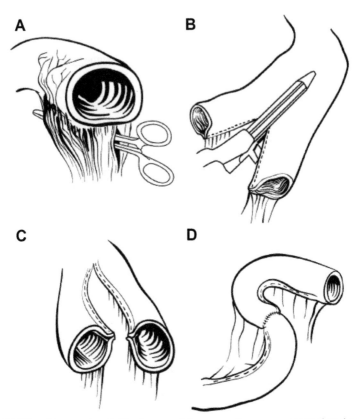

Fig. 4. LILT (Bianchi procedure). The leaves of the mesentery are separated and a tunnel is created to separate the vasculature to alternate sides (*A*). The linear stapler is passed through this tunnel and the bowel is divided longitudinally (*B, C*). A lazy S is then formed to bring the open ends together and hand-sewn anastomosis is performed to restore continuity (*D*). (*From* Thompson J, Sudan D. Intestinal lengthening for short bowel syndrome. *Adv Surg.* 2008;42:49-61; with permission.)

In the setting of CD, there is limited evidence to guide the use of SRSB. CD recurrence at the site of the reversed segment is a concern. In the authors' experience, none of the 3 patients with CD who underwent SRSB developed disease at the reversed segment. Caution must be given, however, prior to undertaking this operation in phenotypically aggressive CD or in patients who have yet to achieve disease control. The authors suggest only those patients who have a strong desire to wean from PN, who are not otherwise candidates for IT, and who have documented rapid intestinal transit time be considered for a 10-cm to 12-cm SRSB if a sustained remission of their CD has been achieved (**Fig. 6**).

Prophylactic Cholecystectomy

Cholelithiasis and its associated complications are common among those with SBS/IF.[46] Long-term need for PN, removal of the terminal ileum, and intestinal length less than 120 cm all predispose patients to the development of gallstones.[47] More than a third of patients with SBS/IF develop cholelithiasis within the first 2 years after their initial resection.[47] Because SBS/IF patients are more likely to develop gallstone-related complications, it is recommended that patients undergo

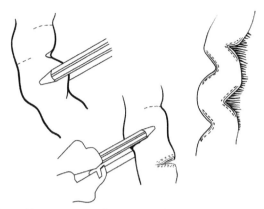

Fig. 5. STEP. The bowel lumen is partially transected using a linear stapler, stopping at the point that leaves the normal luminal diameter (generally 1–2 cm) intact. Subsequent staple firings are displaced the same distance as the remnant lumen (usually 1–2 cm) either proximally or distally along the dilated small bowel loop and alternatively placed at 180° from the first firing. This procedure can be performed either by alternating from side-to-side or from mesenteric to antimesenteric edges. (*From* Thompson J, Sudan D. Intestinal lengthening for short bowel syndrome. *Adv Surg.* 2008;42:49-61; with permission.)

prophylactic cholecystectomy (PC) if feasible at the time of repeat laparotomy. Despite this, PC remains relatively underutilized in SBS/IF, with only a third of patients who are eligible having cholecystectomy.[47] The authors' practice is to consider PC in those with a high risk of cholelithiasis unless surgical risk is prohibitive. PC should be avoided in patients with a prognosis of less than 6 months to 12 months or who are clinically unstable at the time of laparotomy.

Intestinal Transplantation in Inflammatory Bowel Disease

IT, as a component of a multivisceral transplantation or as an isolated graft, offers those with refractory IF an opportunity for regaining enteral autonomy.[48] SBS continues to be the most common indication for IT, representing 60% of all adult patients.[48] Despite improvements in immunosuppression and perioperative care, the use of IT has slowly declined over the past 10 years.[49] In 2017, 109 transplants were performed, 57% of which were in adults.[49]

Survival in patients transplanted since the year 2000 is approximately 77%, 58%, and 47% at 1 year, 5 years, and 10 years, respectively.[48] Even with the growing

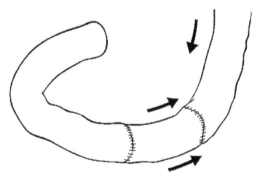

Fig. 6. SRSB. Arrows represent the direction of peristalsis in the adjacent small bowel segment.

experience in IT, patient survival remains inferior to conservative management with PN.[4] Nonetheless, if PN cannot support the health/growth of a patient or if life-threatening complications related to long-term PN develop, IT may represent the only life-sustaining treatment option for patients with SBS/IF.

IT has been performed safely and successfully in IBD. Overall, UC is an uncommon indication for IT, representing less than 1% of patients on home PN and 1.3% of patients who are candidates for IT in Europe.[5,50] CD is the underlying indication for 11% of adult transplants, making it the second most common benign indication for IT.[48,50] A unique consideration for IT in CD is the possibility of IBD recurrence in the transplanted allograft.[51–53] Histologic findings of granulomatous enteritis consistent with CD have been documented on surveillance biopsies of allografts as early as 20 days after IT.[52] Fortunately, the rate of clinically significant CD recurrence seems low, with individual experiences suggesting recurrence occurs in less than 10% of patients.[51–54] It is unclear, however, what effect the presence of recurrent CD in the transplanted graft has on long-term graft and patient survival.

Limketkai and colleagues[53] have investigated the outcomes of IT in CD and non-CD populations. IT in patients with CD was associated with similar rates of histologically confirmed acute rejection at 1 year (36.9 vs. 33.3%) but the rates of graft loss at 1 year, 5 years, and 10 years were significantly higher (18.6%, 38.7%, and 49.2% vs 14.1%, 32.1%, and 41.0%, respectively) compared with patients without CD.[53] Overall survival rates in the CD and non-CD cohort, however, were similar at 5 years (49.7% vs. 51.9%, respectively). The investigators note that in transplants performed after the year 2000, the rate of graft loss in both cohorts is similar, perhaps due to changes in immunosuppression regimens.[53]

Given the few data regarding long-term patient outcomes, IT for IBD should be performed at high-volume centers experienced in IT. Patients with significant liver disease at time of consideration for IT may be best served with multivisceral transplantation. Similarly, given IBD's association with primary sclerosing cholangitis, combined liver-small bowel transplant may be necessary when primary sclerosing cholangitis is present or suspected. Despite the complexity of IT in IBD, it remains a viable treatment option for those who cannot be conservatively managed with medical or surgical adjuncts to SBS care.

SUMMARY

IBD-related SBS/IF remains a rare and challenging disease process. Patient care should take place in a setting familiar with intestinal rehabilitation and IT. Medical therapy should be optimized both to prevent additional bowel loss and enhance the remaining intestinal remnant. Despite few data, surgery to improve absorptive function may be safely performed in IBD. Although IT in IBD offers a chance for regaining enteral autonomy in refractory cases, current data favor conservative strategies unless life-threatening complications of SBS/IF have developed. Further work must be done to outline the optimal treatment regimen for IBD-related SBS/IF.

REFERENCES

1. References, Pironi L, Arends J, et al. ESPEN guidelines on chronic intestinal failure in adults. Clin Nutr 2016;35(2):247–307.
2. Sudan D. Cost and quality of life after intestinal transplantation. Gastroenterology 2006;130(2 Suppl 1):S158–62.
3. Pironi L, Arends J, Baxter J, et al. ESPEN endorsed recommendations. Definition and classification of intestinal failure in adults. Clin Nutr 2015;34(2):171–80.

4. Kesseli S, Sudan D. Small bowel transplantation. Surg Clin North Am 2019;99(1): 103–16.

5. Pironi L, Konrad D, Brandt C, et al. Clinical classification of adult patients with chronic intestinal failure due to benign disease: an international multicenter cross-sectional survey. Clin Nutr 2018;37(2):728–38.

6. Pironi L, Corcos O, Forbes A, et al. Intestinal failure in adults: recommendations from the ESPEN expert groups. Clin Nutr 2018;37(6 Pt A):1798–809.

7. Buchman AL, Scolapio J, Fryer J. AGA technical review on short bowel syndrome and intestinal transplantation. Gastroenterology 2003;124(4):1111–34.

8. Thompson JS, DiBaise JK, Iyer KR, et al. Postoperative short bowel syndrome. J Am Coll Surg 2005;201(1):85–9.

9. Thompson JS. Reversed intestinal segment revisited. Transplant Proc 2016;48(2): 453–6.

10. O'Keefe SJ, Buchman AL, Fishbein TM, et al. Short bowel syndrome and intestinal failure: consensus definitions and overview. Clin Gastroenterol Hepatol 2006; 4(1):6–10.

11. Oley Foundation. North American home parenteral and enteral nutrition patient registry annual report. Albany (NY): Oley Foundation; 1994.

12. Wheeler MJ, Langenfeld SJ, Lyden E, et al. Initial site of Crohn's disease is not an independent predictor of outcome of short bowel syndrome. J Inflamm Bowel Dis Disord 2016;1:2.

13. Thompson JS, Iyer KR, DiBaise JK, et al. Short bowel syndrome and Crohn's disease. J Gastrointest Surg 2003;7:1069–72.

14. Hatoum OA, Spinelli KS, Abu-Hajir M, et al. Mesenteric venous thrombosis in inflammatory bowel disease. J Clin Gastroenterol 2005;39(1):27–31.

15. Jackson CS, Fryer J, Danese S, et al. Mesenteric vascular thromboembolism in inflammatory bowel disease: a single center experience. J Gastrointest Surg 2011;15(1):97–100.

16. Uchino M, Ikeuchi H, Bando T, et al. Risk factors for short bowel syndrome in patients with Crohn's disease. Surg Today 2012;42(5):447–52.

17. Molodecky NA, Soon IS, Rabi DM, et al. Increasing incidence and prevalence of the inflammatory bowel diseases with time, based on systematic review. Gastroenterology 2012;142(1):46–54.e42 [quiz: e30].

18. Shivashankar R, Tremaine WJ, Harmsen WS, et al. Incidence and prevalence of Crohn's disease and ulcerative colitis in olmsted county, minnesota from 1970 through 2010. Clin Gastroenterol Hepatol 2017;15(6):857–63.

19. Coward S, Clement F, Benchimol EI, et al. Past and future burden of inflammatory bowel diseases based on modeling of population-based data. Gastroenterology 2019;156(5):1345–53.e4.

20. Watanabe K, Sasaki I, Fukushima K, et al. Long-term incidence and characteristics of intestinal failure in Crohn's disease: a multicenter study. J Gastroenterol 2014;49(2):231–8.

21. Cosnes J, Gower-Rousseau C, Seksik P, et al. Epidemiology and natural history of inflammatory bowel diseases. Gastroenterology 2011;140(6):1785–94.

22. GATTEX (teduglutide) for injection [package insert]. Lexington, MA: Shire-NPS Pharmaceuticals, Inc; 2019.

23. Wojdemann M, Wettergren A, Hartmann B, et al. Glucagon-like peptide-2 inhibits centrally induced antral motility in pigs. Scand J Gastroenterol 1998;33(8): 828–32.

24. Guan X, Karpen HE, Stephens J, et al. GLP-2 receptor localizes to enteric neurons and endocrine cells expressing vasoactive peptides and mediates increased blood flow. Gastroenterology 2006;130(1):150–64.

25. Tsai CH, Hill M, Asa SL, et al. Intestinal growth-promoting properties of glucagon-like peptide-2 in mice. Am J Physiol 1997;273(1 Pt 1):E77–84.

26. Drucker DJ, Erlich P, Asa SL, et al. Induction of intestinal epithelial proliferation by glucagon-like peptide 2. Proc Natl Acad Sci U S A 1996;93(15):7911–6.

27. Vipperla K, O'Keefe SJ. Study of teduglutide effectiveness in parenteral nutrition-dependent short-bowel syndrome subjects. Expert Rev Gastroenterol Hepatol 2013;7(8):683–7.

28. Schwartz LK, O'Keefe SJ, Fujioka K, et al. Long-term teduglutide for the treatment of patients with intestinal failure associated with short bowel syndrome. Clin Transl Gastroenterol 2016;7:e142.

29. Jeppesen PB, Gilroy R, Pertkiewicz M, et al. Randomised placebo-controlled trial of teduglutide in reducing parenteral nutrition and/or intravenous fluid requirements in patients with short bowel syndrome. Gut 2011;60:902–14.

30. Seidner DL, Joly F, Youssef NN. Effect of teduglutide, a glucagon-like peptide 2 analog, on citrulline levels in patients with short bowel syndrome in two phase III randomized trials. Clin Transl Gastroenterol 2015;6:e93.

31. O'Keefe SJ, Jeppesen PB, Gilroy R, et al. Safety and efficacy of teduglutide after 52 weeks of treatment in patients with short bowel intestinal failure. Clin Gastroenterol Hepatol 2013;11:815–23.

32. Thompson JS, Weseman RA, Mercer DF, et al. Risk of intestinal malignancy in patients with short bowel syndrome. JPEN J Parenter Enteral Nutr 2017;41(4):562–5.

33. Kochar B, Long MD, Shelton E, et al. Safety and efficacy of teduglutide (gattex) in patients with Crohn's disease and need for parenteral support due to short bowel syndrome-associated intestinal failure. J Clin Gastroenterol 2017;51(6):508–11.

34. George AT, Li BH, Carroll RE. Off-lable teduglutide in non-intestinal failure patients with chronic malabsorption. Dig Dis Sci 2019;64(6):1599–603.

35. Buchman AL, Katz S, Fang JC, et al, Teduglutide Study Group. Teduglutide, a novel mucosally active analog of glucagon-like peptide-2 (GLP-2) for the treatment of moderate to severe Crohn's disease. Inflamm Bowel Dis 2010;16(6): 962–73.

36. Jeuring SF, van den Heuvel TR, Liu LY, et al. Improvements in the long-term outcome of Crohn's disease over the past two decades and the relation to changes in medical management: results from the population-based IBDSL cohort. Am J Gastroenterol 2017;112(2):325–36.

37. Burisch J, Kiudelis G, Kupcinskas L, for the Epi-IBD group, et al. Natural disease course of Crohn's disease during the first 5 years after diagnosis in a european population-based inception cohort: an Epi-IBD study. Gut 2019;68:423–33.

38. Limketkai BN, Parian AM, Shah ND, et al. Short bowel syndrome and intestinal failure in Crohn's disease. Inflamm Bowel Dis 2016;22(5):1209–18.

39. McKenna NP, Habermann EB, Glasgow AE, et al. Intra-abdominal sepsis after ileocolic resection in Crohn's disease: the role of combination immunosuppression. Dis Colon Rectum 2018;61(12):1393–402.

40. Thompson JS. Surgical rehabilitation of intestine in short bowel syndrome. Surgery 2004;135(5):465–70.

41. Sudan D, Thompson J, Botha J, et al. Comparison of intestinal lengthening procedures for patients with short bowel syndrome. Ann Surg 2007;246(4):593–601 [discussion: 601–4].

42. Jones BA, Hull MA, Potanos KM, et al. Report of 111 consecutive patients enrolled in the international serial transverse enteroplasty (STEP) data registry: a retrospective observational study. J Am Coll Surg 2013;216(3):438–46.
43. Bianchi A. Intestinal loop lengthening–a technique for increasing small intestinal length. J Pediatr Surg 1980;15(2):145–51.
44. Kim HB, Fauza D, Garza J, et al. Serial transverse enteroplasty (STEP): a novel bowel lengthening procedure. J Pediatr Surg 2003;38(3):425–9.
45. Yannam GR, Sudan DL, Grant W, et al. Intestinal lengthening in adult patients with short bowel syndrome. J Gastrointest Surg 2010;14:1931–6.
46. Beyer-Berjot L, Joly F, Maggiori L, et al. Segmental reversal of the small bowel can end permanent parenteral nutrition dependency: an experience of 38 adults with short bowel syndrome. Ann Surg 2012;256(5):739–44 [discussion: 744–5].
47. Thompson JS, Mercer DF, Vargas LM, et al. Prophylactic cholecystectomy in short bowel syndrome: is it being utilized? Am J Surg 2018;216:73–7.
48. Grant D, Abu-Elmagd K, Mazariegos G, et al. Intestinal transplant registry report: global activity and trends. Am J Transplant 2015;15(1):210–9.
49. Smith JM, Weaver T, Skeans MA, et al. OPTN/SRTR 2017 annual data report: intestine. Am J Transplant 2019;19(Suppl 2):284–322.
50. Pironi L, Hebuterne X, Van Gossum A, et al. Candidates for intestinal transplantation: a multicenter survey in europe. Am J Gastroenterol 2006;101(7):1633–43 [quiz: 1679].
51. Sustento-Reodica N, Ruiz P, Rogers A, et al. Recurrent Crohn's disease in transplanted bowel. Lancet 1997;349(9053):688–91.
52. Harpaz N, Schiano T, Ruf AE, et al. Early and frequent histological recurrence of Crohn's disease in small intestinal allografts. Transplantation 2005;80(12):1667–70.
53. Limketkai BN, Orandi BJ, Luo X, et al. Mortality and rates of graft rejection or failure following intestinal transplantation in patients with vs without Crohn's disease. Clin Gastroenterol Hepatol 2016;14:1574–81.
54. Koritsky DC, Bond G, Shcuster B, et al. Intestinal transplantation for end stage Crohn's disease: therapeutic efficacy and disease recurrence. Inflamm Bowel Dis 2012;18:S3.

Medical Management of Inflammatory Bowel Disease

Derrick D. Eichele, MD*, Renee Young, MD

KEYWORDS

- Inflammatory bowel disease • Treatment • Management • Treat-to-target strategy
- Therapeutic drug monitoring

KEY POINTS

- The goals of inflammatory bowel disease therapy include clinical remission, avoidance of treatment toxicity, improved quality of life, prevention of disease complications, and minimization of cancer risk.
- Biomarkers of intestinal inflammation can predict clinical relapse and provide a noninvasive strategy to manage inflammatory bowel disease.
- Therapeutic drug monitoring has emerged as an indispensable clinical tool to help guide therapeutic decision making in inflammatory bowel disease.
- Newly available classes of biologic agents have led to the consideration of personalized medicine in inflammatory bowel disease.

INTRODUCTION

Inflammatory bowel disease (IBD), including Crohn's disease (CD) and ulcerative colitis (UC), are a group of chronic inflammatory conditions of the gastrointestinal tract related to dysregulation of the immune response to intestinal microbiota in a genetically predisposed host.[1,2] These chronic inflammatory conditions tend to be characterized by periods of relapses and remission and recently have been acknowledged to be progressive diseases. The incidence and prevalence of IBD are increasing (3.1 million adults in the United States [1.3%]), with an increased associated burden on the health care system.[3–5] With the advent of biologic therapies in the early 2000s, there has been a lesser need for surgical intervention. However, only 50% of patients with IBD are reported to be in clinical remission; thus, inadequate care remains for many.[6] Current medical management strategies in IBD have evolved from modest symptom control to maintenance of deep histologic remission with the goal to alter the disease natural history by hindering bowel

Disclosures: The authors have nothing to disclose.
Department of Internal Medicine, Division of Gastroenterology and Hepatology, University of Nebraska Medical Center, Omaha, NE 68198-2000, USA
* Corresponding author.
E-mail address: Derrick.eichele@unmc.edu

Surg Clin N Am 99 (2019) 1223–1235
https://doi.org/10.1016/j.suc.2019.08.011
0039-6109/19/© 2019 Elsevier Inc. All rights reserved.

damage. New therapeutic aims have described treat to target and tight control strategies through therapeutic drug monitoring (TDM) and early intervention. This article reviews the evidence that has brought about the shift in management strategy with a focus on therapeutic positioning in addition to accounting for safety of treatment options available.

TREATMENT STRATEGIES
Treat to Target

The general goals of therapy for IBD are (1) the induction and maintenance of clinical remission, (2) avoidance of treatment toxicity (short and long term), (3) avoidance of long-term corticosteroid use, (4) improved quality of life, and (5) prevention of disease complications, including cancer.[7,8] Historically, therapeutic options were limited to aminosalicylates, corticosteroids and immunomodulators (6-mercaptopurine, azathioprine and methotrexate). With the advent of anti–tumor necrosis factor (TNF)-α agents around the turn of the century, there were now reliably effective medications to induce clinical remission and mucosal healing.[9]

Prior treatment guidelines recommended a "step-up approach" with first-line agents including mesalamine and corticosteroids with subsequent therapy escalation for treatment failures. This escalation started with immunomodulators (azathioprine) and reserved anti–TNF-α therapies for patients who failed conventional therapies.[10] The SONIC trial first indicated that combination therapy with infliximab plus azathioprine was significantly more effective in attaining higher rates of steroid-free remission in CD.[11] Evidence from several subsequent clinical trials has shown that early treatment with combination therapy has led to better clinical outcomes with more rapid induction of remission than the standard step up strategy.[12,13]

Because of this development, the treatment paradigm reversed from a step up to a top-down approach.[14] The top-down approach with the early use of combination therapy resulted in more rapid remission, improved sustained response with longer time to relapse, decreased need for corticosteroids, quicker decrease in clinical symptoms, marked decrease in inflammatory markers, and improved mucosal healing on endoscopic examination.[15]

The concept of "treat-to-target" emerged from research in fields related to other immune-mediated disease, specifically rheumatoid arthritis. The development of this approach arose from the clinical observation that traditional therapeutic strategies failed to significantly alter disease progression in IBD. Frequently, patient-reported symptoms were discordant to objective markers of active disease.[12] The role and objective of Selecting Therapeutic Targets in Inflammatory Bowel Disease (STRIDE) initiative was to provide an international expert consensus that would provide appropriate evidence-based treatment targets for IBD.[16]

STRIDE's target for patient reported outcomes in UC was resolution of hematochezia and normalization of bowel habits. Endoscopic remission was defined as the return of normal vascular pattern with the resolution of friability and ulceration. Histologic remission was not necessary. Patient-reported targets for CD included the resolution of abdominal pain and normalization of bowel habit. Absence of ulceration at ileocolonoscopy and histologic remission was lacking sufficient evidence as a recommended target. Additionally, the committee agreed that there was insufficient evidence to recommend treatment optimization by available biomarkers, including C-reactive protein and fecal calprotectin (FCP), alone because they may reflect residual intestinal inflammation. Rather the available biomarkers serve a role as adjunctive measures of inflammation to monitor disease activity. Through the systematic review of data from randomized clinical trials, it is estimated that one-third to two-thirds of patients with IBD would be able to meet these target endpoints with intensive therapy.[11,17–19]

Tight Control

There is increasing evidence that the use of biomarkers for intestinal inflammation, namely, C-reactive protein and FCP, can predict clinical relapse and provide a noninvasive strategy to manage IBD.[20,21] One meta-analysis showed the pooled sensitivity and specificity of FCP to predict relapse in quiescent IBD was nearly 80%.[22] A limitation with the test in clinical practice is that it has limited accuracy in small bowel CD, but has good accuracy in colonic inflammation in patients with UC or colonic CD.[22] FCP can be used to monitor for postoperative recurrence after ileocolonic resection in CD with a sensitivity of 89%.[23]

The Effect of tight control management on Crohn's disease (CALM study) was designed as a randomized, open-label, active-controlled phase 3 trial to investigate the effectiveness and safety of tight control using clinical symptoms and biomarkers versus patients managed with traditional clinical management.[24] The study findings suggest that tight control with dose escalation of medication based on clinical symptoms and biomarkers lead to improved rates of mucosal healing, deep remission, and steroid-free remission at 48 weeks versus standard clinical management, which was based on symptom-driven decisions alone.[24]

Therapeutic Drug Monitoring

TDM is an integral part of tight control.[25] Optimization of biologic drug levels improves rates of clinical and endoscopic remission. Subtherapeutic drug levels are associated with increased risk of disease flare and reduced clinical efficacy.[12,26] TDM is helpful given several limitations of biologic agents (primary nonresponse, secondary loss of response, or failure to regain response after reinduction in a patient that was previously exposed to the medication).[25] Between 10% and 30% of patients are deemed to be primary nonresponders to anti–TNF-α therapies. The annual risk for loss of response is between 13% and 24%.[27–29] Various pharmacokinetic and pharmacodynamic factors influence response to biologic medication and are related to patient factors (ie, albumin, gender and body mass index), disease (ie, severity, type, and location) and the medication itself (ie, synergism with immunomodulator and immunogenicity).[30]

TDM involves sampling of drug level and antidrug antibody at trough concentrations, which is the point at which the lowest concentration of drug is present before repeat administration[26] (**Table 1**). The optimal therapeutic window concept holds that the trough concentration needs to be at a sufficient level for the medication to exert the desired effect while decreasing the body's response to form antibodies, which is related to the medication immunogenicity.

TDM can be used for target concentration-adjusted dosing and to guide therapy at the time of loss of response to the prescribed biologic medication.[30] TDM avoids escalation of therapy in patients that will not benefit from intensification, allows for escalation in those patients with loss of response with low drug concentrations, and identifies the need to change drug classes in those patients who have a non-TNF-α–driven disease.[30]

TDM is not without controversy because results from clinical trials have been disappointing and the studies have significant limitations including insufficient power and suboptimal design.[12] The Trough Level Adapted Infliximab Treatment (TAXIT) trial found no difference in the primary outcome of clinical remission at 1 year in patients assigned to continuous drug monitoring and conventional therapy.[31] Additionally

Table 1
American Gastroenterological Association Guideline recommendations for TDM in IBD

Trough Concentration	Antidrug Antibodies	Therapeutic Recommendations (Based on Low or Very Low Quality of Evidence)
Optimal	N/A	Restage disease to assess for active inflammation Present - change to a different mechanism of action

Low
Zero
	None
	Low
		Optimize index drug
		  Shorten the dosing interval
		  Increase drug dose
		  Add immunomodulator agent

Zero	High	Consider switching to a different drug
		  Within the same class
		  Different drug class

Data from Feuerstein JD, Nguyen GC, Kupfer SS, Falck-Ytter Y. AGA SECTION. Gastroenterology 2017;153:827-34.

the Tailored Treatment with Infliximab for Active Crohn's Disease (TAILORIX) trial found no difference between study groups for steroid-free clinical remission at 1 year.[32] Based on these limitations, an expert panel concluded that TDM at the end of induction was appropriate in assessment in primary nonresponse, secondary loss of response, restarting medication after drug holiday and again during first year of maintenance.[33]

POSITIONING OF BIOLOGIC THERAPIES

The therapies available for the treatment of IBD have significantly expanded over the last several decades (**Table 2**). Newly available biologic agents have variable safety profiles and rates of efficacy, and there are no head-to-head clinical trials to determine which agents are most suitable for a specific clinical scenario. Instead, the choice of biologic therapy involves physician experience, patient preference, and insurance coverage.

Positioning for Ulcerative Colitis

Current Food and Drug Administration–approved biologic medications for the treatment of UC include 3 anti–TNF-α inhibitors (infliximab, adalimumab, and golimumab), 1 anti-integrin molecule (vedolizumab), and a Janus kinase inhibitor inhibitor (tofacitinib)[34–38] (**Fig. 1**). More data have been generated regarding the efficacy and safety of anti–TNF-α agents with relation to induction and maintenance of clinical remission and mucosal healing in UC. Pooled data across the various anti–TNF-α studies to compare for induction and maintenance of remission showed a trend toward improved rates in infliximab over adalimumab (relative risk, 2.08%; 95% confidence interval, 0.32–12.03), but it did not attain statistical significance.[39] Two additional studies attempted to limit variation in patient populations by examining biologic naïve patients, and in both studies adalimumab was less likely to achieve clinical remission or mucosal healing at 8 weeks.[40,41]

At 52 weeks, infliximab was similar to golimumab and vedolizumab for achieving clinical remission.[41] Both infliximab and adalimumab were effective in reducing hospitalizations, but only infliximab was found to have a reduction in colectomy rates. Data regarding the impact of vedolizumab on hospitalization and colectomy are lacking.[42,43]

Table 2
Available therapies for IBD

	Trade Name	Mechanism of Action	Indication	Route	Common SE
Infliximab[a]	Remicade Inflectra Renflexis	TNF-α	UC/CD	IV	Serious infection, OI, reactivation of TB and Hep B, infusion reaction, DIL, worsening CHF, demyelination, lymphoma, melanoma
Adalimumab[a]	Humira Amjevita Cyletzo	TNF-α	UC/CD	SC	Serious infection, OI, reactivation of TB and Hep B, injection reaction, DIL, worsening CHF, dymelination, lymphoma, melanoma
Certolizumab	Cimzia	TNF-α	CD	SC	Serious infection, OI, reactivation of TB and Hep B, injection reaction, DIL, worsening CHF, dymelination, lymphoma, melanoma
Golimumab	Symponi	TNF-α	UC	SC	Serious infection, OI, reactivation of TB and Hep B, injection reaction, DIL, worsening CHF, dymelination, lymphoma, melanoma
Natalizumab	Tysabri	α4 integrin	CD	IV	PML in positive JC virus
Vedolizumab	Entyvio	α4β7 integrin	UC/CD	IV	Nasopharyngitis
Ustekinumab	Stelara	IL-12 and −23	CD	IV/SC	Arthralgia, headache, nausea, nasopharyngitis, fatigue
Tofacitinib	Xeljanz	JAK 1 and 3	UC	Oral	Serious infection, OI, HSV, PE, nasopharyngitis, arthralgia, NMSC, cholesterol increase

Abbreviations: CHF, congested heart failure; DIL, drug-induced lupus; HSV, herpes simplex virus; IV, intravenous; JAK, Janus kinase inhibitor; NMSC, nonmelanoma skin cancer; OI, opportunistic infection; PE, pulmonary embolism; PML, progressive multifocal leukoencephalopathy; SC, subcutaneous; TB, tuberculosis.
 [a] Including biosimilars of the originator drug.

The data suggest that appropriate first-line agents include infliximab or vedolizumab for the induction and maintenance of remission.[43] Patients at high risk for disease-related complications are more likely to benefit from infliximab because long-term outcomes with vedolizumab are not known.

Positioning for Crohn's Disease

Current Food and Drug Administration–approved biologic medications for the treatment of CD includes 3 anti–TNF-α agents and their biosimilars (infliximab, adalimumab, and certolizumab), 2 anti-integrin molecules (natalizumab, vedolizumab) and an anti-IL agent (ustekinumab)[11,44–49] (**Table 3**). In a recent network meta-analysis

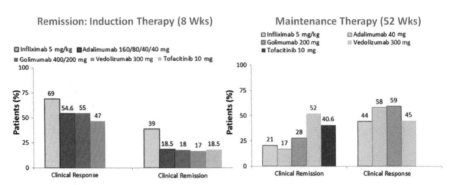

Fig. 1. Efficacy of biologics in remission for UC.

on CD, biologic-naïve patients were found to have better rates of induction and maintenance of clinical remission with anti–TNF-α agents.[50] For patients with exposure to anti–TNF agents and lost response, the meta-analysis found moderate quality evidence to support ustekinumab as a second-line agent to induce clinical remission. For patients intolerant of infliximab, adalimumab had a greater magnitude of benefit over other agents.[50]

In another meta-analysis, infliximab was associated with nearly a 70% decrease in the need for surgery at 1 year.[51] Adalimumab has produced similar results.[52] The newer agents lack data for surgical risk reduction.

Only infliximab has been well-studied with fistula healing as a primary endpoint, and it should remain the first-line agent for fistulizing or penetrating disease. Adalimumab is considered a second-line agent for loss of response to infliximab.[53]

Table 3
Comparative efficacy of biologics in CD

Biologic	Mechanism of Action	Clinical Trial	Remission Rates[a] (%)	% Change with Placebo	Comments
Infliximab	TNF-α	ACCENT I	39	18	CDAI <150 (standard dosing; at 30 wk)
Adalimumab	TNF-α	CHARM	40	23	CDAI <150 (standard dosing; at 26 wk)
Certolizumab	TNF-α	PRECiSE 2	48	19	CDAI <150 (standard dosing; at 26 wk)
Infliximab + AZA	TNF-α + thiopurine	SONIC	57 / 44	13–27[a] / 14–27[b]	Steroid-Free Remission Mucosal Healing (At 26 wk)
Vedolizumab	α4β7 integrin	GEMINI 2	39 / 32	17 / 16	Clinical remission Steroid-free remission (standard dosing, at 52 wk)
Ustekinumab	IL-12 and −23	UNITI	53 / 47	17 / 17	Clinical remission Steroid Free remission (Standard dosing; at 52 wk)

Abbreviation: CDAI, Crohn's Disease Activity Index.
[a] Differences in study design prevent comparison of absolute efficacy.
[b] Represents IFX + Placebo and AZA + Placebo.

The addition of newer agents and evolving treatment strategies provide an opportunity to shift toward a personalized approach to IBD therapy. Ultimately, the appropriate first-line agent takes into account the ability to optimize outcomes for various phenotypes with attention to rapid response, durable remission, and the ability to monitor therapeutic drug levels with enhanced safety in the aim to alter disease progression.

BIOLOGIC AGENTS AND THEIR SIDE EFFECTS

Outside of biologics, it is well-known that corticosteroids are associated with hyperglycemia, fat accumulation, decreased wound healing, infection, and bone metabolism and bone loss.[54] Thiopurines have associated risks including bone marrow suppression, pancreatitis, nonmelanoma skin cancer, and an increased risk of lymphoma.[13,54,55]

Anti–Timor Necrosis Factor-α

A large, prospective, observational long-term registry in North American patients (TREAT registry) with CD was initiated in 1999 to document long-term safety of medications used to treat CD including anti–TNF-α agents and updates have been provided.[13]

Serious infection tends to be at the top of most patient's concerns after viewing direct-to-patient advertisements. The TREAT registry demonstrated an unadjusted relative risk of 2.04 (95% confidence interval, 1.45–2.89).[13] A large meta-analysis showed opportunistic infections in 0.94% of patients on anti–TNF-α compared with 0.31% of those receiving placebo (relative risk, 2.05).[56] Current recommendations to prevent opportunistic infections include baseline hepatitis testing and tuberculosis testing with Quantiferon Gold (Qiagen, Hilden, Germany) before the initiation of therapy.[23,57]

Infusion reactions to infliximab are uncommon (3% of infusions in the TREAT registry with 0.047% being serious reactions).[13] They typically occur within 24 hours of infusion, but can be delayed by up to 14 days. Symptoms include arthralgia, myalgia, urticarial rash, fever, and malaise. Symptoms often resolve with acetaminophen, an antihistamine, and a short course of steroids. Reinfusion is often preceded by a short course of steroids to prevent a second reaction.[58]

The incidence of drug-induced lupus in randomized control trials of anti–TNF-α therapy has been reported as less than 1% (0.76%) and in postmarketing surveillance it ranges from 0.1% in adalimumab to approximately 0.2% in infliximab.[59–61] Typical presentation includes weakness, malaise, arthralgia and/or myalgias, fevers, and rash. Lupus-like reactions occur more often in females with universal findings of arthropathy and positive antinuclear antibody.[62] Treatment of drug-induced lupus includes removal of the offending anti–TNF-α agent; occasionally, patients require corticosteroid therapy to obtain complete clinical resolution.[63] Development of positive antinuclear antibody is common in patients on anti–TNF-α therapy, most will be without symptoms.

Demyelinating disorders have been reported with anti–TNF-α with 0.05% to 0.2% in meta-analysis of randomized clinical trials and in postmarketing surveillance. The pathogenesis is not well understood, but thought to be related to T-cell and humoral attack against peripheral myelin or vasculitis-induced neural ischemia.[64] The treatment in this event again requires withdrawal of offending agent, but unlike drug-induced lupus, this is likely a class effect and it is not recommended to initiate another anti–TNF-α agent. Additionally, patients may require additional therapies of corticosteroids, plasmapheresis, or intravenous immune globulin.[65,66]

The risk of anti–TNF-α induced neoplasia is quite low, and similar to other therapies.[13] The overall incidence of solid tumors was 0.42 events per 100 patient-years, nonmelanoma skin cancer was 0.16 events per 100 patient-years, and lymphoma was 0.05 events per 100 patient-years.[13] In a nested case-controlled study assessing the risk of malignancy in IBD versus patients without IBD results suggested an increased risk of melanoma (Incidence rate ratio, 1.29; 95% confidence interval, 1.09–1.53), which was accentuated with the addition of biologic medication (odds ratio, 1.88; 95% confidence interval, 1.08–3.29).[67]

Anti-IL

Ustekinumab is a fully human monoclonal antibody that targets the p40 subunit of IL-12 and IL-23 that is the first approved medication in its class for the treatment of moderate to severe CD.[1,49] It is generally well-tolerated with overall and serious adverse events comparable between placebo and treatment groups. At week 44 of A Study to Evaluate the Safety and Efficacy of Ustekinumab Maintenance Therapy in Patients With Moderately to Severely Active Crohn's Disease (IM-UNITI), the percentages of serious adverse events were 9.9% to 12.1% for treatment versus 15% for placebo.[1] In a pooled analysis of 7 clinical trials across various disease states with ustekinumab, the risk of serious infection ranged between 2% to 5% based on dosing frequencies versus 2% in the placebo group.[68]

Anti-Integrin

Anti-integrins target membrane-associated antigens, specifically inhibiting T-cell migration into inflamed tissues in the intestinal tract by blocking $\alpha4\beta7$ integrins. There are 2 commercially available molecules used in the treatment of IBD. Vedolizumab is a gut-selective antibody that targets the heterodimer $\alpha4\beta7$ to vascular cell adhesion molecule-1. Natalizumab is a recombinant monoclonal antibody against the cell adhesion molecule a4-integrin that targets the shared a4-integrin of $\alpha4\beta7$ and $\alpha4\beta1$, in which the $\alpha4\beta1$ ligand is mucosal adhesion cell adhesion molecule, which is expressed on the intestinal microvasculature. It has been identified that by inhibition of $\alpha4\beta1$integrin binding to vascular cell adhesion molecule-1 in the central nervous system can decrease immune surveillance and result in risk of development of progressive multifocal leukoencephalopathy in patients who were positive for the JC virus.[69,70] Safety data from 6 randomized controlled trials were examined to determine the long-term safety of vedolizumab in patients with CD and UC.[48] Unexplained neurologic symptoms were experienced in 10% of the patients and owing to the concern for progressive multifocal leukoencephalopathy in the study populations, further evaluation was required, but no events were identified as progressive multifocal leukoencephalopathy. Additionally, infusion related reactions were rare (<5% of patients) and there were no indications of serious opportunistic infection (tuberculosis, candidiasis, herpes zoster, or cytomegalovirus).[48]

Janus Kinase Inhibitors

Janus kinases are located on the cytoplasm of various cytokine receptors and are activated upon receptor-ligand interaction. Janus kinase inhibitors are synthetically derived, orally delivered small molecules that diffuse across cell membranes and work intracellularly.[1] The first oral, small molecule in the class that has been approved for the treatment of UC is tofacitinib. Because the medication is synthetically derived, potential benefit is it portends no immunogenicity and short half-lives as compared with other biologic medications. A dose-dependent risk of herpes zoster has been reported in A Study Of Oral CP-690,550 As A Maintenance Therapy For Ulcerative Colitis (OCTAVE Sustain trial; 3 patients [1.5%] in the 5 mg tofacitinib group, 10 patients [5.1%] in the 10 mg group, and 1 [0.5%] the placebo group), but no cases of herpes zoster were serious enough to warrant discontinuation.[38] It is recommended that recombinant shingles vaccination be administered before the initiation of therapy.

Intestinal perforation was documented in early reports, but no patients in the OCTAVE Sustain trial had intestinal perforation.[38] Across all 3 OCTAVE trials, lipid levels were noted to increase with the initiation of therapy and 5 patients sustained cardiovascular events. Thus, it is recommended that patients have screening cholesterol checked before therapy initiation and during the follow-up period at week 4 to 8. It is also recommended that the patients undergo routine dermatologic examinations on a yearly basis with the risk of nonmelanoma skin cancers having been reported in the OCTAVE trials, but all the cases of nonmelanoma skin cancer had prior exposure to thiopurines.[38] Most recently, the Food and Drug Administration responded to a safety signal of pulmonary embolism in postmarketing data for tofacitinib in rheumatoid arthritis who were taking the 10 mg twice daily dose. The Food and Drug Administration and safety boards continue to monitor this signal.

SUMMARY

IBD has become a growing concern worldwide. The chronic and progressive nature of IBD poses significant challenges to the treatment and management of effected patients with increased strain on health care resources. Fortunately, therapeutic options and our understanding of optimal management strategies in IBD over the last several years has evolved dramatically. The treat-to-target strategy has shifted focus toward identifiable and attainable treatment targets and with ability to optimize tight control through TDM and more reliable determinants of disease activity with the development reliable biomarkers. Advancements in our understanding of the IBD pathophysiology had led to therapeutic mechanisms that have a more narrowed focus toward gut-specific targets, which in turn have improved safety profiles.

REFERENCES

1. Hemperly A, Sandborn WJ, Vande Casteele N. Clinical pharmacology in adult and pediatric inflammatory bowel disease. Inflamm Bowel Dis 2018;24(12): 2527–42.

2. Fiocchi C. Inflammatory bowel disease: etiology and pathogenesis. Gastroenterology 1998;115(1):182–205.

3. Long MD, Hutfless S, Kappelman MD, et al. Challenges in designing a national surveillance program for inflammatory bowel disease in the United States. Inflamm Bowel Dis 2013;20(2):398–415.

4. Kaplan GG, Ng SC. Understanding and preventing the global increase of inflammatory bowel disease. Gastroenterology 2017;152(2):313–21.e2.

5. Dahlhamer JM. Prevalence of inflammatory bowel disease among adults aged≥ 18 years—United States, 2015. MMWR Morb Mortal Wkly Rep 2016;65:1166–9.

6. Frolkis AD, Dykeman J, Negrón ME, et al. Risk of surgery for inflammatory bowel diseases has decreased over time: a systematic review and meta-analysis of population-based studies. Gastroenterology 2013;145(5):996–1006.

7. Hommes D, Colombel J-F, Emery P, et al. Changing Crohn's disease management: need for new goals and indices to prevent disability and improve quality of life. J Crohns Colitis 2012;6:S224–34.

8. Reenaers C, Belaiche J, Louis E. Impact of medical therapies on inflammatory bowel disease complication rate. World J Gastroenterol 2012;18(29):3823.

9. Oussalah A, Danese S, Peyrin-Biroulet L. Efficacy of TNF antagonists beyond one year in adult and pediatric inflammatory bowel diseases: a systematic review. Curr Drug Targets 2010;11(2):156–75.

10. Lichtenstein GR, Hanauer SB, Sandborn WJ. Management of Crohn's disease in adults. Am J Gastroenterol 2009;104(2):465.

11. Colombel JF, Sandborn WJ, Reinisch W, et al. Infliximab, azathioprine, or combination therapy for Crohn's disease. N Engl J Med 2010;362(15):1383–95.

12. Colombel J-F, Narula N, Peyrin-Biroulet L. Management strategies to improve outcomes of patients with inflammatory bowel diseases. Gastroenterology 2017; 152(2):351–61.e5.

13. Lichtenstein GR, Feagan BG, Cohen RD, et al. Serious infection and mortality in patients with Crohn's disease: more than 5 years of follow-up in the TREAT™ registry. Am J Gastroenterol 2012;107(9):1409.

14. D'Haens G, Baert F, Van Assche G, et al. Early combined immunosuppression or conventional management in patients with newly diagnosed Crohn's disease: an open randomised trial. Lancet 2008;371(9613):660–7.

15. Lin MV, Blonski W, Lichtenstein GR. What is the optimal therapy for Crohn's disease: step-up or top-down? Expert Rev Gastroenterol Hepatol 2010;4(2):167–80.

16. Peyrin-Biroulet L, Sandborn W, Sands B, et al. Selecting therapeutic targets in inflammatory bowel disease (STRIDE): determining therapeutic goals for treat-to-target. Am J Gastroenterol 2015;110(9):1324.

17. Colombel JF, Rutgeerts P, Reinisch W, et al. Early mucosal healing with infliximab is associated with improved long-term clinical outcomes in ulcerative colitis. Gastroenterology 2011;141(4):1194–201.

18. Colombel JF, Rutgeerts PJ, Sandborn WJ, et al. Adalimumab induces deep remission in patients with Crohn's disease. Clin Gastroenterol Hepatol 2014; 12(3):414–22.e5.

19. Sandborn W, Colombel JF, D'haens G, et al. One-year maintenance outcomes among patients with moderately-to-severely active ulcerative colitis who responded to induction therapy with adalimumab: subgroup analyses from ULTRA 2. Aliment Pharmacol Ther 2013;37(2):204–13.

20. Sands BE. Biomarkers of inflammation in inflammatory bowel disease. Gastroenterology 2015;149(5):1275–85.e2.

21. Vos MD, Louis EJ, Jahnsen J, et al. Consecutive fecal calprotectin measurements to predict relapse in patients with ulcerative colitis receiving infliximab maintenance therapy. Inflamm Bowel Dis 2013;19(10):2111–7.

22. Mao R, Xiao Y-l, Gao X, et al. Fecal calprotectin in predicting relapse of inflammatory bowel diseases: a meta-analysis of prospective studies. Inflamm Bowel Dis 2012;18(10):1894–9.

23. Lichtenstein GR, Loftus EV, Isaacs KL, et al. ACG clinical guideline: management of Crohn's disease in adults. Am J Gastroenterol 2018;113(4):481.

24. Colombel J-F, Panaccione R, Bossuyt P, et al. Effect of tight control management on Crohn's disease (CALM): a multicentre, randomised, controlled phase 3 trial. Lancet 2017;390(10114):2779–89.

25. Ben-Horin S, Chowers Y. Tailoring anti-TNF therapy in IBD: drug levels and disease activity. Nat Rev Gastroenterol Hepatol 2014;11(4):243.

26. Feuerstein JD, Nguyen GC, Kupfer SS, et al, American Gastroenterological Association Institute Clinical Guidelines Committee. American Gastroenterological Association Institute guideline on therapeutic drug monitoring in inflammatory bowel disease. Gastroenterology 2017;153:827–34.

27. Gisbert JP, Panés J. Loss of response and requirement of infliximab dose intensification in Crohn's disease: a review. Am J Gastroenterol 2009;104(3):760.

28. Billioud V, Sandborn WJ, Peyrin-Biroulet L. Loss of response and need for adalimumab dose intensification in Crohn's disease: a systematic review. Am J Gastroenterol 2011;106(4):674.

29. Allez M, Karmiris K, Louis E, et al. Report of the ECCO pathogenesis workshop on anti-TNF therapy failures in inflammatory bowel diseases: definitions, frequency and pharmacological aspects. J Crohns Colitis 2010;4(4):355–66.

30. Casteele NV, Feagan BG, Gils A, et al. Therapeutic drug monitoring in inflammatory bowel disease: current state and future perspectives. Curr Gastroenterol Rep 2014;16(4):378.

31. Vande Casteele N, Ferrante M, Van Assche G, et al. Trough concentrations of infliximab guide dosing for patients with inflammatory bowel disease. Gastroenterology 2015;148(7):1320–9.

32. D'Haens G, Vermeire S, Lambrecht G, et al. Drug-concentration versus symptom-driven dose adaptation of infliximab in patients with active Crohn's disease: a prospective, randomised, multicentre trial (Tailorix). J Crohns Colitis 2016;10:S24.

33. Melmed GY, Irving PM, Jones J, et al. Appropriateness of testing for anti–tumor necrosis factor agent and antibody concentrations, and interpretation of results. Clin Gastroenterol Hepatol 2016;14(9):1302–9.

34. Rutgeerts P, Sandborn WJ, Feagan BG, et al. Infliximab for induction and maintenance therapy for ulcerative colitis. N Engl J Med 2005;353(23):2462–76.

35. Reinisch W, Sandborn WJ, Hommes DW, et al. Adalimumab for induction of clinical remission in moderately to severely active ulcerative colitis: results of a randomised controlled trial. Gut 2011;60(6):780–7.

36. Sandborn WJ, Feagan BG, Marano C, et al. Subcutaneous golimumab induces clinical response and remission in patients with moderate-to-severe ulcerative colitis. Gastroenterology 2014;146(1):85–95.

37. Feagan BG, Rutgeerts P, Sands BE, et al. Vedolizumab as induction and maintenance therapy for ulcerative colitis. N Engl J Med 2013;369(8):699–710.

38. Sandborn WJ, Su C, Sands BE, et al. Tofacitinib as induction and maintenance therapy for ulcerative colitis. N Engl J Med 2017;376(18):1723–36.

39. Stidham R, Lee T, Higgins P, et al. Systematic review with network meta-analysis: the efficacy of anti-tumour necrosis factor-alpha agents for the treatment of ulcerative colitis. Aliment Pharmacol Ther 2014;39(7):660–71.

40. Thorlund K, Druyts E, Mills EJ, et al. Adalimumab versus infliximab for the treatment of moderate to severe ulcerative colitis in adult patients naive to anti-TNF therapy: an indirect treatment comparison meta-analysis. J Crohns Colitis 2014; 8(7):571–81.

41. Danese S, Fiorino G, Peyrin-Biroulet L, et al. Biological agents for moderately to severely active ulcerative colitis: a systematic review and network meta-analysis. Ann Intern Med 2014;160(10):704–11.

42. Lopez A, Ford AC, Colombel J-F, et al. Efficacy of tumour necrosis factor antagonists on remission, colectomy and hospitalisations in ulcerative colitis: meta-analysis of placebo-controlled trials. Dig Liver Dis 2015;47(5):356–64.

43. Dulai PS, Singh S, Vande Casteele N, et al. How will evolving future therapies and strategies change how we position the use of biologics in moderate to severely active inflammatory bowel disease. Inflamm Bowel Dis 2016;22(4):998–1009.

44. Colombel JF, Sandborn WJ, Rutgeerts P, et al. Adalimumab for maintenance of clinical response and remission in patients with Crohn's disease: the CHARM trial. Gastroenterology 2007;132(1):52–65.

45. Hanauer SB, Feagan BG, Lichtenstein GR, et al. Maintenance infliximab for Crohn's disease: the ACCENT I randomised trial. Lancet 2002;359(9317):1541–9.

46. Schreiber S, Khaliq-Kareemi M, Lawrance IC, et al. Maintenance therapy with certolizumab pegol for Crohn's disease. N Engl J Med 2007;357(3):239–50.

47. Sandborn WJ, Feagan BG, Rutgeerts P, et al. Vedolizumab as induction and maintenance therapy for Crohn's disease. N Engl J Med 2013;369(8):711–21.

48. Colombel J-F, Sands BE, Rutgeerts P, et al. The safety of vedolizumab for ulcerative colitis and Crohn's disease. Gut 2017;66(5):839–51.

49. Feagan BG, Sandborn WJ, Gasink C, et al. Ustekinumab as induction and maintenance therapy for Crohn's disease. N Engl J Med 2016;375(20):1946–60.

50. Singh S, Fumery M, Sandborn W, et al. Systematic review and network meta-analysis: first-and second-line biologic therapies for moderate-severe Crohn's disease. Aliment Pharmacol Ther 2018;48(4):394–409.

51. Costa J, Magro F, Caldeira D, et al. Infliximab reduces hospitalizations and surgery interventions in patients with inflammatory bowel disease: a systematic review and meta-analysis. Inflamm Bowel Dis 2013;19(10):2098–110.

52. Khanna R, Bressler B, Levesque BG, et al. Early combined immunosuppression for the management of Crohn's disease (REACT): a cluster randomised controlled trial. Lancet 2015;386(10006):1825–34.

53. Sands BE, Anderson FH, Bernstein CN, et al. Infliximab maintenance therapy for fistulizing Crohn's disease. N Engl J Med 2004;350(9):876–85.

54. Podolsky D. Inflammatory bowel disease-Reply. N Engl J Med 2002;347(24):1983–4.

55. Kotlyar DS, Osterman MT, Diamond RH, et al. A systematic review of factors that contribute to hepatosplenic T-cell lymphoma in patients with inflammatory bowel disease. Clin Gastroenterol Hepatol 2011;9(1):36–41.e1.

56. Ford AC, Peyrin-Biroulet L. Opportunistic infections with anti-tumor necrosis factor-α therapy in inflammatory bowel disease: meta-analysis of randomized controlled trials. Am J Gastroenterol 2013;108(8):1268.

57. Rahier J-F, Ben-Horin S, Chowers Y, et al. European evidence-based Consensus on the prevention, diagnosis and management of opportunistic infections in inflammatory bowel disease. J Crohns Colitis 2009;3(2):47–91.

58. Cheifetz A, Smedley M, Martin S, et al. The incidence and management of infusion reactions to infliximab: a large center experience. Am J Gastroenterol 2003;98(6):1315.

59. Charles P, Smeenk R, De Jong J, et al. Assessment of antibodies to double-stranded DNA induced in rheumatoid arthritis patients following treatment with infliximab, a monoclonal antibody to tumor necrosis factor α: findings in open-label and randomized placebo-controlled trials. Arthritis Rheum 2000;43(11):2383–90.

60. De Bandt M, Sibilia J, Le Loët X, et al. Systemic lupus erythematosus induced by anti-tumour necrosis factor alpha therapy: a French national survey. Arthritis Res Ther 2005;7(3):R545.

61. Schiff MH, Burmester GR, Kent J, et al. Safety analyses of adalimumab (HUMIRA) in global clinical trials and US postmarketing surveillance of patients with rheumatoid arthritis. Ann Rheum Dis 2006;65(7):889–94.

62. Yanai H, Shuster D, Calabrese E, et al. The incidence and predictors of lupus-like reaction in patients with IBD treated with anti-TNF therapies. Inflamm Bowel Dis 2013;19(13):2778–86.

63. Ramos-Casals M, Diaz-Lagares C, Cuadrado M-J, et al. Autoimmune diseases induced by biological agents: a double-edged sword? Autoimmun Rev 2010; 9(3):188–93.

64. Stübgen JP. Tumor necrosis factor-α antagonists and neuropathy. Muscle Nerve 2008;37(3):281–92.

65. Mohan N, Edwards ET, Cupps TR, et al. Demyelination occurring during anti–tumor necrosis factor α therapy for inflammatory arthritides. Arthritis Rheum 2001;44(12):2862–9.

66. Lozeron P, Denier C, Lacroix C, et al. Long-term course of demyelinating neuropathies occurring during tumor necrosis factor-α–blocker therapy. Arch Neurol 2009;66(4):490–7.

67. Long MD, Martin CF, Pipkin CA, et al. Risk of melanoma and nonmelanoma skin cancer among patients with inflammatory bowel disease. Gastroenterology 2012; 143(2):390–9.e1.

68. Rolston VS, Kimmel J, Hudesman D, et al. Adverse events with use of ustekinumab: a systematic review and meta-analysis. Gastroenterology 2017;152(5): S578–9.

69. Van Assche G, Van Ranst M, Sciot R, et al. Progressive multifocal leukoencephalopathy after natalizumab therapy for Crohn's disease. N Engl J Med 2005;353(4): 362–8.

70. Sandborn WJ, Colombel JF, Enns R, et al. Natalizumab induction and maintenance therapy for Crohn's disease. N Engl J Med 2005;353(18):1912–25.